FUNDAMENTALS OF
Psychopharmacology

FUNDAMENTALS OF
Psychopharmacology

Second edition

BRIAN E. LEONARD

Department of Pharmacology
University College Galway
Ireland

JOHN WILEY & SONS

Chichester · New York · Weinheim · Brisbane · Singapore · Toronto

First published 1992
Reprinted April 1993, July 1993, October 1993, July 1994, October 1994
Second edition 1997
Reprinted July 1997, December 1997, May 1998

Other Wiley Editorial Offices

John Wiley & Sons, Inc., 605 Third Avenue,
New York, NY 10158-0012, USA

VCH Verlagsgesellschaft mbH, Pappelallee 3
D-69469 Weinheim, Germany

Jacaranda Wiley Ltd, 33 Park Road, Milton,
Queensland 4064, Australia

John Wiley & Sons (Canada) Ltd, 22 Worcester Road,
Rexdale, Ontario M9W 1L1, Canada

John Wiley & Sons (Asia) Pte Ltd, 2 Clementi Loop #02-01,
Jin Xing Distripark, Singapore 0512

Library of Congress Cataloging-in-Publication Data
Leonard, B. E.
 Fundamentals of psychopharmacology / Brian E. Leonard. — 2nd ed.
  p. cm.
 Includes bibliographical references and index.
 ISBN 0 471 95115 9 (alk. paper)
 1. Psychotropic drugs. 2. Psychopharmacology. I. Title.
 [DNLM: 1. Psychopharmacology—methods. 2. Psychotropic Drugs—
 pharmacology. 3. Mental Disorders—drug therapy.   QV 77 L581f
 1997]
 RM315.L42   1997
 615′.78—dc21
 DNLM/DLC
 for Library of Congress   96–49182
                                                               CIP

British Library Cataloguing in Publication Data
A catalogue record for this book is available from the British Library

ISBN 0–471–961159

Typeset in 10/12pt Palatino by Dobbie Typesetting Ltd, Tavistock, Devon
Printed and bound in Great Britain by Biddles Ltd, Guildford
This book is printed on acid-free paper responsibly manufactured from sustainable forestation,
for which at least two trees are planted for each one used for paper production.

This book is dedicated to

HELGA

INGRID HEIDE

SAMUEL BENJAMIN

Contents

Preface to the Second Edition

The first edition of *Fundamentals of Psychopharmacology* was completed five years ago and, due to the major advances which have been made in the subject in the intervening years, a thorough revision of the text was necessary. Unfortunately, I did not have the privilege of a sabbatical leave on this occasion to rewrite all the chapters that would ideally be necessary. However, I have tried to compromise by adding several new chapters (on molecular genetics and functional neuroanatomy for example) and to revise intensively those areas (such as the antidepressants, antipsychotics and the importance of serotonin in psychiatric illness) that have undergone major advances in the intervening five years. In addition, I have added two chapters that hopefully will give a flavour to the development of psychopharmacology in the 21st century. One of these deals with the growing area of psychoimmunology and its importance in integrating the immune, endocrine and neurotransmitter systems with behaviour. The second area concerns the role of the enigmatic sigma receptors that appear to play a role in modulating the immune, endocrine and neurotransmitter systems.

Despite my best intentions, I am aware of the deficiencies and limitations that still exist in this volume. I have tried to correct the numerous minor errors in the first edition which undoubtedly reflected my lax proof reading. In this respect I wish to express my sincere thanks to the numerous friends and colleagues who took the time to comment on the strengths and deficiencies of the first edition. Hopefully, the Second Edition has remedied the more glaring errors and omissions. In producing the Second Edition, my intention has been to keep the volume as concise as possible without compromising on the accuracy of the contents.

The last five years have seen the publication of numerous excellent texts and monographs in psychopharmacology many of which are mentioned in the bibliography. Hopefully, the second edition of *Fundamentals of Psychopharmacology* will generate sufficient enthusiasm for the reader to be encouraged to delve more deeply into the subject.

The revision of the Second Edition largely occurred between April and October 1996. As with the first edition, I am particularly indebted to the staff and postgraduate students of the Department of Pharmacology for their help and encouragement for this venture. In particular, I wish to express sincere thanks to my secretary Marie Morrissey for her help in processing some of the new text, to Ambrose O'Halloran for his assistance with all the technical aspects of my word processing, diagrams, etc. and to Dr John Kelly who enabled me to dedicate time and energy to writing by taking over the organization of the research group and many of my departmental activities. Several of the post-doctoral students from the department have also indirectly contributed to the ideas which have been incorporated into the second edition. In particular I wish to thank Maeve Caldwell, Bernadette Earley, Mairead McNamara, Anna Redmond, Cai Song, Alan O'Connell and Michael O'Neill. Michael Davis and Hilary Rowe of John Wiley and Sons have been a constant source of encouragement and monthly faxes to ensure that the Second Edition materialized. Lastly, I thank my long-suffering wife for having endured yet another period of physical and mental absence from our domestic life while I remained obsessed with the fascination of receptors, ion channels and the biochemistry of the brain.

B. E. Leonard
Department of Pharmacology
University College Galway
October 1996   Ireland

Preface to the First Edition

This textbook started life some ten years ago as a collection of lecture notes in neuro- and psychopharmacology. These notes were produced in response to the needs of the undergraduate medical students and postgraduates studying for membership examinations at University College Galway and at the Muhibili Medical Centre, University of Dar es Salaam, where I was involved for several years in teaching under the auspices of an Irish Development Aid programme. Clearly the time had come to completely rewrite the lecture notes or to produce a proper textbook.

The problem was partly solved by my election as a visiting Fellow at Magdalen College, Oxford, during my sabbatical year 1990–1991, and I'm particularly grateful to the Fellows of Magdalen College for having given me this opportunity. The access to the Radcliffe Science Library and the tranquillity of life in Magdalen College provided the ideal setting for this undertaking. Whether the pleasure I achieved in writing this text is reflected in the quality of its content is for the reader to judge. One thing is certain, without the support of Dr Jim O'Donnell and the postgraduates and staff of my department in Galway who undertook many of the vital teaching and administrative duties during my year of absence, the completion of the textbook would have been impossible.

I am particularly grateful to my secretary, Marie Morrissey, for her dedication and determination to ensure that my appallingly bad word-processing was made intelligible to the reader. Ambrose O'Halloran not only taught me what little I know about word-processing but also had the patience and creativity to convert my illiterate sketches of chemical formulae and anatomical drawings into comprehensible figures. Without his enthusiastic support for this project, I'm certain that the text would have been even more mediocre!

My colleagues Drs Ted Dinan and Veronica O'Keane of the Department of Psychiatry, Trinity College, Dublin, kindly offered to read critically the penultimate draft of the text. Their contribution was crucial in highlighting the errors, inconsistencies and lack of clarity in the draft. Their time and energy in helping to improve the text is gratefully acknowledged. Any errors and omissions that remain are, of course, entirely the responsibility of the author!

Michael Davis of John Wiley and Sons has also given invaluable support during the gestation of the text and made many useful suggestions regarding its content.

Finally I express my thanks to my long-suffering wife for having endured my obsessional preoccupation with this enterprise and with my physical and mental absence from our domestic life for the past year.

My sincere wish is that you, the reader, will look upon this modest contribution as merely an introduction to the exciting world of psycho-pharmacology. Your comments and criticisms will be particularly welcome.

B. E. Leonard
Department of Pharmacology
University College Galway
September 1991   Ireland

Introduction

The pain and suffering of those with major psychiatric illness has been appreciated since the dawn of civilization. For over 5000 years, drugs have been used in an attempt to alleviate the suffering of such patients. There is evidence that the Sumerians in the Tigris–Euphrates valley were aware of the mood-elevating effects of the juice of the opium poppy and cultivated these plants for that purpose. The potent analgesic effect of opium was well known to the inhabitants of Asia Minor, Cyprus, Mycenae and Egypt 2000 years BC. Indeed it should not be forgotten that opiates were still being used in the 19th century to relieve depression.

Other plants known to contain psychoactive compounds include hellebore, which was used for centuries in Europe to treat mania, violent temper, mental retardation and epilepsy. However, a drug of major importance in modern psychopharmacology arose from the discovery by medicinal chemists of the alkaloids of *Rauwolfia serpentina*, a root which had been used in the Indian subcontinent for centuries, not only for the treatment of snake bite but also for alleviating "insanity". Understandably, the mechanism of action of reserpine, the alkaloid purified from *Rauwolfia serpentina*, helped to lay the basis to psychopharmacology by demonstrating how the depletion of central and peripheral stores of biogenic amines was correlated with a reduction in blood pressure and tranquillization.

An unexpected discovery also arose during the therapeutic use of reserpine in the treatment of hypotension when it was found that approximately 15% of patients became clinically depressed. As it has been shown that reserpine depletes both the central and peripheral nervous system of noradrenaline, it was postulated that depression would be a consequence of the defective synthesis of noradrenaline and possibly serotonin. This helped to form the basis of the amine therapy of depression.

It is interesting to note that one of the founders of modern psychiatry, Kraepelin, listed only nine substances that were available for the treatment of psychiatric illness in the 1890s. These were: opium, morphine, scopolamine, hashish, chloral hydrate, a barbiturate, alcohol, chloroform and various bromides. Later Bleuler, another founder of modern psychiatry, added paraldehyde and sodium barbiturate to the list. Thus psychopharmacology is a very recent area of medicine and largely arose from the chance discovery of chlorpromazine, by Delay and Deniker in France in 1952, and of imipramine by Kuhn in Switzerland in 1957. Although the chemical structure of the benzodiazepines was first described by Sternbach in the 1930s, the clinical efficacy of these anxiolytics was only fully realized following a clinical trial of chlordiazepoxide by Harris in the USA in 1960.

The purpose of this book is to give the basic neuroscientist and the psychiatrist an overview of psychopharmacology, that relatively recent branch of pharmacology which is concerned with the study of drugs used to treat mental illness. The scope of the subject also covers the use of drugs and other chemical agents as tools that enable the researcher to investigate how the brain functions. This is one of the most rapidly advancing fields of medicine and therefore any short textbook on the subject is bound to omit many aspects of the subject which are fundamentally important.

Nevertheless, based on several years of experience teaching psychopharmacology to undergraduates and to postgraduate clinicians studying for their membership examination for the Royal College of Psychiatrists, I have tried to emphasize the practical advantages of understanding how psychotropic drugs work, not only because this may lead to an improvement in their therapeutic use but also that their side effects may be predicted. A brief glance through this book will persuade the reader that this is not a "cook-book" containing proprietary drug names, doses and a list of side effects. Neither have I attempted to give anything but a brief synopsis of the clinical features of the psychiatric illnesses for which the psychotropic drugs are used. There are many good texts available that cover clinical aspects of psychiatry and most countries have produced excellent formularies to provide practising clinicians with a summary of the therapeutic uses and side effects of the psychotropic drugs in common use. I hope that the reader will not only gain some insight into psychopharmacology as a result of this text but, more importantly, that it will enable the basic and clinical neuroscientist to understand how the brain works in health and disease.

1 Functional Neuroanatomy of the Brain

Understanding the relationship between brain structure and function, and particularly how this relationship becomes disturbed in the mentally ill, is one of the major challenges to clinical and experimental neuroscientists. The brain may be described in terms of its general structure and key anatomical areas. It may also be described in terms of the cellular or subcellular structure of the different types of cells that constitute the brain. Finally it may be considered in terms of its functional importance in terms of memory, consciousness and control of bodily functions. However the brain is described, each level of organization is essentially linked to another level of organization. Conventionally, neuroscientists have concentrated on the structural aspects of the brain and its cellular components while psychologists and psychiatrists have concentrated on the more functional aspects such as consciousness, thought processing and emotional stages. With the advent of sophisticated imaging methods and the introduction of novel drugs that combine therapeutic efficacy with subcellular specificity of action, it is now possible to show how all the levels of brain structure and function are interlinked. This will be illustrated by presenting an overview of brain structure and function and the reader is referred to the key references for further details of neuroanatomy.

Structural and functional subdivision of the brain

Figure 1.1 presents a mid sagittal section through the human brain. In brief, the brain may be divided into the brain stem (consisting of the medulla, pons and midbrain) that is linked to the diencephalon which is composed of the thalamus and the hypothalamus. The two cerebral hemispheres are linked by the corpus callosum, a large tract of nerve fibres that enables the two halves of the brain to communicate, and the brain is permeated by four ventricles, the two largest of which occur beneath the cerebral cortex.

More details of brain structure become evident in the coronal section through the brain (see Figure 1.1). From this figure it is evident that the *basal ganglia* occupies a prominent role. The basal ganglia consists of the corpus striatum (consisting of the caudate nucleus, globus pallidus and putamen)

1

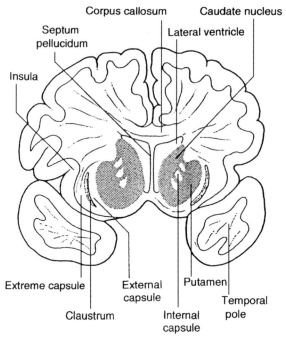

Figure 1.1.   Mid sagittal section through the human brain.

and the substantia nigra. This region is concerned primarily with the control of movement and is malfunctional in Parkinson's disease and Huntington's disease. Figure 1.1 also illustrates the highly indented features of the cerebral cortex which can be visually differentiated into the surface grey matter, consisting of the cell bodies, and the much larger area of white matter which contains the myelinated axons connecting the cells of the cortex to the subcortical regions. The cerebrum contains the largest area of the brain, namely the two cerebral hemispheres.

From this brief description, it is apparent that the brain is really an assembly of organs all of which are structurally and functionally interconnected. Undoubtedly one of the most important areas for the psychopharmacologist is the so-called *limbic system* which is concerned with emotion. This region consists of the hippocampus (concerned with memory processing), the thalamus and hypothalamus (concerned with the control of the endocrine system, temperature regulation, feeding, etc.), the amygdala and septum (the emotional centres of the subcortex), the fornix and the cingulate gyrus of the cortex.

The cerebral cortex is conventionally subdivided into four main regions that may be delineated by the sulci, or large clefts, termed the frontal,

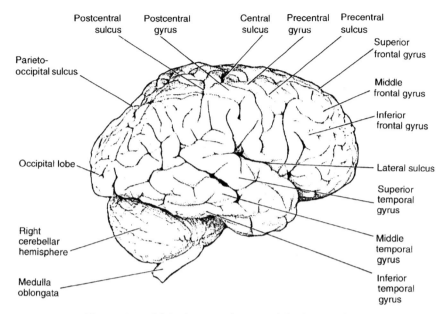

Figure 1.2.   Main functional areas of the human brain.

temporal, parietal and occipital lobes. These names are derived from the bones of the skull which overlay them. Each lobe may be further subdivided according to its cellular structure and composition. Thus Brodmann has divided the cortex into approximately 50 discrete areas according to the specific cellular structure and function. For example, electrical stimulation of the strip of cerebral cortex in front of the central sulcus (see Figure 1.2) is responsible for motor commands to the muscles. This is termed the *primary motor cortex* and can be further subdivided according to which muscles are controlled in different parts of the body.

Similar maps exist in other parts of the brain; for example, the areas concerned with sensory input such as the *primary somatosensory cortex* (see Figure 1.2). Such brain maps of the body are important because information from various organs converge on the brain in a highly organized fashion and can therefore be reflected at all levels of information processing. Such integration also allows the brain to obtain a true representation of the external environment as projected by the sensory organs.

The functional importance of specific cortical and subcortical regions of the brain may also be elucidated by studying the consequences of specific neurological lesions. For example, it has been shown by imaging methods that blood flow to the hippocampus of patients with Alzheimer's disease is dramatically reduced, the reduction paralleling the degree of short-term

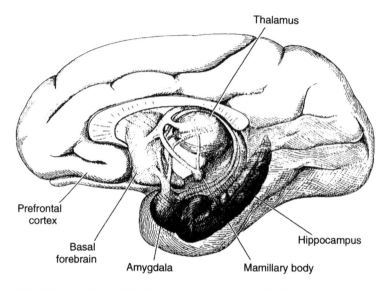

Figure 1.3.   Main regions of the human brain concerned with memory, emotion and intellect.

memory impairment. In addition, blood flow to the parietotemporal association cortex is also greatly reduced. Such changes in the functional activity of these brain areas may account for the memory and cognitive deficits that are symptomatic of the disease, the main function of the parietotemporal association cortex being the integration of sensory and cognitive processes in the brain.

Figures 1.3 and 1.4 show the main structures of the human brain and the areas of the brain which are primarily affected in different types of neurological disease.

In SUMMARY, areas of the cerebral cortex can be identified according to the bodily functions which they control. For example, the motor cortex for muscle control, somatosensory cortex for sensory input, visual cortex for visual input, an area concerned with speech, etc. In addition to these specific areas, the cortex also contains highly developed association areas which are probably involved in the complex synthesis of information.

Blood supply to the brain and the role of the blood–brain barrier

Although the brain constitutes only 2% of body weight, it receives approximately 15% of the blood supply and consumes nearly 20% of the

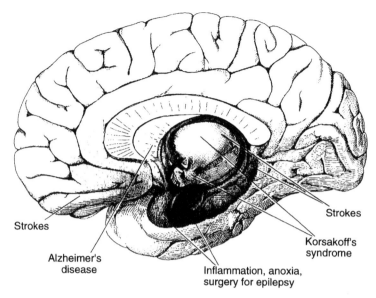

Figure 1.4. Areas of the human brain likely to be affected in some types of neurological dementing diseases.

total oxygen and glucose available to the body. In order to supply these essential nutrients for brain function, there must be a consistent and rapid blood supply to the brain in order that the brain cells may function. This is supplied by the cerebral arteries derived from the internal carotid arteries which branch over the surface of the brain and send smaller branches into the deeper subcortical structures. The capillaries are highly branched and it has been calculated that every nerve cell is no more than 40–50 μm from a capillary.

Because of the unique dependence of the brain on oxygen and glucose to enable the extensive oxidative metabolism to take place with the nerve cells, it is essential that the composition of nutrients, electrolytes, etc. in the fluid surrounding the brain cells is controlled. The composition of the blood varies to some extent according to the composition of the diet and therefore a mechanism has evolved to ensure that the composition of the extracellular fluid surrounding the brain cells is constant. The extracellular fluid is in equilibrium with the cerebrospinal fluid which fills the four ventricles of the brain, and covers the surface of the brain and the spinal cord.

Cerebrospinal fluid is formed from the blood and may be considered as an ultra filtrate of plasma. Thus cerebrospinal fluid contains most of the electrolytes and low molecular weight nutrients but is low in protein. It is formed from a network of capillaries in the ventricles termed the *choroid*

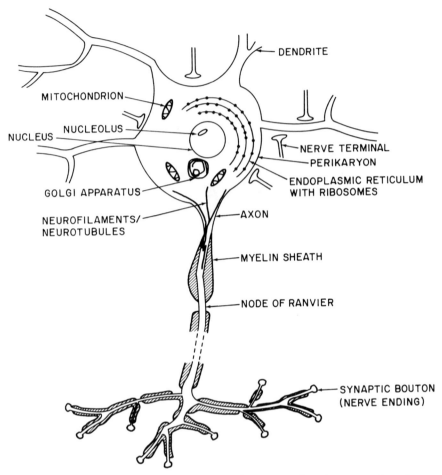

Figure 1.5. Diagrammatic representation of a nerve cell and nerve ending from mammalian brain.

plexus but the cerebral capillaries also contribute to the production of cerebrospinal fluid. The extracellular fluid and the cerebrospinal fluid compartment is separated from the blood by the *blood–brain barrier*. This is a barrier formed by tight junctions that exist between the endothelial cells lining the capillaries and the epithelial cells at the choroid plexus. Such a barrier prevents the influx of large molecular weight molecules but enables small molecular weight substances such as glucose, amino acids, fatty acids, electrolytes, etc., which are essential for normal brain function, to enter. In addition to the structural nature of the blood–brain barrier, there also exists specific transport sites that assist the transport of glucose and essential amino acids into the extracellular fluid. Thus the blood–brain barrier has both a structural and a metabolic role to play in maintaining homeostasis.

Cellular structure of the brain

It has been calculated that the human brain contains approximately 10^{-12} neurons of which the cortex probably contains 10^{-10}. Such complexity is further magnified by the neuronal interconnections. Structurally the neuronal cell body contains a number of organelles that are characteristic of all cells types (see Figure 1.5). The most important features are the *nucleus*, which contains the deoxyribonucleic acid (DNA) together with specific proteins that form chromosomes, and which functions to control the synthesis of all molecules within the neuron, and the *nucleolus* which is involved in ribosome synthesis and in the transfer of ribonucleic acid (RNA) to the cytosol. There is now evidence that the messenger RNA forming specific proteins is targeted to specific parts of the nerve cell. For example, the messenger RNA for microtubule associated protein-2 (MAP-2) targets the dendrites. This provides a mechanism for maintaining the structural integrity and differentiation of the neuron. The mitochondria, as in all types of cells, provides energy to the nerve cell in the form of adenosine triphosphate (ATP). The *smooth endoplasmic reticulum* is involved in lipid synthesis and in protein glycosylation whereas the *rough endoplasmic reticulum* is formed from the attachment of ribosomes to the smooth endoplasmic reticulum. These ribosomes are the main sites of membrane protein synthesis.

The Golgi apparatus is situated near the nucleus and is responsible for protein glycosylation, membrane assembly and protein sorting. *Lysosomes* are responsible for the degradation of all types of cellular debris. *The plasma membrane* surrounds the neuron and consists of a phospholipid bilayer, inserted into which are intrinsic and extrinsic membrane proteins and cholesterol. The plasma membrane provides an impermeable barrier for many large molecular weight and charged molecules. The plasma membrane is transversed by different types of proteins that act as neurotransmitter receptors and voltage-sensitive ion channels.

The *cytosol* is the fluid compartment of the cell and contains the enzymes responsible for cellular metabolism together with free ribosomes concerned with local protein synthesis. In addition to these structures which are common to all cell types, the neuron also contains specific organelles which are unique to the nervous system. For example, *the neuronal skeleton* is responsible for monitoring the shape of the neuron. This is composed of several fibrous proteins that strengthen the axonal process and provide a structure for the location of specific membrane proteins. The axonal cytoskeleton has been divided into the internal cytoskeleton, which consists of microtubules linked to filaments along the length of the axon, which provides a track for the movement of vesicular material by fast axonal transport, and the cortical cytoskeleton.

The cytoskeleton is found near the axonal membrane and consists of microfilaments linked internally to microtubules and the plasma membrane by a network of filamentous protein that includes the brain-specific protein fodrin. This protein forms attachment sites for integral membrane proteins either by means of the neuronal cell adhesion molecule (N-CAM) or indirectly by means of a specific protein called ankyrin in the case of the sodium channels. This may provide a means whereby the sodium channels are concentrated in the region of the nodes of Ranvier. Thus the cortical cytoskeleton plays a vital role in neuronal function by acting as an attachment site for various receptors and ion channels, but also for synaptic vesicles at nerve terminals, thereby providing a mechanism for concentrating the vesicles prior to the release of the neurotransmitter.

There is also interest in the involvement of the cytoskeleton in such degenerative diseases as Alzheimer's disease (see Chapter 13) which is characterized by tangles (paired behind filaments). It seems likely that one of the microtubule-associated proteins (tau protein) is an important component of the tangles found in Alzheimer's disease.

Another unique feature of the neuron is the presence of synaptic and coated vesicles. The former are small smooth-coated vesicles 30–100 nm in diameter and containing the neurotransmitters. The latter are rough-coated vesicles that contain the protein clathrin. These are thought to be involved in the retrieval and recycling of membrane components including the synaptic vesicles once they have liberated their neurotransmitter into the synaptic cleft.

Other types of cell that are important to brain function

The neurons are surrounded by *neuroglia* (or glia) cells. These differ from the neurons in that they do not have electrically excitable membranes. They comprise nearly half the brain volume and function to separate and support the neurons. There are two main types of neuroglial cells, termed the *macroglia* and *microglia*. The macroglia are divided into the astrocytes, oligodendrocytes and ependymal cells. The astrocytes are characterized by long narrow cellular processes which give them a star-like structure; through their feet-like endings they can make contact with both the capillaries and neurons. It has been suggested that the astrocytes play a role in conducting nutrients from the blood to the neurons. Other roles include the removal by active transport of released neurotransmitters (particularly the inhibitory transmitter gamma-aminobutyric acid – GABA), the provision of precursors for transmitter synthesis (e.g. glutamine for the synthesis of GABA) and the buffering of the neuron against excessive concentrations of potassium ions formed following depolarization. Thus the astrocytes appear to play a critical role both in terms of physical protection of the neurons and in providing a metabolic buffer to ensure homeostasis. The *oligodendrocytes* occur in both grey and white matter. In white matter they form the insulating myelin sheath around the axon, whereas in grey matter they probably provide myelin for axons coursing through the grey matter. In the peripheral nervous system, these functions are fulfilled by the Schwann cells. The myelin is formed by the outgrowth of the plasma membrane of the oligodendrocyte which is wrapped several times around the axon thereby excluding extracellular fluid from between the layers of the plasma membrane and thereby generating a highly insulating coat. This insulating coat, which is interrupted at the nodes of Ranvier, is important for the efficient transmission of the electrical impulses down the axon.

The *ependymal* cells line the inner surfaces of the ventricles and, together with the neuroglial cells, appear to be involved in the exchange of material with the surrounding cerebrospinal fluid. The *microglia* can be considered as the macrophage cells of the brain whose function is to remove cell debris by a process of phagocytosis following neuronal damage. There is also evidence that the macroglia are involved in localized inflammatory processes within the brain and may play an important role in the cause of neurodegenerative diseases such as Alzheimer's disease (see Chapter 13). Damage to brain tissue is associated with the proliferation of neuroglia. This is termed *gliosis* and is associated with an increase in the number of macroglia and microglia. Scar tissue is frequently associated with gliosis.

Structure and function of nerve cells

Nerve cells have two distinct properties that distinguish them from all other types of cells in the body. First, they conduct bioelectrical signals for relatively long distances without any loss of signal strength. Second, they possess specific, intracellular connections with other cells and with tissues that they innervate such as muscles and glands. These connections determine the type of information a neuron can receive and also the nature of the responses it can yield.

It is not within the scope of this text to give a detailed account of the anatomical structure of the central nervous system; this has been very adequately covered in a number of excellent textbooks, some of which are listed in the Appendix. However, to understand the physiological mechanisms which form the basis of psychopharmacology, a brief outline of the subject will be given.

Essentially all nerve cells have one or more projections termed *dendrites* whose primary function is to receive information from other cells in their vicinity and pass this information on to the cell body. Following the analysis of this information by the nerve cell, bioelectrical changes occur in the nerve membrane that result in the information being passed to the nerve terminal situated at the end of the *axon*. The change in membrane permeability at the nerve terminal then triggers the release of the *neurotransmitter*.

There is now evidence that the mammalian central nervous system contains several dozen neurotransmitters such as acetylcholine, noradrenaline, dopamine and 5-hydroxytryptamine (5-HT), together with many more cotransmitters, which are mainly small peptides such as met-enkephalin and neuromodulators such as the prostaglandins. It is well established that any one nerve cell may be influenced by more than one of these transmitters at any time. If, for example, the inhibitory amino acids GABA or glycine activate a cell membrane then the activity of the membrane will be depressed, whereas if the excitatory amino acid glutamate activates the nerve membrane, activity will be increased. The final response of the nerve cell that receives all this information will thus depend on the balance between the various stimuli that impinge upon it.

The structure of the nerve cell and nerve terminal is shown in Figure 1.5.

Although different neurotransmitters can be produced at different synapses within the brain, the individual neuron seems capable of releasing only one major neurotransmitter from its axonal terminal, for example noradrenaline or acetylcholine. This view was originally postulated by Sir Henry Dale in 1935 and was subsequently called *Dale's Law*, not incidentally by Dale himself! It is now known that in addition to such "classical transmitters", peptides and/or prostaglandins may also be coreleased, and Dale's Law has been modified in the light of such evidence. The nature of the physiological response to any transmitter will depend on the function of the target *receptor* upon which it acts. For example, acetylcholine released from a motor neuron will stimulate the nicotinic receptor on a muscle end-plate and cause muscle contraction. When the same neurotransmitter is released from the vagus nerve innervating the heart, however, it acts on muscarinic receptors and slows the heart.

Recently it has become apparent that neurotransmitters can also be released from dendrites as well as axons. For example, in dendrites found on the cells of the substantia nigra dopamine may be released which then diffuses over considerable distances to act on receptors situated on the axons and dendrites of GABAergic and dopaminergic neurons in other regions of the basal ganglia. Another means of communication between nerve cells involves dendrodendritic contacts, where the dendrites from one cell communicate directly with those of an adjacent cell. In the olfactory bulb, for example, such synapses appear to utilize GABA as the main transmitter. Thus any neuron responding to inputs that may converge from several sources may inhibit, activate or otherwise modulate the cells to which it projects and, because many axons are branched, the target cells may be widely separated and varied in function. In this way, one neuron may project to an inhibitory or excitatory cell which may then excite, inhibit or otherwise modulate the activity of the original cell. As most neurons are interlinked in an intricate network the complexity of such transmitter interactions becomes phenomenal! In brief, neurons can be conceived as complex gates which integrate the data they receive and, via their specific collection of transmitters and modulators, have a large repertoire of effects which they impose upon their target cells.

Neuronal plasticity

Neuronal plasticity is an essential component of neuronal adaptability and there is increasing evidence that this is primarily a biochemical rather than a morphological process. The neuron is not a fixed entity in terms of the quantity of transmitter it releases, and transmitters which are co-localized in a nerve terminal may be differentially secreted under different conditions. This, together with the repeated firing of some neurons that appear to have "leaky" membranes, may underlie the rhythmicity of neuronal activity within the brain.

Plasticity is also evident at the level of the neurotransmitter receptors. These are fluid structures that can be internalized into the membrane so that their density, and affinity for a transmitter, on the outer surface of the nerve membrane may change according to functional need.

Perhaps it is not surprising to find that our knowledge of how the brain works and where defects that lead to abnormal behaviour can arise is so deficient. The approach to understanding the biochemical basis of psychiatric disease is largely based on the assumption that the brain is chemically homogeneous, which is improbable! Nevertheless, there has been some success in recent years in probing the changes that may be causally related to schizophrenia, depression and anxiety. It should be apparent to anyone interested in the neurosciences that the brain is more than a sophisticated computer that follows a complicated programme, and any dogmatic approach to unravelling the complexities of this dynamic, plastic collection of organs which we call "brain" is doomed to failure.

In CONCLUSION, it can be seen that the adaptability of the organism to external and internal environmental changes is largely dependent on the functional flexibility of the cellular structure of the different brain areas. It is too often assumed that the brain is structurally homogeneous and that, like the heart or liver, once a drug penetrates the blood–brain barrier, it has access to most central compartments. Clearly this is not the case and the pharmacokinetic properties of a psychotropic drug (lipophilicity, molecular size, etc.), as well as the relative blood perfusion rate of a specific brain region which will depend on the metabolic activity at the time of day the drug is administered, could profoundly affect its concentration in a part of the brain. In support of this view, it is known that following its parenteral administration, the concentration of chlorpromazine in the left hemisphere is higher than in the right hemisphere, which presumably reflects the increased functional activity of the left hemisphere. Hopefully this chapter will provide a basis for understanding the physical substrate upon which psychotropic drugs act to produce their effects on the brain.

2 Basic Aspects of Neurotransmitter Function

Introduction

The concept of chemical transmission in the nervous system arose in the early years of the century when it was discovered that the functioning of the autonomic nervous system was largely dependent on the secretion of acetylcholine and noradrenaline from the parasympathetic and sympathetic nerves respectively. The physiologist Sherrington proposed that nerve cells communicated with one another, and with any other type of adjacent cell, by liberating the neurotransmitter into the space, or *synapse*, in the immediate vicinity of the nerve ending. He believed that transmission across the synaptic cleft was unidirectional and, unlike conduction down the nerve fibre, was delayed by some milliseconds because of the time it takes the transmitter to diffuse across the synapse and activate a specific neurotransmitter receptor on the cell membrane.

While it was generally assumed that the brain also contained acetylcholine and noradrenaline as transmitters, it was only in the early 1950s that experimental evidence accumulated that there were also many other types of transmitters in the brain. The indoleamine neurotransmitter 5-hydroxytryptamine (5-HT), or serotonin, which is now recognized as an important component of mental function, was first studied by Erspamer in Italy and by Page in the United States in enterochromaffin tissue and platelets, respectively. It was left to Gaddum and colleagues in Edinburgh to show that 5-HT was present in the mammalian brain where it may have neurotransmitter properties. The potential importance of 5-HT to psychopharmacology arose when Woolley and Shaw in the United States suggested that lysergic acid diethylamide (LSD) owed its potent hallucinogenic properties to its ability to interfere in some way with brain 5-HT, the similarity in chemical structure of these molecules suggesting that they might compete for a common receptor site on the cell membrane.

There are several criteria which must be fulfilled for a substance to be considered as a transmitter:

1. The substance is present in neurons, together with the enzymes involved in its synthesis. Most transmitters are stored in storage vesicles in the nerve terminals.

13

2. The substance is released from the terminals following depolarization; this process is calcium dependent.
3. Specific receptors are located on the postsynaptic membrane which on activation by the putative transmitter causes a depolarization or hyperpolarization of the postsynaptic membrane.
4. When the substance is applied to the receptor by microiontophoresis the effect observed is the same as that initiated by stimulating its release physiologically.
5. Specific antagonists block the effect of the putative transmitter whether it is released physiologically or by microiontophoretic application.
6. The action of the substance must be terminated by a specific mechanism, for example, by a degrading enzyme such as monoamine oxidase or acetyl cholinesterase, or a transport mechanism for rapidly removing the substance from the synaptic cleft as occurs for the biogenic amine transmitters.
7. For most transmitters, specific receptors are located on presynaptic terminals which on stimulation by the transmitter reduce its release. Such inhibitory presynaptic (or auto-) receptors thereby regulate the concentration of the transmitter in the synaptic cleft.

These criteria should be regarded as general guidelines not specific rules.

How do neurotransmitters produce their physiological effects?

Neurotransmitters can either excite or inhibit the activity of a cell with which they are in contact. When an excitatory transmitter such as acetylcholine, or an inhibitory transmitter such as gamma-aminobutyric acid (GABA), is released from a nerve terminal it diffuses across the synaptic cleft to the postsynaptic membrane where it activates the receptor site. Some receptors such as the nicotinic receptor, are directly linked to sodium ion channels so that when acetylcholine stimulates the nicotinic receptor, the ion channel opens to allow an exchange of sodium and potassium ions across the nerve membrane. Such receptors are called *ionotropic* receptors.

The generation of action potentials by nerve axons and muscle fibres was first described by the German physiologist Emil DuBois-Reymond in 1849. However, it was not until over a century later that the underlying mechanism was explained in terms of the properties of specific membrane proteins, the voltage-gated ion channels of sodium and potassium ions. Most of these experimental studies were carried out on the giant axon of the squid. In the late 1940s, Hodgkin and Katz showed that the amplitude of the action potential was reduced when the external sodium ion concentration was reduced. This observation led to the concept that the process of *depolarization* that initiates the action potential and causes a transient change in the membrane

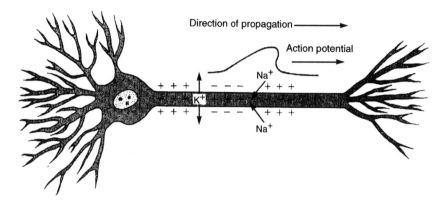

Figure 2.1. Diagram showing propagation of an action potential.

that briefly switches its permeability from potassium to sodium ions. These permeability changes occur because of the opening of voltage-sensitive channels in the membrane that allow sodium ions to move down its concentration gradient into the cell. These sodium channels are normally kept closed by a voltage-sensitive gating mechanism (see Figure 2.1). Depolarization opens these channels, allowing an increased sodium ion influx into the cell thereby producing the rising phase of the action potential. The falling phase of the action potential is caused by the subsequent closing of the sodium channels, which reduces the sodium ion influx, and by the opening of voltage-gated potassium channels which allows increased efflux of potassium ions from the cell. In most nerve cells, action potentials are followed by a transient hyperpolarization. This brief increase in membrane potential occurs because the potassium channels that open during the latter phase of the action potential take a few milliseconds to return to the closed state. During this time, the efflux of potassium ions from the cell is greater than during the resting state and, as a consequence, the membrane is hyperpolarized with respect to its normal resting value. The action potential is followed by a refractory period during which it is only possible to trigger an action potential by applying a stimulus that is stronger than normal. This period of refractoriness, which lasts for a few milliseconds, is caused by the residual inactivation of sodium channels and the opening of potassium channels. All excitatory neurotransmitters produce excitatory postsynaptic potentials (EPSPs) which last for about 5 ms. The understanding of the process of depolarization, which was largely due to the experimental studies of Hodgkin and Huxley in the early 1950s using the giant axon of the squid, has subsequently been found to be applicable to cell bodies, dendrites and presynaptic terminals of vertebrates.

The major inhibitory transmitters in the vertebrate brain are GABA and glycine. The postsynaptic receptors for these transmitters form channels permeable to chloride ions. Gating of these channels premits the influx of chloride and potassium ions into the cell. This increases the membrane potential to approximately $-90\,mV$ and is termed *hyperpolarization*. Two important classes of drugs, the benzodiazepines and barbiturates, enhance the action of GABA on inhibitory GABA receptors and thereby enhance the chloride (and potassium) ion flux through these channels in response to GABA. An inhibitory postsynaptic potential (IPSP) results from the hyperpolarization caused by GABA or any other inhibitory transmitter. In practice, the activity of a neuron depends on a balance between a number of excitatory and inhibitory processes which can occur simultaneously so that the membrane potential of any nerve cell may be in a constant state of flux.

Repolarization of an excitable membrane is associated with the re-establishment of a resting state of the membrane, a state whereby the concentration of sodium ions is greater outside and potassium ions greater inside the membrane. This is achieved by the energy-dependent removal of sodium ions against the concentration gradient from inside the cell and their replacement by potassium ions. The enzyme sodium, potassium-dependent adenosine triphosphatase (Na^+K^+-ATPase) is responsible for this process of repolarization, the energy being provided by adenosine triphosphate (ATP) which is generated by the oxidative metabolism of sugars, etc. within the mitochondria.

Conduction of sodium and potassium ions across excitable membranes may be inhibited by drugs that block sodium or potassium channels or in a selective manner and thereby slow or prevent depolarization. Thus the naturally occurring animal toxins tetrodotoxin and saxitoxin selectively block sodium channels and thus paralyse conduction. Conversely tetraethyl ammonium, and an increasing number of other compounds that may eventually have therapeutic use in conditions such as multiple sclerosis, selectively block potassium channels. Another mechanism whereby conduction across excitable membranes may be affected relies on the prevention of repolarization. The cardiac glycosides (for example, digoxin and ouabain) inhibit Na^+K^+-ATPase and thereby slow the repolarization process. Such drugs have found therapeutic application in the treatment of congestive heart failure by facilitating the duration of muscle contraction and thereby improving cardiac emptying.

When receptors are directly linked to ion channels, fast EPSPs or IPSPs occur. These receptors are called *ionotropic* or *fast receptors*. However, it is well established that slow potential changes also occur and that such changes are due to the receptor being linked to the ion channel indirectly via a *second messenger system*. For example, the stimulation of beta adrenoceptors by noradrenaline result in the activation of adenylate cyclase on the inner side of the nerve membrane. This enzyme catalyses the breakdown of ATP to the very labile high energy compound cyclic 3,5-adenosine monophosphate (cyclic AMP). Cyclic AMP then activates a protein kinase which, by phosphorylating specific membrane proteins, opens an ion channel to cause an efflux of potassium and an influx of sodium ions. Such receptors are termed *metabotropic* or *slow receptors*. Many monoamine neurotransmitters are now thought to work by this receptor-linked secondary messenger system. In some cases, however, stimulation of the postsynaptic receptors can cause the inhibition of adenylate cyclase activity. For example, D_2 dopamine receptors inhibit while D_1 receptors stimulate the activity of the cyclase. Such differences have been ascribed to the fact that the cyclase is linked to two distinct guanosine triphosphate (GTP) binding proteins in the cell membrane termed G_i and G_s. The former protein inhibits the cyclase, possibly by reducing the effects of the G_s protein which stimulates the cyclase. The relationship between the postsynaptic receptor and the secondary messenger system is illustrated diagrammatically in Figure 2.2.

In addition to their functional differences, the structure of fast receptors (which respond to an agonist within a few milliseconds) differ from slow receptors which take hundreds of milliseconds to elicit a response. Thus fast receptors consist of five subunits which form an oligomeric protein containing a receptor binding site around an ion channel (see Figure 2.3). By contrast, the slow receptor consists of seven or more membrane spanning units linked to a second messenger system (see Figure 2.4).

Recently there has been much interest in the possible role of the family of protein kinases which translate information from the secondary messenger to the membrane proteins. Many of these kinases are controlled by free calcium ions within the cell. It is now established that some 5-HT receptors, for example, are linked via G proteins to the phosphatidyl inositol pathway which, by mobilizing membrane-bound diacylglycerol and free calcium ions, can activate a specific protein kinase C. This enzyme can cause a number of intracellular changes by affecting the concentration of calmodulin, a calcium sequestering protein that plays a key role in many intracellular processes.

Some examples of fast and slow receptors are given in Table 2.1.

The functional response of a nerve cell to a transmitter can change as a result of the receptor becoming sensitized or desensitized following a decrease or increase, respectively, in the concentration of the transmitter at the receptor site. Among those receptors that are directly coupled to ion channels, receptor desensitization is often rapid and pronounced. Most of the experimental evidence came initially from studies of the frog motor end-plate where it was shown that the desensitization of the nicotinic receptor caused by continuous short pulses of acetylcholine was associated with a slow conformational change in the receptor. This resulted in the ion channel remaining closed despite the fact that the transmitter was bound to the

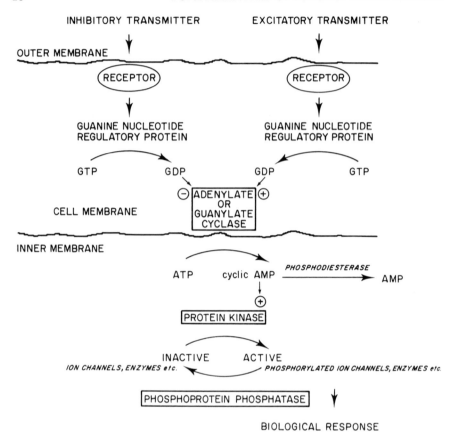

Figure 2.2. Relationship between the postsynaptic receptor and the secondary messenger system. GTP=guanosine triphosphate; GDP=guanosine diphosphate; ATP=adenosine triphosphate; AMP=adenosine monophosphate.

receptor surface. A similar mechanism has also been shown to occur in brain cells. For example, continuous exposure of beta adrenoceptors on rat glioma cells *in vitro* results in a rapid reduction in the responsiveness of the receptors. This is followed by a secondary stage of desensitization whereby the number of beta receptors decreases. It seems likely that the receptors are not lost but move into the cell and are therefore no longer accessible to the transmitter. The importance of the changes in receptor sensitivity to our understanding of the chronic effects of psychotropic drugs will be discussed later.

In SUMMARY, neurotransmitters can control cellular events by two basic mechanisms either by being linked directly to sodium (for example,

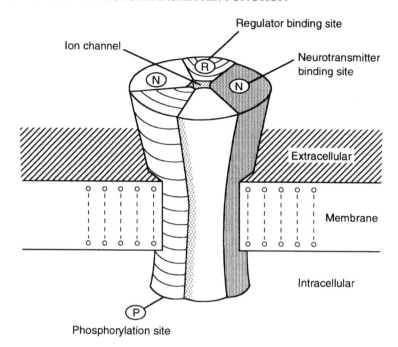

Figure 2.3. Ion channel linked receptor.

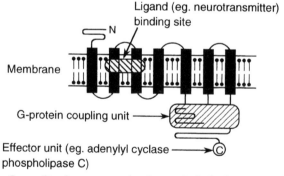

Figure 2.4. Generalized structure of a G protein linked receptor showing the single subunit containing the binding site for the neurotransmitter N. Also shown are the G protein and effector molecule, e.g. adenylyl cyclase, phospholipase C, or ion channel making up the transmembrane signalling unit.

acetylcholine acting on nicotinic receptors or excitatory amino acids such as glutamate acting on glutamate receptors) or chloride (as exemplified by GABA) ion channels thereby leading to the generation of fast EPSPs or IPSPs respectively. Alternatively, the receptor may be linked to a secondary messenger system that mediates slower postsynaptic changes. These

Table 2.1.   Classification of fast and slow receptors in the mammalian brain

---

Fast ion channel linked receptors (ionotropic receptors)
Cholinergic nicotinic
GABA-A
Glutamate/aspartate
Glycine
5-HT$_3$

Slow receptors linked to G proteins (metabotropic receptors)
Cholinergic muscarinic
Adrenergic (alpha$_1$, alpha$_2$, beta$_1$, beta$_2$)
GABA-B
Glutamate (metabotropic)
Dopamine (D$_1$, D$_2$)
Histamine (H$_1$, H$_2$, H$_3$)
5-HT$_{1A}$, 5-HT$_{1B}$, 5-HT$_{1D}$, 5-HT$_{2A}$, 5-HT$_{2C}$
Peptide receptors (e.g. angiotensin II, cholecystokinin, neuropeptide-Y, somatostatin, opiate, vasopressin)

---

different mechanisms whereby neurotransmitters may change the activity of a postsynaptic membrane by fast voltage-dependent mechanisms or slower second messenger mediated mechanisms provides a physiological mechanism for functional plasticity within its nervous system.

Presynaptic mechanisms

Another important mechanism whereby the release of a neurotransmitter may be altered is by *presynaptic inhibition*. Initially, this mechanism was thought to be restricted to noradrenergic synapses but it is now known to occur at GABAergic, dopaminergic and serotonergic terminals also. In brief, it has been shown that at noradrenergic synapses the release of noradrenaline may be reduced by the presence of high concentrations of the transmitter in the synaptic cleft. Conversely, some adrenoceptor antagonists such as phenoxybenzamine have been found to enhance the release of the amine. It is now known that the subclass of adrenoceptors responsible for this process of auto-inhibition are distinct from the alpha$_1$ adrenoceptors which are located on blood vessels, on secretory cells and in the brain. These auto-inhibitory receptors, or alpha$_2$ adrenoceptors, can be identified by the use of specific agonists and antagonists, for example clonidine and yohimbine respectively; drugs acting as specific agonists or antagonists on alpha$_1$ receptors, for example, the agonist methoxamine and the antagonist prazosin, do not affect noradrenaline release by this mechanism. The inhibitory effect of alpha$_2$ agonists on noradrenaline release involves a hyperpolarization of the presynaptic membranes by opening potassium ion channels. The reduction in the release of noradrenaline following the administration of an alpha$_2$ agonist is ultimately due to a reduction in the concentration of free cytosolic calcium which is an essential component of the mechanism whereby the synaptic vesicles containing noradrenaline fuse to the synaptic membrane prior to their release. There is evidence that a number of closely related phosphoproteins associated with the synaptic vesicles, called *snapsins*, are involved in the short-term regulation of neurotransmitter release. These proteins also appear to be involved in the regulation of synapse formation that allows the nerve network to adapt to long-term passage of nerve impulses.

Experimental studies have shown that the release of a transmitter from a nerve terminal can be decreased or increased by a variety of other neurotransmitters. For example, stimulation of 5-HT receptors on noradrenergic terminals can lead to an enhanced release of noradrenaline. While the physiological importance of such a mechanism is unclear, this could be a means whereby drugs could produce some of their effects. Such receptors have been termed *heteroceptors*. In addition to the physiological process of autoinhibition, another mechanism of presynaptic inhibition has been identified in the periphery although its precise relevance to the brain is unclear. In the dorsal horn of the spinal cord, for example, the axon terminal of a local neuron makes axo-axonal contact with a primary afferent excitatory input which leads to a reduction in the neurotransmitter released. This is due to the local neuron partly depolarizing the nerve terminal so that when the axon potential arrives, the change induced is diminished, thereby leading to a smaller quantity of transmitter being released. In the brain, it is possible that GABA can cause presynaptic inhibition in this way.

In SUMMARY, it seems that the release of a transmitter from its nerve terminal is not only dependent upon the passage of an action potential but also on the intersynaptic concentration of the transmitter and the modulatory effects of other neurotransmitters that act presynaptically on the nerve terminal. The inter-relationship between these different processes is illustrated in Figure 2.5.

Co-transmission

During the mid-1970s, studies on such invertebrates as the mollusc *Aplysia* showed that at least four different types of transmitters could be liberated from the same nerve terminal. This was the first evidence that Dale's Law (i.e. a neuron can only release one type of neurotransmitter) does not always apply. Extensive histochemical studies of the mammalian peripheral and central nervous systems followed and it was shown that transmitters such as

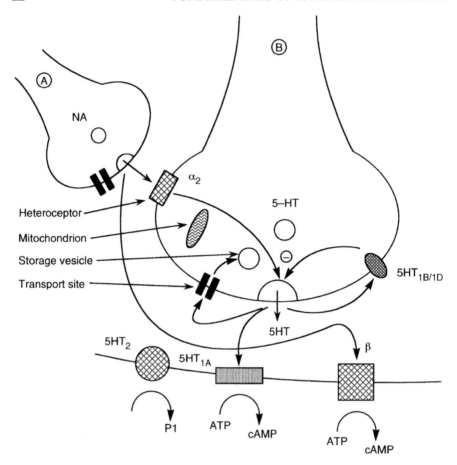

Figure 2.5. Modulation of 5-HT release by alpha-adrenergic heteroceptors.

acetylcholine, noradrenaline and dopamine can coexist with such peptides as cholecystokinin, vasoactive intestinal peptide and gastrin-like peptides. It is now evident that nerve terminals in the brain may contain different types of storage vesicles that store the peptide co-transmitters. Following their release, these peptides activate specific pre- or postsynaptic receptors and thereby modulate the responsiveness of the membrane to the action of the traditional neurotransmitters such as acetylcholine or noradrenaline. In the mammalian and human brain, acetylcholine has been found to co-localize with vasoactive intestinal peptide; dopamine with cholecystokinin-like peptide and 5-HT with substance P. In addition, there is increasing evidence that a number of peptides may act as neurotransmitters in the mammalian brain in their own right. These include the enkephalins, thyrotropin releasing hormone, angiotensin II, vasopressin, substance P, neurotensin, somatostatin and corticotropin, amongst many others. With the advent of specific and sensitive immunocytochemical techniques several more peptides are being added to this list every year! The similarities and differences between the peptide transmitters/co-transmitters and the "classical" transmitters such as acetylcholine may be summarized as follows:

1. Both neurotransmitters and peptides show high specificity for their specific receptors.
2. Neurotransmitters produce physiological responses in nano- or micro-molar $(10^{-9}-10^{-6})$ concentrations whereas peptides are active in picomolar (10^{-12}) concentrations.
3. Neurotransmitters bind to their receptors with high affinity but low potency whereas peptides bind with very high affinity and high potency.
4. Neurotransmitters are synthesized at a moderate rate in the nerve terminal whereas the rate of synthesis of peptides is probably very slow.
5. Neurotransmitters are generally of low molecular weight (200 or below) whereas peptides are of intermediate molecular weight (1000 to 10 000 or occasionally more).

Table 2.2. summarizes the different types of neurotransmitter that have been found in the human brain. These are broadly classified into "classical" transmitters, which fulfil the well-established physiological functions in the peripheral and central nervous systems, and the neuropeptides. The

Table 2.2. Neurotransmitters in the brain

"Classical" neurotransmitters
Fast transmitters (Milliseconds): acetylcholine*, GABA*, glutamate*, aspartate, glycine, 5-HT (serotonin)
Slow transmitters (Milliseconds–seconds): acetylcholine*, adenosine, adrenaline, dopamine, GABA*, glutamate*, histamine, 5-HT, noradrenaline

Neuropeptide neurotransmitters**
Angiotensin II, bombesin, bradykinin, carnosine, cholecystokinin (CCK), corticotrophin (ACTH), corticotropin releasing factor (CRF), dymorphin, beta-endorphin, gastrin, leucine enkephalin, luteinizing hormone releasing hormone (LHRH), melanotropin (alpha MSH), methionine enkephalin, neurokinins A and B, neuropeptide Y (NPY), neurotensin, somatostatin, substance P, TRH, vasopressin, vasoactive intestinal peptide (VIP)

---

*Several classical neurotransmitters are either "fast" or "slow" depending upon the subtype of receptor they activate. For example, acetylcholine is a fast transmitter when it activates the ion channel linked nicotinic receptor but is a slow transmitter when activating on the muscarinic receptors.
**Many neuropeptides are slow transmitters and it is not proven that all these listed are transmitters. Many neuropeptides (e.g. substances P, NPY, vasopressin, the enkephalins, somatostatin and CCK) coexist in neurons with some of the classical transmitters, where they may function as co-transmitters.

neuropeptides can act as neurotransmitters in their own right or act as modulators of "classical" neurotransmitters.

Measuring neurotransmitter receptors in the brain

Little was known about the identity of neurotransmitter receptors in the brain until the early 1970s when several laboratories independently reported that a potent snake venom, alpha-bungarotoxin, could bind with high affinity to nicotinic receptors that occurred in the electric organs of certain species of fish. This laid the basis for *ligand receptor binding studies*. Such studies rely on the use of radiolabelled (generally with tritium or carbon-14) drugs or chemicals which have a high affinity for a specific receptor. Such ligands may be either agonists or antagonists that bind to the receptor, thereby enabling the number of receptors on a tissue to be determined by measuring the quantity of radioactive ligand that has been specifically bound.

In practice, pieces of brain tissue (e.g. membrane preparations or crude tissue homogenates) are incubated with the radioligand in a physiological buffer solution. The tissue is then filtered or centrifuged to separate the tissue from the incubation medium. The quantity of ligand bound to the tissue can then be estimated by solubilizing the tissue and counting the radioactivity in a liquid scintillation counter. As most radioligands also bind non-specifically to brain tissue, to the walls of the incubation tube and even to the filters used to separate the tissue from the incubation medium, it is essential to determine the amount of radioligand bound specifically to the receptor. This is done by incubating the tissue preparation in tubes containing the specific radioligand alone and also with the ligand together with another drug or compound which is not radioactively labelled but which also binds with high affinity to the same receptor. For example, to study the number of beta adrenoceptors in a brain or lymphocyte preparation, tritiated dihydroalpre-nolol ([^{3}H]DHA) is used as the radioligand and DL-propranolol as the non-radioactive displacing agent. Thus propranolol will tend to displace all of the [^{3}H]DHA bound to the beta receptor but is less effective in displacing any radioligand that is bound non-specifically, and possibly irreversibly, to other types of receptor or to non-receptor sites. The amount of radioactivity present in the tissue preparation that has been incubated with the radioligand alone and that remaining after the specifically bound ligand has been displaced by propranolol is then counted. The difference between the total (i.e. the radioactivity in the tube containing the radioligand alone) and the non-specifically bound activity (i.e. the radioactivity in the tube containing the radioligand and the displacing agent) gives a measure of the amount of radioactivity specifically bound to the beta adrenoceptor. This is illustrated in Figure 2.6.

The number of receptors in a tissue preparation may be determined by plotting the ratio of the bound to free radioligand against the total bound ligand. For one population of receptors in a tissue, this plot yields a straight line, the number of binding sites (termed the B_{max}) being determined from the point of intersection of the y axis. This is illustrated in Figure 2.7.

This method of expressing the results of radioligand binding assays is known as a *Scatchard plot*, after the chemist who used it to study the binding of small molecules to proteins. A non-linear Scatchard plot often implies that there are two or more binding sites, one of these sites to which the ligand binds with high affinity and low capacity (shown as B_{max1} in Figure 2.8) and the other to which the ligand binds with low affinity and high capacity (shown as B_{max2} in Figure 2.8).

The affinity of a ligand for a receptor can be calculated from the slope of the plot, $1/slope$ being known as the K_d value or the binding affinity.

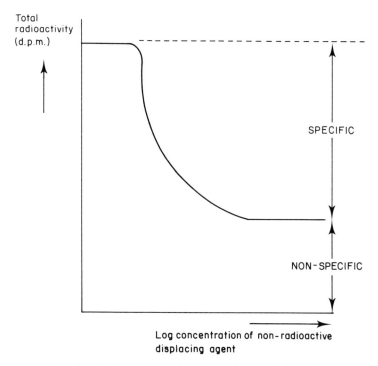

Figure 2.6. Scatchard plot of the binding of a radioligand to a membrane preparation containing two binding sites. In this diagram, B_{max1} represents a high affinity (K_{d1}) low capacity site, whereas B_{max2} represents a low affinity (K_{d2}) high capacity site.

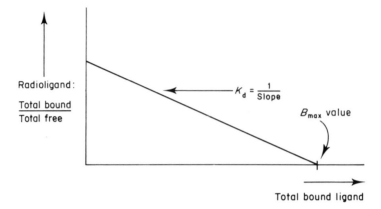

Figure 2.7. Diagrammatic representation of the binding of a radioactive ligand to a membrane preparation.

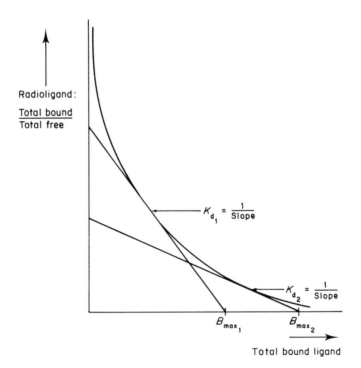

Figure 2.8. Method used to determine the receptor number and the ligand affinity for the receptor by the Scatchard plot.

Thus by means of this relatively simple technique it is possible to determine the number of binding sites in a piece of brain tissue, their homogeneity and the affinity of the ligand for these sites. This enables changes in the density of specific receptors to be determined following drug treatment or as a result of disease. However, it must be emphasized that a binding site for a radioligand is not necessarily a receptor. To classify a binding site as a receptor it is essential to show that the binding site is linked to an ion channel or secondary messenger system or that an electro-physiological response occurs as a direct consequence of the activation of the binding site. It is possible, for example, that the ligand binds to a portion of the nerve membrane that is not involved in neurotransmission. Following the discovery that tritiated benzodiazepines bind with high specificity to nerve membranes it took several years of further research to show that occupation of the benzodiazepine-binding site could lead to the enhanced sensitivity of the GABA-A receptor to the effects of GABA. Only when the functional activity of the benzodiazepine receptor was established could the binding site be justifiably called a receptor site.

The application of ligand binding techniques to the quantification of receptor sites in the brain has had important implications for psychopharmacology. It has now been possible to correlate the therapeutic potencies of some drugs with their receptor occupancy. Neuroleptics are known to block dopamine receptors in the brain. By studying the binding of a series of neuroleptics to the different types of dopamine receptor in nerve membrane preparations, it has been found that there is a good correlation between the occupancy of the D_2 receptor subtype and the therapeutic potency. There does not appear to be a direct correlation between the binding of these drugs to adrenoceptors, histamine, 5-HT or acetylcholine receptors and their therapeutic potency. However, by considering the interaction of psychotropic drugs with these various receptors, it is possible to predict their side effects. For example, antagonism of alpha$_1$ adrenoceptors, histamine$_1$ and muscarinic receptors is associated with postural hypotension, sedation and anticholinergic side effects respectively. Thus by using this relatively simple technique it is possible to gain an insight into the site(s) of action of most classes of psychotropic drug and to predict with reasonable accuracy what their side effects will be. Whether the receptor affinity of a drug *in vitro* necessarily provides information about its mode of action in the brain is quite another issue.

Quantitative autoradiography

In this method, thin tissue sections of the brain are incubated with a specific radioligand, the unbound ligand removed by washing and the resulting tissue section placed on a sensitive photographic film. The sites where the radioligand binds to the tissue fog the film, and following its development grain counts, densitometric analysis and photometric techniques can be used to quantify the extent of the binding of the radioligand to specific cell structures. More recently, the application of computerized image analysis has simplified the problem of visualization and quantification. The system most widely used consists of a television camera linked to an IBM personal computer. This system can colour code images to enhance contrast, modify images, subtract one image from another and average densities in specific regions of the visual field. The ability of this system to include and process autoradiographic standards enables the density of the radioligand binding to be quantified. Finally, the system can tabulate, store and calculate the B_{max} and K_d values of the radioligand.

One of the most important uses of autoradiography in psychopharmacology lies in enabling the sites in the brain where a drug acts to be identified. For example, the brain region or specific neuronal circuit that is affected by a drug may be visualized. Since most psychotropic drugs have multiple effects in the brain, autoradiographic methods have helped to explain the complexity of the effects by identifying the receptors and their distribution in the brain. Changes in receptor density may reflect neuronal function. Receptor mapping has therefore been applied to biopsy and autopsy samples from patients with parkinsonism, Alzheimer's disease, schizophrenia and depression. The results of such studies have already begun to throw light on the possible biochemical changes that underlie such diseases. There are practical limitations to the autoradiographic technique however. The resolution using the light micro-scope is limited and it is seldom possible to readily identify specific cell structures that contain the receptors or to distinguish between functional and non-functional receptors to which the ligand is bound. It should be emphasized that this is also a problem with conventional radioligand techniques as applied to membrane preparations or to tissue homogenates. To overcome the problem of resolution, electron microscopic autoradiography may eventually prove to be of value, particularly when this is combined with immunohistochemical techniques to improve the resolution.

Positron emission tomography scanning of receptors

Positron emission tomography (PET) is a technique whereby receptors may be visualized in the living human or animal brain. The distribution of the positron emitting isotope (i.e. non-radioactive isotopes such as oxygen-15, nitrogen-13, carbon-11 and fluorine-12) can be accurately calculated by detecting the positrons emitted from the brain after administration of a labelled drug that binds specifically to the receptor. This technique enables the distribution and density of receptors in the living brain to be determined and has been invaluable in studying the receptor changes that arise during the progression of a disease or in response to drug treatment. A major problem with PET scanning is the cost involved, as a cyclotron is needed to produce the ultra-short-lived isotopes. The isotopes in common use have half-lives of between 2 and 110 minutes. Furthermore, the resolution is currently limited to 1 mm thick brain slices.

More recently, PET has been combined with magnetic resonance imaging (MRI) so that the precise anatomical location and receptor density may be obtained in the same area of the brain. Clearly such techniques are of crucial importance in developing our understanding of the receptor changes in psychiatric disease and in identifying the primary site(s) of action of psychotropic drugs in the human brain.

Single photon emission computed tomography

Another novel brain imaging technique that has recently been introduced combines computed tomography with the measurement of cerebral blood flow. This is known as single photon emission computerized tomography (SPECT) and employs radiochemicals which emit a single gamma ray (e.g. iodine-123, xenon-133 or technetium-99m) that can be detected by means of a rotating gamma ray sensitive camera. While the resolution is inferior to that of PET, a major advantage of SPECT over PET is the cost, as a cyclotron is not required for SPECT studies. Clearly this is an imaging technique which will find extensive use in psychiatric research in the near future.

Biochemical pathways leading to the synthesis and metabolism of the major neurotransmitters in the mammalian brain

No attempt will be made to give an overview of the main pathways of the several dozen neurotransmitters, neuromodulators and cotransmitters which are possibly involved in the aetiology of mental illness. Instead a summary is given of the relevant pathways involved in the synthesis and metabolism of those transmitters which have conventionally been considered to be involved in the major psychiatric and neurological diseases and through which the psychotropic drugs used in the treatment of such diseases are believed to operate.

Acetylcholine

Acetylcholine has been implicated in learning and memory in all mammals, and the gross deficits in memory found in patients suffering from Alzheimer's disease have been ascribed to a defect in central cholinergic transmission. This transmitter has also been implicated in the altered mood states found in mania and depression, while many different classes of psychotropic drugs are known to have potent anticholinergic properties which undoubtedly have adverse consequences for brain function.

Acetylcholine is synthesized within the nerve terminal from choline (from both dietary and endogenous origins) and acetyl coenzyme A (acetyl CoA) by the enzyme choline acetyltransferase. Acetyl CoA is derived from glucose and other intermediates via the glycolytic pathway and ultimately the pyruvate oxidase system, while choline is selectively transported into the cholinergic nerve terminal by an active transport system. There are believed to be two main transport sites for choline, the high affinity site being dependent on sodium ions and ATP and which is inhibited by membrane depolarization, while the low affinity site operates by a process of passive diffusion and is therefore dependent on the intersynaptic concentration of choline. The uptake of choline by the high affinity site controls the rate of acetylcholine synthesis, while the low affinity site, which occurs predominantly in cell bodies, appears to be important for phospholipid synthesis. As the transport of choline by the active transport site is probably optimal, there seems little value in increasing the dietary intake of the precursor in an attempt to increase acetylcholine synthesis. This could be one of the reasons why feeding choline-rich diets (e.g. lecithin) to patients with Alzheimer's disease has been shown to be ineffective.

As with all the major transmitters, acetylcholine is stored in vesicles within the nerve terminal from which it is released by a calcium-dependent mechanism following the passage of a nerve impulse. The inter-relationship between the intermediary metabolism of glucose, phospholipids and the uptake of choline is summarized in Figure 2.9.

It is well established that acetylcholine can be catabolized by both *acetylcholinesterase* (ACHE) and *butyrylcholinesterase* (BCHE); these are also known as "true" and "pseudo" cholinesterase, respectively. Such enzymes may be differentiated by their specificity for different choline esters and by their susceptibility to different antagonists. They also differ in their anatomical distribution, with ACHE being associated with nervous tissue while BCHE is largely found in non-nervous tissue. In the brain there does not seem to be a good correlation between the distribution of cholinergic terminals and the presence of ACHE, choline acetyltransferase having been found to be a better marker of such terminals. An assessment of cholinesterase activity can be made by examining red blood cells, which contain only ACHE, and plasma, which contains only BCHE. Of the *anticholinesterases*, the organophosphorus derivatives such as diisopropylfluorophosphonate are specific for BCHE, while drugs such as ambenonium inhibit ACHE.

Most cholinesterase inhibitors inhibit the enzyme by acylating the esteratic site on the enzyme surface. Physostigmine and neostigmine are examples of *reversible anticholinesterases* which are in clinical use. Both act in similar ways but they differ in terms of their lipophilicity, the former being able to

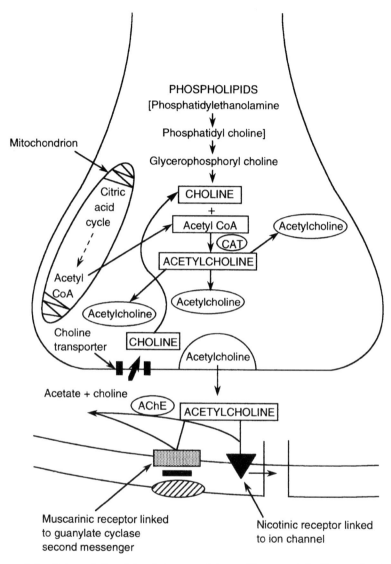

Figure 2.9. Inter-relationship between intermediary metabolism of glucose, phospholipids and acetylcholine synthesis. Acetyl CoA=acetyl coenzyme A; CAT=catechol-*O*-methyltransferase; AChE=acetylcholinesterase.

penetrate the blood–brain barrier while the latter cannot. The main clinical use of these drugs is in the treatment of glaucoma and myasthenia gravis.

Irreversible anticholinesterases include the organophosphorus inhibitors and ambenonium, which irreversibly phosphorylate the esteratic site. Such drugs

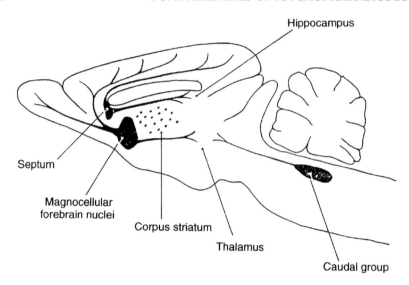

Figure 2.10.   Cholinergic pathways in the rat brain.

have few clinical uses but have been developed as insecticides and nerve gases. Besides blocking the muscarinic receptors with atropine sulphate in an attempt to reduce the toxic effects that result from an accumulation of acetylcholine, the only specific treatment for organophosphate poisoning would appear to be the administration of 2-pyridine aldoxime methiodide, which increases the rate of dissociation of the organophosphate from the esteratic site on the enzyme surface.

Anatomical distribution of the central cholinergic system

The cholinergic pathways in the mammalian brain are extremely diffuse and arise from cell bodies located in the hindbrain and the midbrain. Of these areas, there has been considerable interest of late in the nucleus basalis magnocellularis of Meynert because this region appears to be particularly affected in some patients with familial Alzheimer's disease. As the projections from this area innervate the cortex, it has been speculated that a disruption of the cortical cholinergic system may be responsible for many of the clinical features of the illness. The use of cholinomimetic drugs of various types to treat such diseases is discussed in a later chapter.

    Figure 2.10 illustrates the distribution of the main cholinergic tracts in the rat brain.

The catecholamines

Much attention has been paid to the catecholamines noradrenaline and dopamine following the discovery that their depletion in the brain leads to profound mood changes and locomotor deficits. Thus noradrenaline has been implicated in the mood changes associated with mania and depression, while an excess of dopamine has been implicated in schizophrenia and a deficit in Parkinson's disease.

Noradrenaline is the main catecholamine in postganglionic sympathetic nerves and in the central nervous system; it is also released from the adrenal gland together with adrenaline. Recently *adrenaline* has also been shown to be a transmitter in the hypothalamic region of the mammalian brain so, while the terms "noradrenergic" and "adrenergic" are presently used interchangeably, it is anticipated that they will be used with much more precision once the unique functions of adrenaline in the brain have been established.

The catecholamines are formed from the dietary amino acid precursors phenylalanine and tyrosine, as illustrated in Figure 2.11.

The rate-limiting step in the synthesis of the catecholamines from tyrosine is tyrosine hydroxylase, so that any drug or substance which can reduce the activity of this enzyme, for example by reducing the concentration of the tetrahydropteridine cofactor, will reduce the rate of synthesis of the catecholamines. Under normal conditions tyrosine hydroxylase is maximally active, which implies that the rate of synthesis of the catecholamines is not in any way dependent on the dietary precursor tyrosine. Catecholamine synthesis may be reduced by *end product inhibition*. This is a process whereby catecholamine present in the synaptic cleft, for example as a result of excessive nerve stimulation, will reduce the affinity of the pteridine cofactor for tyrosine hydroxylase and thereby reduce synthesis of the transmitter. The experimental drug alpha-methyl-*para*-tyrosine inhibits the rate-limiting step by acting as a false substrate for the enzyme, the net result being a reduction in the catecholamine concentrations in both the central and peripheral nervous systems.

Drugs have been developed which specifically inhibit the L-aromatic amino acid decarboxylase step in catecholamine synthesis and thereby lead to a reduction in catecholamine concentration. Carbidopa and benserazide are examples of decarboxylase inhibitors which are used clinically to prevent the peripheral catabolism of L-dopa (levodopa) in patients being treated for parkinsonism. As these drugs do not penetrate the blood–brain barrier they will prevent the peripheral decarboxylation of dopa so that it can enter the brain and be converted to dopamine by dopamine beta-oxidase (also called dopamine beta-hydroxylase).

Dopamine beta-oxidase inhibitors are only of limited clinical use at the present time, probably due to their relative lack of specificity. Diethyldithiocarbamate

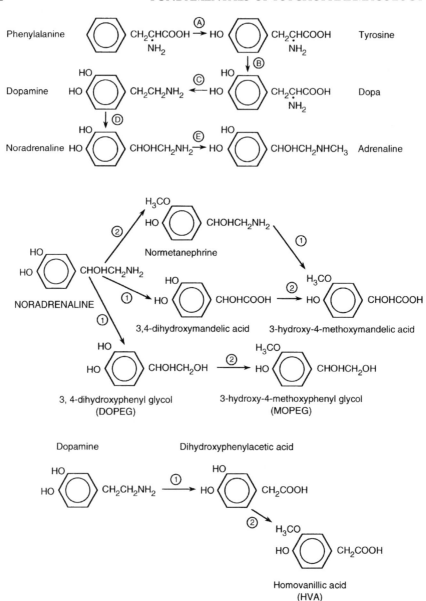

Figure 2.11. Pathways for the synthesis and metabolism of the catecholamines. A=phenylalanine hydroxylase+pteridine cofactor+O_2; B=tyrosine hydroxylase+tetra-hydropteridine+Fe^{++}+O_2; C=dopa decarboxylase+pyridoxal phosphate; D=dopamine beta-oxidase+ascorbate phosphtate+Cu^{++}+O_2; E=phenylethanolamine N-methyl-transferase+S-adenosylmethionine; 1=monoamine oxidase and aldehyde dehydrogenase; 2=catechol-O-methyltransferase+S-adenosylmethionine.

and disulfiram are examples of drugs that inhibit dopamine beta-oxidase by acting as copper-chelating agents and thereby reducing the availability of the cofactor for this enzyme. Whether their clinical use in the treatment of alcoholism is in any way related to the reduction in brain catecholamine concentrations is uncertain. The main action of these drugs is to inhibit liver aldehyde dehydrogenase activity, thereby leading to an accumulation of acetaldehyde, and the onset of nausea and vomiting, should the patient drink alcohol.

Two enzymes are concerned in the metabolism of catecholamines, namely *monoamine oxidase*, which occurs mainly intraneuronally, and *catechol-O-methyltransferase*, which is restricted to the synaptic cleft. The importance of the two major forms of monoamine oxidase, A and B, will be considered elsewhere.

The process of oxidative deamination is the most important mechanism whereby all monoamines are inactivated (i.e. the catecholamines, 5-HT and the numerous trace amines such as phenylethylamine and tryptamine). Monoamine oxidase occurs in virtually all tissues, where it appears to be bound to the outer mitochondrial membrane. Whereas there are several specific and therapeutically useful monoamine oxidase inhibitors, inhibitors of catechol-O-methyltransferase have found little application. This is mainly due to the fact that at most only 10% of the monoamines released from the nerve terminal are catabolized by this enzyme. The main pathways involved in the catabolism of the catecholamines are shown in Figure 2.11.

Anatomical distribution

One of the first demonstrations of the central monoamine pathways in the mammalian brain was by a fluorescence technique in which thin sections of the animal brain were exposed to formaldehyde vapour which converted the amines to their corresponding fluorescent isoquinolines. The distribution of these compounds could then be visualized under the fluorescent microscope. Using this technique it has been possible to map the distribution of the noradrenergic, dopaminergic and serotonergic pathways in the animal and human brain.

The central noradrenergic system. This is not so diffusely distributed as the cholinergic system. In the lower brain stem, the neurons innervate the medulla oblongata and the dorsal vagal nucleus, which are thought to be important in the central control of blood pressure. Other projections arising from cell bodies in the medulla descend to the spinal cord where they are believed to be involved in the control of flexor muscles. However, the most important noradrenergic projections with regard to psychological functions arise from a dense collection of cells in the locus ceruleus and ascend from

the brain stem to innervate the thalamus, dorsal hypothalamus, hippocampus and cortex. The ventral noradrenergic bundle occurs caudally and
ventrally to the locus ceruleus and terminates in the hypothalamus and the
subcortical limbic regions. The dorsal bundle arises from the locus ceruleus
and innervates the cortex. Both the dorsal and ventral noradrenergic systems
appear to be involved psychologically in drive and motivation, in
mechanisms of reward and in rapid eye movement (REM) sleep. As such
processes are severely deranged in the major affective disorders it is not
unreasonable to speculate that the central noradrenergic system is defective
in such disorders.

The central dopaminergic systems.   These are considerably more complex than
the noradrenergic system. This may reflect the greater density of dopamine-
containing cells, which have been estimated to be 30–40 000 in number
compared with 10 000 noradrenaline-containing cells. There are several
dopamine-containing nuclei as well as specialized dopaminergic neurons
localized within the retina and the olfactory bulb. The dopaminergic system
within the mammalian brain can be divided according to the length of the
efferent fibres into the intermediate and long length systems.

The intermediate length systems include the tuberoinfundibular system,
which projects from the arcuate and periventricular nuclei into the
intermediate lobe of the pituitary and the median eminence. This system is
responsible for the regulation of such hormones as prolactin. The
interhypothalamic neurons send projections to the dorsal and posterior
hypothalamus, the lateral septal nuclei and the medullary periventricular
group, which are linked to the dorsal motor nucleus of the vagus; such
projections may play a role in the effects of dopamine on the autonomic
nervous system.

The *long length fibres* link the ventral tegmental and substantia nigra
dopamine-containing cells with the neostriatum (mainly the caudate and the
putamen), the limbic cortex (the medial prefrontal, cingulate and entorhinal
areas) and with limbic structures such as the septum, nucleus accumbens,
amygdaloid complex and piriform cortex. These projections are usually
called the *mesocortical* and *mesolimbic dopaminergic systems*, respectively, and
are functionally important in psychotic disorders and in the therapeutic
effects of neuroleptic drugs. Conversely, changes in the functional activity of
the dopaminergic cells in the neostriatum are primarily responsible for
movement disorders such as parkinsonism and Huntington's chorea.

The central adrenergic system.   It is only recently that immunohistochemical
methods have been developed to show that adrenaline-containing cells occur
in the brain. Some of these cells are located in the lateral tegmental area,
while others are found in the dorsal medulla. Axons from these cells

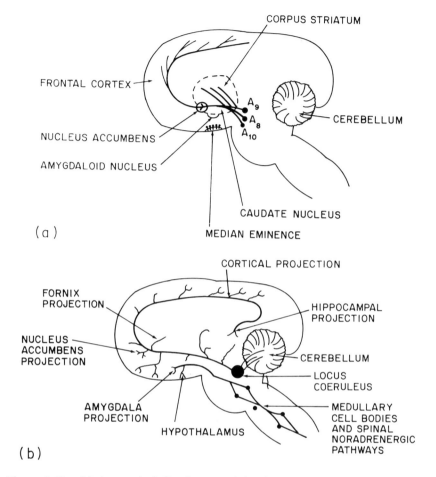

Figure 2.12. (a) Anatomical distribution of the dopaminergic pathways in human brain. (b) Anatomical distribution of the noradrenergic pathways in human brain.

innervate the hypothalamus, the locus ceruleus and the dorsal motor nucleus of the vagus nerve. While the precise function of adrenergic system within the brain is uncertain, it may be surmised that adrenaline could play a role in endocrine regulation and in the central control of blood pressure. There is evidence that the concentration of this amine in cerebrospinal fluid is reduced in depression, which might imply that it is also concerned in the control of mood.

The distribution of the main catecholaminergic pathways in the brain is shown diagrammatically in Figure 2.12.

5-HT

5-HT, together with noradrenaline, has long been implicated in the aetiology of depression. Indirect evidence has been obtained from the actions of drugs which can either precipitate or alleviate the symptoms of depression and from the analysis of body fluids from depressed patients. Recently, the development of novel anxiolytic drugs which appear to act as specific agonists for a subpopulation of 5-HT receptors (the 5-HT_{1A} type) suggests that this amine may also play a role in anxiety. To add to the complexity of the role of 5-HT, there is evidence that impulsive behaviour as exhibited by patients with obsessive–compulsive disorders and bulimia may also involve an abnormality of the serotonergic system. Whether 5-HT is primarily involved in this disparate group of disorders or whether it functions to "fine tune" other neurotransmitters which are causally involved is presently unclear.

5-HT is an indoleamine transmitter which is synthesized within the nerve ending from the amino acid L-tryptophan. Tryptophan, which is obtained from dietary and endogenous sources, is unique among the amino acids concerned in neurotransmitter synthesis in that it is about 85% bound to plasma proteins. This means that it is only the unbound portion that can be taken up by the brain and is therefore available for 5-HT synthesis. In the periphery, tryptophan may be metabolized in the liver via the *kynurenine* pathway, and it must be emphasized that the pathway that leads to the synthesis of 5-HT in the periphery (e.g. in platelets and the enterochromaffin cells of the gastrointestinal tract) or as a neurotransmitter in the brain is relatively minor. It is known that the activity of the kynurenine pathway, also known as the tryptophan pyrrolase pathway, in the liver can be increased by steroid hormones. Thus natural or synthetic glucocorticoids can induce an increase in the activity of this pathway and thereby increase the catabolism of plasma free tryptophan. Other steroids, such as the oestrogens used in the contraceptive pill, can also induce pyrrolase activity. This has been proposed as a mechanism whereby the contraceptive pill, particularly the high oestrogen type of pill which has now largely been withdrawn, may predispose some women to depression by reducing the availability of free tryptophan for brain 5-HT synthesis. Despite the plausible belief that the availability of plasma free tryptophan determines the rate of brain 5-HT synthesis, it now seems unlikely that such an important central transmitter would be in any way dependent on the vagaries of diet to sustain its synthesis! Nevertheless, changes in liver tryptophan pyrrolase activity, which may be brought about by endogenous steroids, insulin, changes in diet and by the circadian rhythm, may play a secondary role in regulating brain 5-HT synthesis. Furthermore, there is evidence that a tryptophan-deficient diet can precipitate depression in depressed patients who are in remission. Thus when such patients are given a drink containing high concentrations of amino acids but which lacks tryptophan, a depressive episode rapidly occurs.

Free tryptophan is transported into the brain and nerve terminal by an active transport system which it shares with tyrosine and a number of other essential amino acids. On entering the nerve terminal, tryptophan is hydroxylated by tryptophan hydroxylase, which is the rate-limiting step in the synthesis of 5-HT. Tryptophan hydroxylase is not bound in the nerve terminal and optimal activity of the enzyme is only achieved in the presence of molecular oxygen and a pteridine cofactor. Unlike tyrosine hydroxylase, tryptophan hydroxylase is not usually saturated by its substrate. This implies that if the brain concentration rises then the rate of 5-HT synthesis will also increase. Conversely, the rate of 5-HT synthesis will decrease following the administration of experimental drugs such as *para*-chlorophenylalanine, a synthetic amino acid which irreversibly inhibits the enzyme. *Para*-chloramphetamine also inhibits the activity of this enzyme, but this experimental drug also increases 5-HT release and delays its reuptake thereby leading to the appearance of the so-called "serotonin syndrome", which in animals is associated with abnormal movements, body posture and temperature.

Following the synthesis of 5-hydroxytryptophan (5-HTP) by tryptophan hydroxylase, the enzyme aromatic amino acid decarboxylase (also known as 5-HTP or dopa decarboxylase) then decarboxylates the amino acid to 5-HT. L-aromatic amino acid decarboxylase is approximately 60% bound in the nerve terminal and requires pyridoxal phosphate as an essential enzyme.

There is evidence that the compartmentalization of 5-HT in the nerve terminal is important in regulating its synthesis. It appears that 5-HT is synthesized in excess of normal physiological requirements and that some of the amine which is not immediately transported into the storage vesicle is metabolized by intraneuronal monoamine oxidase. Another autoregulatory mechanism governing 5-HT synthesis relies on the rise in the intersynaptic concentration of the amine stimulating the autoreceptor of the nerve terminal.

5-HT is metabolized by the action of monoamine oxidase by a process of oxidative deamination to yield 5-hydroxyindoleacetic acid (5-HIAA). In the *pineal gland*, 5-HT is o-methylated to form melatonin. While the physiological importance of this transmitter in the regulation of the oestrus cycle in ferrets would appear to be established, its precise role in man is unknown. Nevertheless, it has been speculated that melatonin plays some role in regulating the circadian rhythm, which may account for the occurrence of low plasma melatonin levels in depressed patients.

A summary of the major steps that lead to the synthesis of 5-HT, and of the minor pathway whereby the trace amine tryptamine is synthesized from tryptophan by the action of tryptophan hydroxylase, is shown in Figure 2.13.

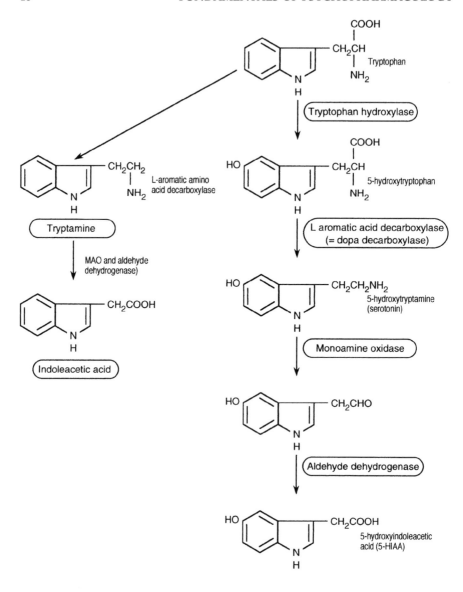

Figure 2.13. The major pathway leading to the synthesis and metabolism of 5-hydroxytryptamine (5-HT). Metabolism of tryptophan to tryptamine is a minor pathway which may be of functional importance following administration of a monoamine oxidase (MAO) inhibitor. Tryptamine is a trace amine. L-Aromatic amino acid decarboxylase is also known to decarboxylate dopa and therefore the term "L-aromatic amino acid decarboxylase" refers to both "dopa decarboxylase" and "5-HTP decarboxylase".

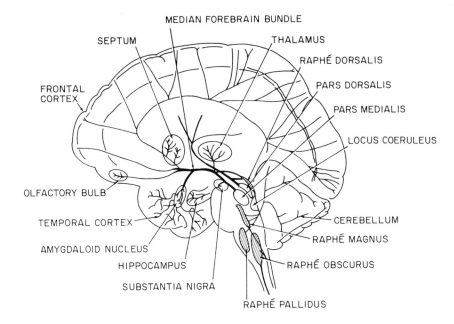

MEDIAN FOREBRAIN BUNDLE

SEPTUM

THALAMUS

RAPHÉ DORSALIS

FRONTAL
CORTEX

PARS DORSALIS

PARS MEDIALIS

LOCUS COERULEUS

OLFACTORY BULB

TEMPORAL CORTEX

CEREBELLUM

RAPHÉ MAGNUS

AMYGDALOID NUCLEUS

HIPPOCAMPUS

RAPHÉ OBSCURUS

SUBSTANTIA NIGRA

RAPHÉ PALLIDUS

Figure 2.14.   Anatomical distribution of the serotonergic pathways in human brain.

Anatomical distribution of the central serotonergic system

Neurons containing 5-HT are restricted to clusters of cells around the midline of the pons and upper brain stem; this is known as the raphé area of the midbrain. In addition, according to studies of rat brain, cells containing 5-HT are located in the area postrema and in the caudal locus ceruleus, which forms an anatomical basis for a direct connection between the serotonergic and noradrenergic systems. The more caudal groups of cells in the raphé project largely to the medulla and the spinal cord, the latter projections being physiologically important in the regulation of pain perception at the level of the dorsal horn. Conversely, the more rostral cells of the dorsal and median raphé project to limbic structures such as the hippocampus and in particular, to innervate extensively the cortex. Unlike the noradrenergic cortical projections, there does not appear to be an organized pattern of serotonergic terminals in the cortex. In general, it would appear that the noradrenergic and serotonergic systems are colocalized in most limbic areas of the brain, which may provide the anatomical basis for the major involvement of these transmitters in the affective disorders.

The distribution of the serotonergic system in the human brain is shown in Figure 2.14.

Amino acid neurotransmitters

Unlike for the "classical" neurotransmitters such as acetylcholine and noradrenaline, it has not been possible to map the distribution of the amino acid transmitters in the mammalian brain. The reason for this is that these transmitters are present in numerous metabolic pools in the brain and are not restricted to one particular type of neuron as occurs with the "classical" transmitters. As an example, glutamate is involved in peptide and protein synthesis, in the detoxification of ammonia in the brain (by forming glutamine), in intermediary metabolism, as a precursor of the inhibitory transmitter GABA and as an important excitatory transmitter in its own right. While the evidence in favour of the amino acids glutamate, aspartate, glycine and GABA as transmitters is good, it is not yet possible to describe their anatomical distribution in detail.

With regard to the possible role of these neurotransmitters in psychiatric and neurological diseases, there is growing evidence that glutamate is causally involved in the brain damage that results from cerebral anoxia, for example following stroke, and possibly in epilepsy. Conversely, GABA deficiency has been implicated in anxiety states, epilepsy, Huntington's chorea and possibly parkinsonism. The roles of the excitatory amino acid aspartate and the inhibitory transmitter glycine in disease are unknown.

The principal amino acid transmitters and their metabolic inter-relationships are shown in Figure 2.15.

Glycine

Glycine is structurally the simplest amino acid. There is evidence that it acts as an inhibitory transmitter in the hindbrain and spinal cord. The seizures that occur in response to strychnine poisoning are attributable to the convulsant-blocking glycine receptors in the spinal cord. Recent evidence also suggests that glycine can modulate the action of the excitatory transmitter glutamate on the major excitatory amino acid receptor complex in the brain, the so-called N-methyl-D-aspartate (NMDA) receptor. As the density of NMDA receptor sites is high in the cortex, amygdala and basal ganglia, this might explain the relatively high concentration of glycine which also occurs in these brain regions.

Aspartate and glutamate

Aspartate and glutamate are the most abundant amino acids in the mammalian brain. While the precise role of aspartate in brain function is obscure, the importance of glutamate as an excitatory transmitter and as a precursor of GABA is well recognized. Despite the many roles which glutamate has been shown to play in intermediary metabolism and

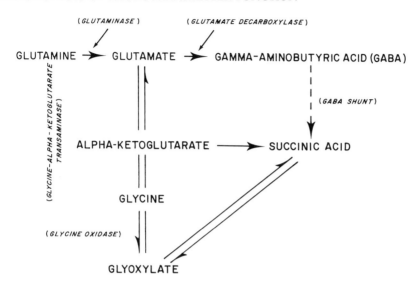

Figure 2.15. Metabolic inter-relationship between the amino acid transmitters glutamate, GABA and glycine. The diagram shows how glutamate and glycine synthesis are linked via the succinic acid component of the citric acid cycle. GABA, formed by the decarboxylation of glutamate, may also be metabolized to succinate via the "GABA shunt". Alpha-ketoglutarate acts as an intermediate between glutamate and glycine synthesis; the transfer of the $-NH_2$ group from glycine to alpha-ketoglutarate leads to the synthesis of glutamate and glyoxylate.

transmitter function, studies on the dentate gyrus of the hippocampal formation, where glutamate has been established as a transmitter, have shown that the synthesis of glutamate is regulated by feedback inhibition and by the concentration of its precursor glutamine. Thus the neuronal regulation of glutamate synthesis would appear to be similar to that of the "classical" transmitters. In the brain, there appears to be an inverse relationship between the concentration of glutamate and of GABA, apart from the context where both amino acids are present in low concentrations.

GABA

GABA is also present in very high concentrations in the mammalian brain, approximately 500 μg/g wet weight of brain being recorded for some regions! Thus GABA is present in a concentration some 200–1000 times greater than neurotransmitters such as acetylcholine, noradrenaline and 5-HT.

GABA is one of the most widely distributed transmitters in the brain and it has been calculated that it occurs in over 30% of all synapses. Nevertheless, its distribution is quite heterogeneous, with the highest concentrations being

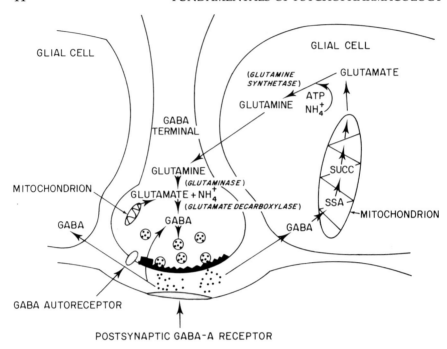

Figure 2.16. Inter-relationship between a GABAergic terminal and the glia: the GABA shunt. The diagram shows the synthesis of GABA in the nerve terminal from glutamine and glutamate. Glutamine synthesis is essential for the transport of the GABA precursor from the glial cell to the nerve terminal. Glutamate is synthesized in mitochondria by the action of GABA transaminase. Following its release from the nerve terminal, GABA can be transported into the nerve terminal by a specific active transport system or taken up into glial cells where, under the influence of GABA transaminase, it is converted to glutamate. Glutamate is also synthesized from citric acid cycle intermediates in the mitochondria. SSA=succinic semi-aldehyde; SUCC=succinic acid; ATP=adenosine triphosphate.

present in the basal ganglia, followed by the hypothalamus, the periaqueductal grey matter and the hippocampus; approximately equal concentrations are present in the cortex, amygdala and thalamus.

GABA is present in storage vesicles in nerve terminals and also in the glia that are densely packed around nerve terminals, where they probably act as physical and metabolic "buffers" for the nerve terminals. Following its release from the nerve terminal, the action of GABA may therefore be terminated either by being transported back into the nerve terminal by an active transport system or by being transported into the glia. This is shown diagrammatically in Figure 2.16.

The rate of synthesis of this transmitter is determined by glutamate decarboxylase, which synthesizes it from glutamate. A feedback inhibitory mechanism also seems to operate whereby an excess of GABA in the synaptic cleft triggers the GABA autoreceptor on the presynaptic terminal, leading to a reduction in transmitter release. Specific GABA-containing neurons have been identified as distinct pathways in the basal ganglia, namely in interneurons in the striatum, in the nigrostriatal pathway and in the pallidonigral pathway.

Gaseous neurotransmitters

Perhaps one of the most surprising discoveries in neuroscience in recent years has been the discovery that small gaseous molecules such as nitric oxide and carbon monoxide, which are generally considered to be atmospheric pollutants, are biologically active in the mammalian brain. It is now known that nitric oxide is synthesized by the vascular endothelium where it is responsible for maintaining the vascular tone. This process is crucial for the regulation of *blood flow and blood pressure*. The quest for the identification of endothelium-dependent vascular relaxation factor, later known as the endothelium-derived relaxing factor (EDRF), led to the discovery of the enzyme nitric oxide synthase in the blood vessel wall. This enzyme was found to be responsible for the synthesis of nitric oxide from the amino acid L-arginine. It was also shown that this enzyme was calcium and calmodulin dependent and that it released picomoles of nitric oxide in response to physical tension in the vessel wall. The discovery of nitric oxide in the vascular endothelium for the first time provided an explanation for the pharmacological action of drugs such as glyceryl trinitrate and sodium nitroprusside which have been known to be clinically effective in relaxing vascular smooth muscle. The organic and inorganic nitrates, which are converted into nitric oxide *in vivo*, behave like endogenous nitric oxide in that they stimulate soluble guanyl cyclase which acts as a second messenger in vascular smooth muscle cells and thereby causes their relaxation. Nitric oxide is inactivated by binding to the ferrous iron portion of haemoglobin. Other physiological roles of nitric oxide include the inhibition of platelet aggregation and leucocyte activation. It would appear that nitric oxide can therefore act as an important factor in the general homeostatic control of the vasculature.

In the *brain* it has also been shown that nitric oxide is released following the activation of NMDA receptors. Subsequently, it was shown that a calcium-dependent nitric oxide synthase was also present in brain and was responsible for the synthesis of the transmitter from arginine. The connection between the functional activity of the NMDA receptor and memory suggested that one of the physiological actions of nitric oxide was in memory formation. Experimental studies suggest that the transmitter, when released from postsynaptic sites, acts on presynaptic terminals to increase the release of glutamate and thereby cause long-term potentiation which is believed to be the basis of memory formation. In support of the role of nitric oxide in memory formation, it has been shown that inhibition of nitric oxide synthase can impair learning in animals. Other physiological functions of nitric oxide include the reception and transmission of vision, feeding behaviour, nociception and olfaction.

For well over 20 years it has been postulated that the excessive release of glutamate is linked with convulsions and some forms of neurotoxicity. The possible link between stimulation of glutamate receptors and the activation of nitric oxide synthase led to the suggestion that overproduction of nitric oxide might be causally involved in conditions such as cerebral ischaemia and epilepsy. In addition to the neurons, microglia, which form part of the immune system in the brain and show macrophage activity, are known to express an inducible form of nitric oxide synthase. The microglia have been implicated in the pathogenesis of multiple sclerosis, Alzheimer's disease, Parkinson's disease and acquired immune deficiency syndrome dementia. Thus the possibility arises that such chronic neurodegenerative diseases may arise as a consequence of the increased synthesis of nitric oxide.

The two forms of nitric oxide synthase, the constitutive and the inducible forms, have now been purified from many sources including the brain. The inducible form of the enzyme has been cloned from macrophages, and found to have a molecular weight in the region of 135 to 155 kDa. The constitutive form of the enzyme is activated by calcium ions and calmodulin whilst the inducible form is calcium independent. It is now known that glucocorticoids inhibit the induction of the calcium-independent form of the enzyme and as this inhibitory effect occurs at concentrations that are therapeutically relevant it seems likely that some of the therapeutic actions of these drugs are due to the inhibition of nitric oxide formation. The inducible form of the enzyme is also highly regulated by cytokines which, depending on their properties, may either inhibit or induce the enzyme. Thus the physiological role of nitric oxide provides further evidence of the close link between central neurotransmission and the regulation of the immune system.

Table 2.3 presents a summary of the properties and possible functions of nitric oxide and carbon monoxide in the mammalian brain.

Classification of neurotransmitter receptors

The British physiologist Langley, in 1905, was the first to postulate that most drugs, hormones and transmitters produce their effects by interacting with specific sites on the cell membrane which we now call *receptors*. Langley's

Table 2.3. Nitric oxide and carbon monoxide as mediators

	Nitric oxide (NO)	Carbon monoxide (CO)
Formation		
Precursor	Arginine	Haem
Enzyme	NO Synthase (NOS)	Haem oxygenase
Inhibited by	L-NMMA	Zn protoporphyrin
	L-NAME	
Activated by	Intracellular Ca^{2+}	Not known
Effect	Activates soluble guanylate cyclase	Activates soluble guanylate cyclase
	Increases cGMP	Increases cGMP
Inactivated by	Haemoglobin	Haemoglobin
Implicated in	Vasodilatation	?LTP
	Smooth muscle relaxation	
	LTP/LTD	
	Neuroprotection/neurotoxicity	

L-NMMA=N^G-monomethyl-L-arginine; L-NAME=N^G-monomethyl-L-arginine; LTP=long-term potentiation; LTD=long-term depression
(These phenomena are probably important in memory formation and are discussed on page 60.)

postulate was based on his observation that drugs can mimic both the specificity and potency of endogenous hormones and neurotransmitters, while others appear to be able selectively to antagonize the actions of such substances. Thus substances which stimulate the receptor, or mimic the action of natural ligands for the receptor, are called *agonists* while those substances blocking the receptor are called *antagonists*. This was a conceptually revolutionary hypothesis which was later extended by Hill, Gaddum and Clarke who quantified the ways in which agonists and antagonists interacted with receptors both *in vitro* and *in vivo*. More recently, the precise structure of a large number of different types of transmitter receptors have been determined using cloning and other techniques so that it is now possible to visualize precisely how an agonist or antagonist interacts with certain types of receptor.

To date, different types of cholinergic, beta adrenergic, and serotonergic receptors have been cloned and their essential molecular features identified. In addition, a number of peptide receptors such as the insulin, gonadotropin, angiotensin, glucagon, prolactin and thyroid stimulating hormone receptors have also been identified and their key structures determined. The location and possible functional importance of the different types of neurotransmitter receptors which are of relevance to the psychopharmacologist can be summarized as follows. It must be emphasized that this list is by no means complete and that many of these receptor types are likely to be further subdivided as a result of the development of highly selective ligands.

Cholinergic receptors

Sir Henry Dale noticed that the different esters of choline elicited responses in isolated organ preparations which were similar to those seen following the application of either of the natural substances muscarine (from poisonous toadstools) or nicotine. This led Dale to conclude that, in the appropriate organs, acetylcholine could act on either *muscarinic* or *nicotinic receptors*. Later it was found that the effects of muscarine and nicotine could be blocked by atropine and tubocurarine respectively. Further studies showed that these receptors differed not only in their molecular structure but also in the ways in which they brought about their physiological responses once the receptor had been stimulated by an agonist. Thus nicotinic receptors were found to be linked directly to an ion channel and that their activation always caused a rapid increase in cellular permeability to sodium and potassium ions. Conversely, the responses to muscarinic receptor stimulation were slower and involved the activation of a second messenger system which was linked to the receptor by so-called G proteins.

Following further studies of the actions of specific agonists and antagonists on the nicotinic receptors from the skeletal muscle and sympathetic ganglia, it was soon apparent that not all nicotinic receptors were the same. The heterogeneity of the nicotinic receptors was further revealed by the application of molecular cloning techniques. This has led to the classification of nicotinic receptors into N-m receptors and N-n receptors, the former being located in the neuromuscular junction, where activation causes end-plate depolarization and muscle contraction, while the latter are found in the autonomic ganglia (involved in ganglionic transmission), adrenal medulla (where activation causes catecholamine release) and in the brain, where their precise physiological importance is currently unclear. Of the specific antagonists that block these receptor subtypes, and which have clinical application, tubocurarine and related neuromuscular blockers inhibit the N-m type receptor while the antihypertensive agent trimethaphan blocks the N-n receptor.

So far, five subtypes of muscarinic receptor have been described but, unlike the nicotinic receptors, these subtypes act through different secondary messenger systems. The diversity of muscarinic receptor subtypes only became apparent following the discovery that the antagonist pirenzepine blocked gastric secretion at doses that did not affect the activity of muscarinic receptors in the heart. By contrast, atropine blocked both the gastric and cardiac activity of acetylcholine. This led to the classification of these receptors into the M_1 and M_2 types, pirenzepine being specific for M_1 receptors. Anatomically, M_1 receptors are found in ganglia and secretory glands while M_2 receptors are present in the myocardium and on smooth muscle. An additional muscarinic receptor, the M_3 receptor, has also been identified by using the selective antagonist hexahydrosiladifenidol which, in smooth muscle, appears to be involved in contraction and in the secretory glands in facilitating secretion. Cloning techniques have led to the identification of at least five subtypes, the first three of which are identical with the M_1 M_2 and M_3 receptors; all the subtypes are present in the brain but their precise physiological function is unknown. Muscarinic receptors are glycoproteins with molecular weights of about 80 000. It is now known that these receptors contain at least seven membrane spanning units.

Differences between the muscarinic receptors occur not only in their anatomical distribution but also in the nature of their secondary messenger systems. The M_1, M_3 and M_5 receptor subtypes activate a G protein which, via the phosphatidyl inositol pathway, which will be described later, activates phospholipase C activity. The importance of the phosphatidyl inositol pathway lies in the formation of inositol triphosphate which mobilizes calcium from intracellular sources and therefore aids in the facilitation of smooth muscle contraction and in glandular secretion. By contrast, the M_2 and M_4 receptors are linked to another group of G proteins (G_s and G_i, see later) which lead to the inhibition of adenylate cyclase activity. This results in a closing of potassium channels and, together with a reduction in available free calcium ions, leads to reduced cardiac activity. Other changes that occur following muscarinic receptor activation include the release of arachidonic acid (the precursor of the prostenoids such as the prostaglandins) and the second messenger guanylate cyclase. The precise importance of such mechanisms in brain function has not yet been elucidated.

Adrenergic receptors

Ahlquist, in 1948, first proposed that noradrenaline could produce its diverse physiological effects by acting on different populations of adrenoceptors which he termed *alpha* and *beta* receptors. This classification was based upon the relative selectivity of adrenaline for the alpha receptors and isoprenaline for the beta receptors; drugs such as phentolamine were found to be specific antagonists of the alpha and propranolol for the beta receptors. It later became possible to further separate these main groups of receptors into alpha$_1$ and alpha$_2$ based on the selectivity of the antagonists prazosin, the antihypertensive agent that blocks alpha$_1$ receptors, and yohimbine that is an antagonist of alpha$_2$ receptors. At one time it was though that alpha$_1$ receptors were postsynaptic and the alpha$_2$ type were presynaptic and concerned with the inhibitory control of noradrenaline release. Indeed, novel antidepressants like mianserin, and more recently the highly selective alpha$_2$ receptor antagonist idazoxan, were thought to act by stimulating the release of noradrenaline from central noradrenergic synapses. It is now established however that the alpha$_2$ receptors also occur postsynaptically and that their stimulation by specific agonists such as clonidine leads to a reduction in the activity of the vasomotor centre thereby leading to a decrease in blood pressure.

Alpha$_1$ receptors are excitatory in their action while alpha$_2$ receptors are inhibitory, these activities being related to the different types of secondary messengers or ion channels to which they are linked. Thus, alpha$_2$ receptors hyperpolarize presynaptic membranes by opening potassium ion channels and thereby reduce noradrenaline release. Conversely, stimulation of alpha$_1$ receptors increases intracellular calcium via the phosphatidyl-inositol cycle which causes the release of calcium from its intracellular stores; protein kinase C activity is increased as a result of the free calcium which then brings about further changes in the membrane activity. Both types of receptor occur in the brain as well as in vascular and intestinal smooth muscle; alpha$_1$ receptors are found in the heart whereas the alpha$_2$ receptors occur on the platelet membrane (stimulation induces aggregation) and nerve terminals (stimulation inhibits release of the transmitter). It is now recognized that there are several subtypes of alpha$_1$ and alpha$_2$ receptors but their precise function is unclear.

So far three subtypes of beta receptors have been identified and cloned. They differ in their distribution, the beta$_1$ type being found in the heart, the beta$_2$ in lung, smooth muscle, skeletal muscle and liver while the beta$_3$ type occurs in adipose tissue. There is evidence that beta$_2$ adrenoceptors also occur on the lymphocyte membrane but the precise function there is unknown. The antihypertensive drug metoprolol is a clinically effective example of a beta$_1$ antagonist. All the beta receptor subtypes are linked to adenylate cyclase as the second messenger system. It seems that both beta$_1$ and beta$_2$ receptor types occur in the brain and that their activation leads to excitatory effects. Of particular interest to the psychopharmacologist is the finding that chronic antidepressant treatment leads to a decrease in the functional responsiveness of the beta receptors in the brain, and in the density of these receptors on lymphocytes, which coincides with the time necessary for the therapeutic effects of the drugs to be manifest. Such changes have been ascribed to the drugs affecting the activity of the G proteins which couple the receptor to the cyclase subunit. The adrenergic receptors have been purified and their genes cloned. They have seven membrane spanning units which are involved in binding the selective agonists and antagonists.

Dopamine receptors

Two types of dopamine receptors have been characterized in the mammalian brain termed D$_1$ and D$_2$. The existence of these subtypes largely arose in response to the finding that while all types of clinically useful neuroleptics inhibit dopaminergic transmission in the brain, there was a poor correlation between the reduction in adenylate cyclase activity, believed to be the second messenger linked to dopamine receptors, and the clinical potency of the drugs. This was particularly true for the butyrophenone (e.g. haloperidol) series which are known to be potent neuroleptics and yet are relatively inactive in inhibiting adenylate cyclase. Detailed studies of the binding of [3H]haloperidol to neuronal membranes showed that there was a much better correlation between the therapeutic potency of a neuroleptic and its ability to displace this ligand from the nerve membrane. This led to the discovery of two types of dopamine receptor that are both linked to adenylate cyclase but whereas the D_1 receptor is positively linked to the cyclase, the D_2 receptor is negatively linked. It was also shown that the D_1 receptor is approximately 15 times more sensitive to the action of dopamine than the D_2 receptor; conversely, the D_1 receptor has a low affinity for the butyrophenones and atypical neuroleptics such as clozapine whereas the D_2 receptor appears to have a high affinity for most therapeutically active neuroleptics.

There is still some controversy over the precise anatomical location of the dopamine receptor subtypes but there is now evidence that the D_2 receptors are located presynaptically on the corticostriatal neurons and postsynaptically in the striatum and substantia nigra. Conversely, the D_1 receptors are found presynaptically on nigroneostriatal neurons and also occur post-synaptically in the striatum. It is possible to differentiate these receptor types on the basis of their agonist and antagonist affinities. In addition to these two subtypes, there is also evidence that the release of dopamine is partially regulated by feedback inhibition operating via the dopamine autoreceptor.

With the development of D_1 and D_2 agonists however, emphasis has become centred on the pharmacological characteristics of the specific drug in order to determine whether an observed effect is mediated by D_1 or D_2 receptors. It is now apparent that dopamine receptors with the same pharmacological characteristics do not necessarily produce the same functional responses at the same receptor. For example, D_2 receptors are present in both the striatum and the nucleus accumbens but the D_2 receptors cause an inhibition of adenylate cyclase only in the striatum. Furthermore, recent studies indicate that dopamine receptors can influence cellular activities through mechanisms other than adenylate cyclase. These may include direct effects on potassium and calcium channels, as well as modulation of the phosphatidyl-inositol cycle. To further complicate the picture, D_1 and D_2 receptors have opposite effects on some behaviours (for example, chewing behaviour in the rat) but are synergistic in causing other behaviours (for example, locomotor activity and some types of stereotypy).

The densities and functional activities of dopamine receptors have been shown to change in response to chronic drug treatment and in disease states.

Thus an increase in the dopamine receptor density in the nigrostriatal pathway appears to be related to the behavioural supersensitivity observed following unilateral destruction of the dopaminergic system in the striatum. Dopamine receptor antagonists, for example the "classical" neuroleptics such as chlorpromazine, are also known to increase the density of dopamine receptors in the striatal region. This contributes to the extrapyramidal side effects of such drugs which frequently follow their prolonged use and reflect the drug-induced functional deficit of dopamine in the brain.

Abrupt withdrawal of a neuroleptic following its prolonged administration is frequently associated with tardive dyskinesia, a disorder which may be partly due to the sudden activation of supersensitive dopamine receptors. Despite the appeal of this hypothesis, it should be emphasized that many other factors, such as brain damage and prior exposure to tricyclic antidepressants, may also predispose patients to this condition.

In regard to the change in dopamine receptor activity in disease, there is some evidence from post-mortem studies that the density of D_2 receptors is increased in the mesocortical areas of the schizophrenic brain, and in the putamen and caudate nucleus, in neuroleptic-free patients. Subsequent PET studies in schizophrenic patients have, however, failed to confirm these findings. There is also evidence that the link between the D_1 and D_2 receptors is defective in some patients in which the dopaminergic system might be involved. Thus the well-known loss of dopaminergic function in patients with Parkinson's disease is associated with a compensatory rise in the density of postsynaptic D_1 and D_2 receptors. The long-term treatment of Parkinson's disease with L-dopa reduces the receptor density to normal (so-called receptor "down-regulation"). Similarly, the densities of D_1 and D_2 receptors are reduced in the striata of patients with Huntington's chorea, as is the linkage between these receptors.

Recent developments in molecular biology have shown that there are at least four subtypes of dopamine receptor in the mammalian brain. The subtype of the D_2 receptor, the D_3 receptor, has been identified and found to exhibit some unique properties. Thus it differs in its distribution from the D_1 and D_2 receptors in the brain and appears to be present in a high density in limbic regions. It may be differentiated from the D_2 receptor by the fact that it has 100 times greater affinity for the dopamine receptor agonist quinpirole. More recently, an additional subtype of the D_2 receptor has been discovered and termed the D_4 receptor. While the general pharmacological properties of the D_4 receptor resemble the D_2 and D_3 types, the D_4 receptor is of particular interest to psychopharmacologists because of its high affinity for the novel antipsychotic drug, clozapine. Furthermore, as the density of the D_4 receptor is highest in the frontal cortex and amygdala, but relatively low in the basal ganglia, an explanation can now be provided for the efficacy of clozapine in attenuating the symptoms of schizophrenia without causing the extrapyramidal side effects which characterize most conventional neuroleptics.

The subtypes of the D_2 receptor (termed D_{2A} and D_{2B}) were formed by cloning and shown to consist of seven membrane-spanning domains similar to those found in the beta receptor. Differences in the binding of specific agonists and antagonists of the receptor subtypes are presumed to be related to the variations in their amino acid sequences within the membrane-spanning domains. The atypical neuroleptic remoxipride may partly owe its low propensity to cause extrapyramidal effects to its selectivity to block D_{2B} receptors which are predominantly located in the limbic cortex.

The D_1 receptor from both the rat and man has also been cloned. There is recent evidence that a subtype of the receptor, the D_5 receptor, also exists which has a five-fold greater affinity for dopamine than the D_1 receptor. It is located on the neurons in limbic regions of the brain but, unlike the D_1 receptor is not found in the parathyroid, kidney or in the adrenal glands.

The importance of the discoveries of different subtypes of dopamine receptor lies in the possibility of developing drugs which combine selectivity of action with a low incidence of adverse effects. The plausibility of this approach has been assisted by the discovery that clozapine, which for over a decade has been recognized as an atypical neuroleptic, has a selective affinity for the D_4 receptor.

5-HT receptors

Gaddum and Picarelli, in 1957, were the first investigators to provide evidence for the existence of two different types of 5-HT receptor in peripheral smooth muscle. These receptors were termed D (for dibenzyline, an alpha$_1$ adrenoceptor antagonist which also blocked 5-HT receptors) and M (for morphine which blocked the contractile response mediated through the myenteric plexus in the intestinal wall). Receptor binding studies undertaken in the 1980s revealed the existence of multiple binding sites for 5-HT receptors. The 5-HT$_D$ receptor was shown to have the characteristics of the 5-HT$_2$ receptor while the M receptor has been shown to be identical to the 5-HT$_3$ receptor in the brain and gastrointestinal tract.

Ligand binding studies, and more importantly molecular biology techniques, have identified at least 14 different types of 5-HT receptors in the mammalian brain but the main difficulty is to decide on the physiological function of these receptor subtypes. The 5-HT receptors in the brain have been divided into three major groups, namely the 5-HT$_1$-like (which is subdivided into 1A, 1B and 1D), 5-HT$_{2A}$, 5-HT$_{2B}$ and 5-HT$_{2C}$ and 5-HT$_3$. In addition, there is experimental evidence for the existence of a 5-HT$_4$ receptor which may be associated with the 5-HT$_1$ family of receptors. At present, the precise physiological role of this receptor in man is unclear but there is experimental evidence that $5\text{-}HT_4$ receptor agonists can enhance the release of acetylcholine from the guinea-pig ileum which, if this also happens in the brain, could indicate a use for such compounds in the treatment of memory impairment.

Recently $5\text{-}HT_{5A}$ and $5\text{-}HT_{5B}$ receptors have also been identified in mouse brain but so far only the $5\text{-}HT_{5B}$ receptor has been cloned. Both these receptors are labelled by LSD but serotonin only binds to these receptors with a moderate affinity. Pharmacologically the $5\text{-}HT_5$ receptor has many similarities to the $5\text{-}HT_{1D}$ receptor. Potential therapeutic roles for drugs occupying the $5\text{-}HT_5$ receptors include their use in the treatment of anxiety and depression, in motor control and possibly feeding behaviour.

$5\text{-}HT_6$ receptors have been identified in the corpus striatum and in various cortical and limbic regions of the brain. This receptor has now been cloned and several ergolines such as LSD bind to the receptor with a high affinity. Both $5\text{-}HT_5$ and $5\text{-}HT_6$ receptors stimulate cyclic AMP synthesis. Interest in the possible function of these receptors arise from the finding that many atypical neuroleptics (for example, clozapine) and antidepressants (for example, tricyclic antidepressants and amoxapine) bind with high affinity. This suggests that compounds acting on such receptors may be of value in the treatment of psychotic disorder and depression.

Lastly, $5\text{-}HT_7$ receptors have been identified and, like $5\text{-}HT_6$ receptors, are positively linked to adenylylcyclase activity. Many typical (for example, chlorpromazine and spiperone) and atypical (for example, clozapine) neuroleptics bind with a high affinity to these receptors as do LSD, lisuride and mianserin. It has been speculated that $5\text{-}HT_7$ receptors may play a role in the control of mood and that ligands for these receptors may be useful in the treatment of psychotic disorders.

There is some evidence to show that some of these receptor subtypes have physiological correlates. Thus $5\text{-}HT_{1A}$ receptors, located presynaptically on cell bodies and dendrites but not on nerve terminals, mediate the inhibitory effects of 5-HT on raphé neurons and hippocampal pyramidal cells. A potent and selective agonist of the $5\text{-}HT_{1A}$ receptor is 8-hydroxy-dipropylamino tetralin (8OH-DPAT). It now seems likely that the atypical anxiolytic drugs as exemplified by buspirone, gepirone and ipsapirone act in a somewhat similar manner to 8OH-DPAT and may owe their therapeutic activity to their ability to reduce the firing of the raphé nuclei. The $5\text{-}HT_{2A}$ receptors appear to mediate excitatory effects particularly in the cortex. These receptors are also found on the platelet membrane and a decrease in the functional activity of these receptors (e.g. decreased aggregation response to 5-HT) appears to be associated with the symptoms of depression. Ritanserin is a specific antagonist and there is some evidence that it has anxiolytic properties.

Little can be said at present regarding the possible functional importance of the other 5-HT receptor subtypes. The 5-HT$_{1B}$ receptors occur both pre- and postsynaptically on serotonergic terminals while the 5-HT$_{2C}$ receptors appear to be confined to the choroid plexus. At least three of the subtypes have now been cloned (5-HT$_{1A}$, 5-HT$_{2C}$ and 5-HT$_{2A}$). The 5-HT$_{1A}$, 5-HT$_{1B}$ and 5-HT$_{1D}$ receptors are linked to adenylate cyclase which is inhibited by selective agonists. 5-HT$_{2C}$ and 5-HT$_{2A}$ receptors are linked to the phosphatidyl-inositol pathway which is stimulated by agonists, while the 5-HT$_3$ receptors are directly linked to an ion channel which is opened by specific agonists.

There has been considerable interest in the therapeutic potential of the 5-HT$_3$ receptor antagonists, as exemplified by ondansetron, in recent years. While such drugs are undoubtedly useful in the treatment of nausea and emesis, possibly due in part to their action on 5-HT$_3$ receptors in the gastrointestinal tract, there is also evidence that they have anxiolytic properties. Experimental studies have shown that ondansetron has neuroleptic-like properties in animal models of schizophrenia and improves memory in ageing rodents. Whether such findings can be extrapolated to man presently seems uncertain.

Clearly much remains to be learned about the distribution and functional activity of these receptor subtypes before their possible roles in mental illness can be elucidated. A summary of the distribution of the different types of 5-HT receptors and their agonists and antagonists is discussed in more detail in Chapter 5.

Amino acid receptors

There are two amino acid neurotransmitters, namely GABA and glutamate, which have been of major interest to the psychopharmacologist because of the potential therapeutic importance of their agonists and antagonists. The receptors upon which GABA and glutamate act to produce their effects differ from the "classical" transmitter receptors in that they seem to exist as receptor complexes that contain sites for other agonists in addition to the amino acid transmitters which, when occupied, modulate the responsiveness of the receptor to the amino acid. For example, the benzodiazepines have long been known to facilitate inhibitory transmission, and their therapeutic properties as anxiolytics and anticonvulsants are attributable to such an action. It is now apparent that benzodiazepines occupy a receptor site on the GABA receptor complex which enhances the responsiveness of the GABA receptor to the inhibitory action of GABA. Similarly, it has recently been shown that the inhibitory transmitter glycine can act on a strychnine insensitive site on the NMDA receptor, and thereby modify its responsiveness to glutamate. Knowledge of the mechanisms whereby the amino acid transmitters produce their effects have been valuable in the development of psychotropic drugs that may improve memory, reduce anxiety or even counteract the effects of post-stroke hypoxia on brain cell survival. Some of these aspects will be considered later.

GABA receptors

Ligand binding and electrophysiological studies have now clearly established that there are two major classes of GABA receptors, termed GABA-A and GABA-B. The GABA-A receptors have been cloned and the structure of some of the 10 subtypes of this receptor have been described. As these subtypes appear to be heterogeneously distributed throughout the brain it may ultimately be possible to develop drugs that will affect only one specific species of GABA-A receptor, thereby optimizing the therapeutic effect and reducing the possibility of non-specific side effects. It seems likely that this will be an important area for psychotropic drug development in the near future.

The GABA-A receptor is directly linked to chloride ion channels which on activation, results in an increase in the membrane permeability to chloride ions thereby hyperpolarizing cell bodies. GABA-A receptors are also found extrasynaptically where, following activation, they can depolarize neurons. The convulsant drug bicuculline acts as a specific antagonist of GABA on its receptor site, while the convulsant drug picrotoxin binds to an adjacent site on the GABA-A receptor complex and directly decreases chloride ion flux; barbiturates have the opposite effect on the chloride channel and lock the channel open (see Figure 2.17).

The inhibitory effect of GABA is mediated by the chloride ion channel. When the GABA-A receptor is activated by GABA or a specific agonist such as muscimol, the frequency of opening of the channel is increased and the cell is hyperpolarized. Barbiturates, such as phenobarbitone, and possibly alcohol also facilitate the chloride ion influx but these drugs increase the duration, rather than the frequency of the channel opening. Recently, novel benzodiazepine receptor ligands have been produced which, like the typical benzodiazepines, increase the frequency of chloride channel opening. The cyclopyrrolone sedative-hypnotic zopiclone is an example of such a ligand. Some glucocorticoids are also known to have sedative effects which may be ascribed to their ability to activate specific steroid receptor facilitatory sites on the GABA-A receptor.

In addition to the benzodiazepine receptor agonists which, depending on the dose administered have anxiolytic, anticonvulsant, sedative and amnestic properties, benzodiazepines have also been developed which block the action of agonists on this receptor. Such antagonists may be exemplified by flumazenil. Other compounds have a mixture of agonist and antagonist properties and are termed partial agonists or antagonists. However, the

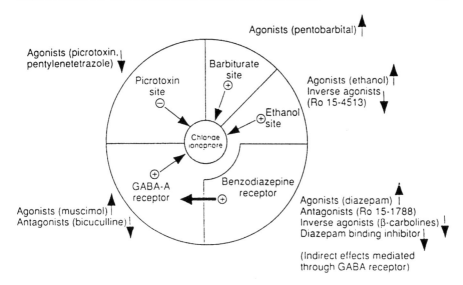

Figure 2.17. Diagrammatic representation of the GABA-benzodiazepine supramolecular complex. Compounds that increase inhibitory transmission may do so either by directly activating the GABA receptor site (e.g. muscimol) or by acting directly on the chloride ionophore (e.g. barbiturates). Benzodiazepines (e.g. diazepam) enhance the sensitivity of the GABA-A receptor to GABA. Compounds that decrease inhibitory transmission may do so by activating the picrotoxin site, which closes the chloride ionophore, or by blocking the GABA-A receptor.

complexity of the benzodiazepine receptor only became fully apparent recently when a series of compounds were discovered that had the opposite effects of the "classical" benzodiazepines when they activated the receptor. These inverse agonists were found to have anxiogenic, proconvulsant, stimulant, spasmogenic and promnesic properties in man and animals. Such compounds were found to decrease GABA transmission.

Naturally occurring inverse agonists called the beta-carbolines have been isolated from human urine but it now seems probable that these compounds are by-products of the extraction procedure. Thus the benzodiazepine receptor is unique in that it has a bidirectional function. This may be of considerable importance in the design of benzodiazepine ligands which act as partial agonists or partial inverse agonists. Such drugs may combine the efficacy of the conventional agents with a lack of unwanted side effects, such as sedation, amnesia and dependence. The presence of a specific benzodiazepine site in the mammalian brain also raises the possibility that endogenous substances are present that modulate the activity of the site. While the precise identity of such natural ligands remains an enigma, there is evidence that substances like tribulin, nephentin and the diazepam-binding inhibitor could have a physiological and pathological function. There is also evidence that trace amounts of benzodiazepines (such as nordiazepam and lorazepam) occur in human brain, human breast milk and also in many plants including the potato! Such benzodiazepines have been found in post-mortem brains from the 1940s and 1950s, before the discovery of the benzodiazepine anxiolytics.

Whereas the GABA-A receptors are widely distributed in the limbic regions of the brain in particular, GABA-B receptors appear to be widely distributed in the brain and at autonomic nerve terminals in the periphery. These receptors differ substantially from the GABA-A receptors in that they are not linked to chloride channels but seem to act by increasing potassium and decreasing calcium conductance. Whereas stimulation of the GABA-A receptors leads to the generation of fast inhibitory potentials, GABA-B activation causes slow inhibitory potentials and directly depolarizes nerve membranes. Other differences between these receptor types are associated with their agonists and antagonists; baclofen, the antispastic drug, is a specific agonist on the B receptors while isoguvacine is a specific agonist for A receptors. While the functional importance of the B receptors is controversial, their ability to facilitate monoamine release in the cortex may form the basis for the possible involvement of these receptors in depression. It is known, for example, that chronic antidepressant treatment reduces the density of these receptors in the brains of experimental animals.

In addition the GABA-A and GABA-B receptors, a new class of GABA receptors has recently been recognized. These GABA-C receptors are unique in that they are activated by very low concentrations of GABA and are unlikely to be desensitized by prolonged exposure to GABA. Once activated, the chloride ion channel which is linked to these receptors remains open for a long time. So far the activity of these receptors has only been investigated in the retina but the GABA-C receptors do occur in the cerebellum and spinal cord. The functional relevance of GABA-C receptors outside the retina has yet to be established.

Excitatory amino acid receptors

It has long been recognized that glutamic and aspartic acids occur in uniquely high concentrations in the mammalian brain and that they can cause excitation of nerve cells. However, these amino acids have only recently been identified as excitatory neurotransmitters because of the difficulty that arose in dissociating their transmitter from their metabolic role in the brain. For example, glutamate is an important component of brain proteins, peptides and a precursor of GABA. As a result of microdialysis and microiontophoretic techniques, in which the release and effect of local application could be demonstrated, and the synthesis and isolation of

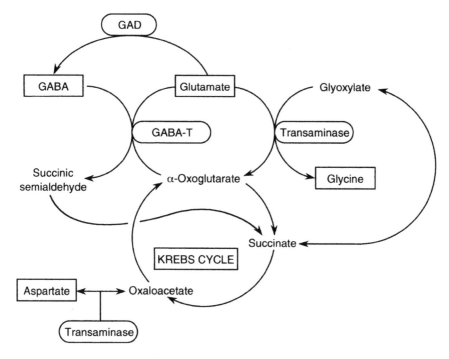

Figure 2.18 Metabolism of transmitter amino acids in the brain. GABA=gamma-aminobutyric acid; GAD=glutamic acid decarboxylase; GABA-T=GABA transaminase. Transmitter substances are marked.

specific agonists for the different types of excitatory amino acid receptor (for example, quisqualic, ibotenic and kainic acids) it is now generally accepted that glutamic and aspartic acids are excitatory transmitters in the mammalian brain. The inter-relationship between the amino acid neurotransmitters and intermediary metabolism is shown in Figure 2.18.

Glutamate and aspartate depolarize neurons by interacting with at least three types of receptors, although it is presently unclear whether they preferentially activate any one of the receptor subtypes *in vivo*. In the excitatory amino acid pathways in the brain, depolarization of postsynaptic membranes occurs within 1–2 msec of stimulation and lasts for 5–10 sec. The excitatory amino acid receptors are selectively permeable to sodium and other cations. The excitatory amino acid receptors have been classified according to the synthetic agonists which specifically activate them. These include the synthetic amino acid N-methyl-D-aspartate (NMDA), kainate and alpha-amino-3-hydroxy-5-methyl-4-isoxazole proprionic acid (AMPA). The AMPA receptor was previously known as the quisqualate receptor. There are also excitatory amino acid receptors that are coupled to adenylate cyclase or inositol phosphate second messenger systems unlike the NMDA, AMPA and kainate receptors which are linked to ion channels. These metabotropic receptors, classified as mGluR1–mGluR6 receptors, either stimulate the synthesis of inositol phosphate (mGluR1 and 5) or decrease the synthesis of cyclic AMP (mGluR3 and 4). Of the various excitatory amino acid receptors which have been identified, the NMDA receptor has been the subject of particular attention. A summary of the properties and possible functional importance of the different types of excitatory amino acid receptor is shown in Table 2.4.

The NMDA receptor consists of multiple regulatory sites that can be manipulated to control the passage of potassium, calcium and sodium ions through the ion channel. This is illustrated in Figure 2.19. In addition to the glutamate, glycine and polyamine (for example, spermine and spermidine) sites which open the ion channel, there are sites in the ion channel to which drugs such as the anticonvulsant dizocilpine (MK801), phencyclidine, ketamine and dextromethorphan bind to block the flow of ions through the channel. The channel is also blocked by magnesium ions. The action of these drugs on the ion channel depends on the extent of depolarization of the nerve membrane; the magnitude of the block is reduced when the membrane is depolarized.

The NMDA receptors are present in the highest densities in the hippocampus, a region of the brain primarily concerned with short-term memory formation. This led Bliss and his colleagues in London to investigate the effects of electrical stimuli to the CA1 region of the hippocampus. They showed that repeated electrical stimulation of this region of the hippocampus resulted in an enhanced postsynaptic depolarization. This increase in the efficacy of synaptic transmission lasted for up to 72 hours and has been called *long-term potentiation* (LTP). It has been hypothesized that LTP is the physiological correlate of memory. In support of this hypothesis it has been shown that drugs which block the NMDA receptor ion channel (such as the dissociation anaesthetic ketamine) block memory formation. The NMDA receptors are also involved in excitotoxic neuronal death. This excitotoxicity is probably linked to a dramatic influx of calcium ions through the NMDA linked ion channel which leads to activation of intracellular proteases and lipases, impaired mitochondrial function and the generation of free radicals. The net result of these changes is destruction of the neuron. Such an event probably accounts for the damage to the brain occurring after a stroke and possibly also in a severe epileptic attack. Indeed it has been suggested that other forms of neurodegenerative disease such as Huntington's chorea and possibly Alzheimer's disease result from an excessive calcium overload mediated by NMDA receptors. A further discussion of the role of NMDA receptors in epilepsy and the neurodegenerative diseases is discussed later (see Chapters 11 and 13).

Table 2.4. Excitatory amino acid receptors

| | Receptor type | | | |
	NMDA	AMPA (quisqualate)	Kainate	Metabotropic
Agonists	Glutamate Aspartate Homocysteate Glycine*	Glutamate Quisqualate	Glutamate Kainate	Glutamate Quisqualate
Antagonists	AP5 CPP 7-chlorokynurenate*	CNQX	CNQX Gamma-DGG Kynurenate	
Channel blockers	Ketamine Phencyclidine MK801 Mg^{2+}			
Effector mechanism	High conductance channels $(Ca^{2+}/Na^+/K^+)$	Low conductance channels (Na^+/K^+)	Low conductance channels (Na^+/K^+)	Activation of PLC→IP3 DAG
Possible functions	Slow epsp Synaptic plasticity/ LTP Excitotoxicity ? Role in epilepsy	Fast synaptic transmission	Fast synaptic transmission	? May be involved in excitotoxicity, plasticity

*Act on glycine modulatory site. AP5=2-amino-5-phosphonovaleric acid; CNQX=6-cyano-7-nitroquinoxaline-2,3-dione; CPP=carboxy-piperazinylpropyl-phosphonic acid.

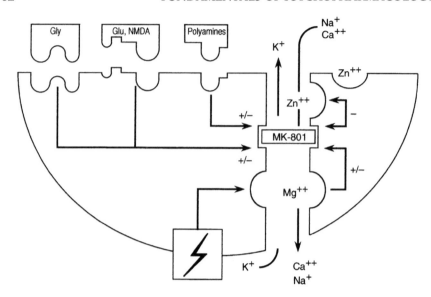

Figure 2.19. Schematic model of the NMDA receptor. The flow of ions through the channel of the NMDA receptor can be regulated by a variety of factors. Glycine (Gly) and glutamate (Glu) must both bind to the NMDA receptor to cause opening of the ion channel. Polyamines bind to a distinct recognition site on the receptor to regulate the opening of the ion channel. Compounds such as MK-801 appear to bind in the open channel. At physiological concentrations of Mg^{++}, the channel is blocked unless the membrane is depolarized. Zn^{++} also regulates the opening of the ion channel.

Less is known about the physiological roles of the AMPA and kainate receptors. It is known however that the AMPA receptors mediate most of the rapid excitatory synaptic responses and that these receptors are widely distributed throughout the brain. Both the AMPA and the kainate receptors often coexist with the NMDA in the brain. A summary of the properties of the main excitatory amino acid receptors is given in Table 2.4 and the structures of some of the agonists and antagonists acting on these receptors in Figure 2.20.

How can psychotropic drugs affect the neurotransmission in the brain?

The "classical" neurotransmitters such as acetylcholine, noradrenaline, dopamine, 5-HT and GABA are presumed to be of fundamental importance in the aetiology of major psychiatric and neurological disease and have therefore been the target of attention of those seeking to explain how

Agonists

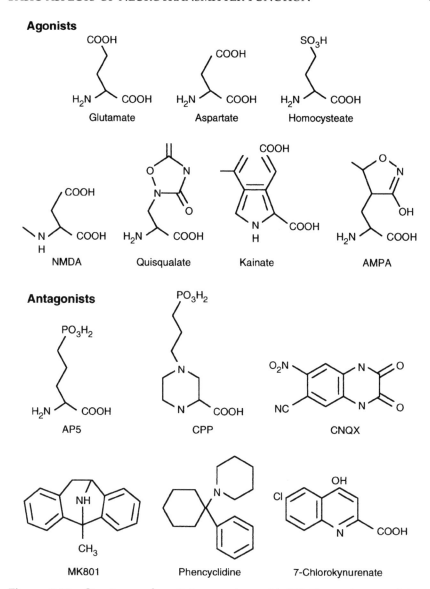

Figure 2.20. Structures of excitatory amino acid (EAA)-receptor agonists and antagonists.

psychotropic drugs act. A detailed account of the biochemical processes involved in the synthesis, release and metabolism of these transmitters is given earlier in this chapter. As common mechanisms appear to exist regarding the storage and release of these transmitters, the actions of psychotropic drugs can be explained in general terms by their effects on some of these processes.

Presynaptic effects of psychotropic drugs

These can arise when, for example, a drug specifically affects the *reuptake* of a transmitter into the nerve terminal. Many different types of antidepressants affect the reuptake of the biogenic amine neurotransmitters (i.e. noradrenaline, dopamine and 5-HT), either specifically (e.g. fluoxetine for 5-HT, maprotiline for noradrenaline, and nomifensine to a lesser extent for dopamine) or non-specifically, as in the case of most tricyclic antidepressants. While this mechanism has been used to explain the therapeutic actions of antidepressants, it is now widely accepted that the long delay in the onset of their therapeutic effects cannot be attributed to such a mechanism. This will be considered in more detail in a later chapter.

A specific reduction in the *availability of the precursor* of the transmitter, for example tyrosine for noradrenaline, tryptophan for 5-HT and choline for acetylcholine, is theoretically a means whereby psychotropic drugs could affect neurotransmission. However, apart from the use of hemicholinium to inhibit the uptake of choline, the acetylcholine precursor, in an animal model of myasthenia gravis, this would not appear to be a mechanism of fundamental importance. It is possible that the acute effects of lithium are, nonetheless, ascribable to an enhanced uptake of both tryptophan and noradrenaline into the nerve terminal. A change in the precursor availability might also be a predisposing factor in some women who develop depression following the use of the high oestrogen containing contraceptive pill. There is evidence that an oestrogen-dependent induction of liver tryptophan pyrrolase can result in a reduction in plasma free tryptophan, which could contribute to a reduction in brain 5-HT synthesis.

Psychotropic drugs can also inhibit the *synthesis* of a transmitter and thereby selectively reduce transmitter function. For example, the peripheral dopa decarboxylase inhibitor carbidopa, by inhibiting the enzyme that catalyses dopa to dopamine, prevents the peripheral breakdown of this amino acid, thereby allowing most of the orally administered drug to reach the brain where it can be converted to dopamine. This is an example of one of the few cases where a knowledge of the basic biochemical mechanism has led to the rational development of a drug to treat a disease of the brain! Other examples of drugs that affect neurotransmitter synthesis include the experimental compounds *para*-chlorophenylalanine and alpha-methyl-*para*-tyrosine, which inhibit tryptophan and tyrosine hydroxylase, respectively, thereby causing a reduction in the synthesis of 5-HT and noradrenaline. It would appear that no psychotropic drugs in current use specifically increase the synthesis of a neurotransmitter, although the rationale behind the use of tryptophan to treat depression was the assumption that it could increase the brain 5-HT concentration, a hypothesis that has not been borne out in practice.

The *storage* of a neurotransmitter in the storage vesicle may be specifically affected by drugs such as reserpine that appear to inhibit the transport to biogenic amine transmitters into the vesicle, thereby rendering the transmitter vulnerable to intraneuronal catabolism by monoamine oxidase. The hypertensive crisis that can occur as a consequence of a patient on a monoamine oxidase inhibitor taking tyramine-containing foods can be explained by the ability of tyramine to displace noradrenaline from peripheral vesicular stores.

Lastly, psychotropic drugs may enhance or impede the *release* of transmitters from the nerve terminal. Stimulants of the amphetamine type, for example, can release catecholamines by a calcium-independent mechanism, which probably explains their marked stimulant properties in both animals and man. Other centrally acting drugs can modify the physiological release of transmitters like noradrenaline by either activating (e.g. the antihypertensive drug clonidine) or inhibiting (e.g. yohimbine or the novel antidepressant mianserin) the presynaptic alpha$_2$ noradrenergic receptor, thereby modifying the calcium flux within the nerve terminal and leading to a decrease or increase in the calcium-dependent fusion of the vesicles with the synaptic membrane. More recently, the introduction of calcium channel inhibitors such as verapamil in the treatment of mania suggests that such drugs may act by reducing the calcium flux across specific types of nerve membrane.

Postsynaptic effects

The most frequent action of psychotropic drugs that modify synaptic transmission involves an activation or inhibition of postsynaptic receptors. For example, neuroleptics are antagonists at dopamine receptors, and it is generally assumed that the therapeutic effects of these drugs is attributable to their ability to reduce dopaminergic transmission by this action. Conversely, drugs such as apomorphine and bromocriptine are dopamine agonists, which accounts for their pharmacological activity (emesis and stereotypy in animals) and their use in the treatment of parkinsonism. Another example of a means whereby psychotropic drugs modify postsynaptic receptor activity is given by the action of the benzodiazepines. These drugs do not act directly on postsynaptic receptors but, by occupying a specific benzodiazepine receptor site which forms part of the GABA-A receptor complex, cause a conformational change in the GABA receptor, thereby increasing its sensitivity to the action of the transmitter. Other novel anxiolytics such as buspirone and ipsapirone apparently owe their

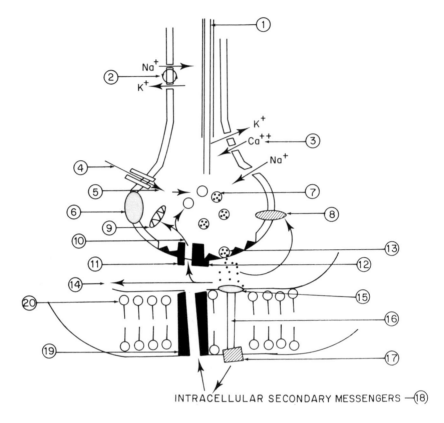

Figure 2.21.   *(Caption opposite).*

pharmacological activity to their agonist action on postsynaptic 5-HT$_{1A}$ receptors.

A general mechanism which appears to be of major importance in regard to the long-term effects of psychotropic drugs on neurotransmission involves *receptor adaptation*. It is evident that most psychotropic drugs only produce their optimal therapeutic effects following their chronic administration, even though it can be shown in patients that they can profoundly affect neurotransmitter function after a single dose. This has led to the suggestion that most psychotropic drugs work by producing subtle changes in receptor function that occur secondarily to their initial biochemical effects. For example, it has been shown that all classes of antidepressants reduce the functional sensitivity of postsynaptic beta adrenoceptors in the frontal cortex of the rat brain (and presumably in the brain of the depressed patient)

Figure 2.21. *(Figure opposite)* Possible sites of action of psychotropic drugs on nerve terminals in the central nervous system. **1**: Axonal transport via neurofilaments. **2**: Sodium potassium ATPase; lithium may slow repolarization processed by this mechanism and by exchange diffusion of ions. **3**: Influx of calcium impeded by calcium channel antagonists, e.g. verapamil, nifedipine. **4**: Precursors of many neurotransmitters transported into nerve terminal by an active transport mechanism. Availability of precursor affected by plasma free concentration. Some drugs (e.g. hemicholinium) may selectively block uptake of precursor (e.g. choline). **5**: Synthesis of transmitter may be selectively inhibited; for example, α-methyl-*para*-tyrosine inhibits tyrosine hydroxylase, the rating-limiting step, and thereby reduces the catecholamine concentration. **6**: Heteroceptor agonists may stimulate or inhibit the release of transmitter from the terminal upon which it is located; for example, baclofen may stimulate cortical noradrenaline release by acting as an agonist at GABA-B heteroceptors. **7**: Storage vesicles. Some "false transmitters" (e.g. tyramine) displace monoamines from their vesicle stores thereby leading to increased activity of the peripheral sympathetic system. **8**: Autoreceptors when stimulated by endogenous or exogenous agonist inhibit neurotransmitter release. Antagonists may have the opposite effect on neurotransmitter release; for example, yohimbine increases release of noradrenaline. **9**: Monoamine oxidase associated with mitochondria in nerve terminal. MAOIs inhibit intraneuronal metabolism of all monoamine neuro-transmitters. **10**: Following reuptake, transmitters with metabolized monoamines are restored in vesicles. Uptake into vesicles is an energy-dependent process which is inhibited by reserpine. **11**: Many transmitters are inactivated by an energy-dependent, high-affinity reuptake process. Many antidepressants inhibit this reuptake process while lithium possibly increases the reuptake of noradrenaline. Cocaine is an inhibitor of most transmitter uptake processes. **12**: Imipramine-binding site that regulates the rate of transport of some monoamine transmitters. Endogenous substances (e.g. tryptolines) may act as modulators of this site. Many antidepressants may act via such binding sites. **13**: Vesicular release of transmitter, usually dependent on intracellular calcium. Amphetamines stimulate amine release by a calcium-independent process. **14**: Some transmitters are metabolized in the synaptic cleft by specific enzymes, e.g. acetylcholinesterase and catechol-*o*-methyltransferase. **15**: Postsynaptic receptor. Many different classes of psychotropic drugs act as antagonists on postsynaptic receptors, e.g. neuroleptics on dopamine receptors. **16**: G protein regulatory unit that is responsible for signal transduction from receptor to second messenger system. Possible that lithium may "incomplete" receptor from second messenger unit. **17**: Secondary messenger unit (e.g. adenylate and guanylate cyclase) whose activity is largely responsible for the physiological response to postsynaptic receptor stimulation. **18**: Intracellular secondary messengers, usually high-energy phosphate compounds such as cyclic AMP. Phosphodiesterase inhibitors (e.g. xanthines) may owe some of their activity to preventing the inactivation of such messengers. **19**: Ion channel may be linked to receptor via a second messenger system (a metabotropic receptor) or directly to a receptor site (an iontropic receptor). Nicotinic receptors are directly blocked by toxins such as alpha-bungarotoxin. **20**: Alcohols and general anaesthetics may produce their pharmacological effects by acting directly on the membrane lipids. The pharmacological effects thus result from a change in membrane fluidity.

following 2–3 weeks' administration, even though there is no evidence that these drugs have a direct effect on beta receptors. The time of onset of this receptor desensitization (or down-regulation) approximately parallels the time it takes for the therapeutic effects of the antidepressant to become apparent. While the precise mechanism whereby this occurs is still the subject of intense research, it would appear that the primary change either occurs in the G protein coupling unit that links the postsynaptic receptor to the secondary messenger unit or is due to a change in the activity of the phosphokinase that enables cyclic AMP to phosphorylate the membrane proteins and thus open the ion channel and depolarize the membrane.

Enzyme inhibition

The two major enzymes concerned with the catabolism of "classical" neurotransmitters are monoamine oxidase and ACHE, the former being largely found in the nerve terminal while the latter is confined to the synaptic cleft. These enzymes are involved in the catabolism of the biogenic amines, such as noradrenaline, dopamine and 5-HT, and acetylcholine, respectively. In addition, catechol-o-methyltransferase occurs in the synaptic cleft, but only plays a minor role in the catabolism of the biogenic amines; it forms o-methylated metabolites of noradrenaline and dopamine such as normetanephrine and homovanillic acid (HVA), respectively. Inhibition of monoamine oxidase by drugs such as phenelzine or pargyline leads to an increase not only in the concentrations of the biogenic amines but also of such "trace" amines as tryptamine and phenylephrine, which may be important in the stimulant properties of some centrally acting drugs. This could have a bearing on the therapeutic effects of monoamine oxidase inhibitors in depression.

Inhibition of ACHE by drugs like physostigmine leads to enhanced cholinergic function. This causes increased gastrointestinal activity, decreased heart rate, etc., which can be attenuated by the concurrent administration of a drug such as atropine methylnitrate, which blocks the peripheral effects of the ACHE inhibitor without affecting its central effects. ACHE inhibitors have been used experimentally to treat Alzheimer's disease. More recently, tetrahydroaminoacridine (THA, tacrine) has been investigated because of its greater selectivity in inhibiting ACHE in the brain. The rationale behind the use of such drugs in the treatment of Alzheimer's disease is based upon the evidence that the cholinergic system is defective, particularly in the familial form of the disease. To date there is little evidence that catechol-o-methyltransferase inhibitors are of any therapeutic value due to their toxicity and lack of efficacy in potentiating central catecholaminergic function.

Neurotransmitter turnover

The net effect of a psychotropic drug on brain transmitter function can be expressed by the turnover index. This index, expressed as the quantity of neurotransmitter synthesized per unit of time, is usually reflected in the amount of transmitter released and catabolized per unit of time. Thus by measuring the effect of a psychotropic drug on the turnover of a transmitter it is possible to quantify its functional effects. While measurement of the turnover rate is largely restricted to studies on animals, it has been of value in predicting how such drugs may affect central transmission in man. An indication of the turnover of 5-HT and dopamine in man may be obtained by measuring the rate of accumulation of the acid metabolites (i.e. 5-HIAA and HVA respectively) in the cerebrospinal fluid following the administration of probenecid. Probenecid blocks the acid carrier mechanism and thereby prevents the efflux of these metabolites from the cerebrospinal fluid.

A schematic representation of the sites at which psychotropic drugs act on central neurotransmission is given in Figure 2.21.

3 Pharmacokinetic Aspects of Psychopharmacology

Introduction

Pharmacokinetics is concerned with the bioavailability, distribution and excretion of drugs. For many classes of drugs there is a direct relationship between the pharmacological and toxicological effects of a drug and its concentration in the body. For most lipophilic drugs, which would include psychotropic agents, there is a positive relationship between the concentration of the drugs in the blood and its concentration at the site of action. Pharmacokinetics also enables the relationship between the efficacy of the drug and the dose administered to the patient to be determined.

The *bioavailability* of a drug is defined as the fraction of the unchanged drug that reaches the systemic circulation following administration by any route. For an intravenously administered drug this equals unity, whereas for an orally administered drug this will be less than unity. This is due to factors such as incomplete absorption, metabolism by the liver and incomplete reabsorption of the drug following enterohepatic cycling.

When assessing the bioavailability of a drug it is also possible to determine the rate at which a given dose reaches the general circulation. Thus by plotting a graph of the blood concentration against the time following administration, the rate at which the peak drug concentration is reached may be calculated from the graph and the bioavailability can be calculated from the area under the curve. The duration of the pharmacological effect is a function of the length of time that the blood concentration is above the minimum effective concentration, while the intensity of the pharmacological effect is directly related to the degree to which the drug concentration exceeds the minimum effective concentration.

There are two further terms which are important in pharmacokinetics – the *clearance* and the *volume of distribution*. The volume of distribution (V_d) relates the quantity of drug in the body to that in the blood or plasma. This factor reflects the space available in the general circulation or within the tissues. Depending on the dissociation constant (pK_a) of the drug in the various body fluids, the lipophilicity, the degree of protein binding to serum and tissue proteins, the V_d of drugs may vary widely. For example, the antimalarial drug quinacrine (mepacrine) has an apparent V_d of 50 000 litres,

71

while drugs that are extensively plasma protein bound have V_d values of as little as 7 litres. The tricyclic antidepressants have a high V_d value despite their strong protein binding; this may be related to their lipophilicity and to the fact that their binding to brain proteins is greater than to plasma proteins.

The clearance of a drug is usually defined as the rate of elimination of a compound in the urine relative to its concentration in the blood. In practice, the clearance value of a drug is usually determined for the kidney, liver, blood or any other tissue, and the total systemic clearance calculated from the sum of the clearance values for the individual tissues. For most drugs clearance is constant over the therapeutic range, so that the rate of drug elimination is directly proportional to the blood concentration. Some drugs, for example phenytoin, exhibit saturable or dose-dependent elimination so that the clearance will not be directly related to the plasma concentration in all cases.

The rate of elimination of a drug from a specific organ can be calculated from the blood flow to and from the organ and the blood concentration. If a drug is largely metabolized in the liver, the clearance of the drug will be largely dependent on the hepatic blood flow; many classes of psychotropic drug are almost completely metabolized by the liver. Small changes in the hepatic circulation or in the rate of liver metabolism will therefore have a dramatic effect on the drug clearance.

Once the clearance rate for a drug is known, the frequency of dosing may be calculated. It is usually desirable to maintain drug concentrations at a steady-state level within a known therapeutic range. This will be achieved when the rate of drug administration equals the total rate of clearance.

Another term which is important in pharmacokinetics is the *half-life* ($t_{1/2}$) of a drug. This value is related to the V_d and the total clearance. If it is assumed that the body is a single compartment in which the size of the compartment equals the V_d, the $t_{1/2}$ may be calculated from the equation:

$$t_{1/2} = 0.693 \, \frac{V_d}{Cl}$$

where Cl is the total clearance. The $t_{1/2}$ is defined as the time required for the drug to obtain 50% of the steady-state level, or to decay 50% from the steady-state concentration after the drug administration has ceased. It must be emphasized that disease states can profoundly affect both the V_d and the clearance, so the $t_{1/2}$ value of a drug is not a reliable indicator of drug disposition unless the functional state of the liver, kidneys, etc. is normal.

This short introduction to the terms used in pharmacokinetics is intended to provide a general overview of the subject. Those wishing to obtain a proper grounding in this important subject are recommended to consult a standard textbook of pharmacology.

Relationship between plasma neuroleptic concentrations and the therapeutic response

Controversy still rages regarding the value of measuring the plasma drug concentrations of psychotropic drugs as a means of assessing the therapeutic response of the patient to treatment. A number of factors determine the value of such information. These include:

1. The reliability of the assay method used to determine the concentration of the drug and its possible metabolites.
2. The homogeneous nature of the patient population and the number of patients in the sample.
3. The use of fixed doses of the drugs so that the plasma levels remain independent of clinical impression or improvement.
4. The use of double-blind conditions and ensuring that the drug is administered for an adequate period of time.
5. Ensuring that other drugs or treatments are not administered which may interact with the psychotropic drug under investigation (e.g. lithium, electroconvulsive therapy).
6. Use of appropriate statistical methods for the analysis of the data.

Unfortunately, few of the studies that have attempted to relate the blood concentrations of neuroleptics to therapeutic response have fulfilled all these criteria. There is a suggestion that a *"therapeutic window"* exists for some phenothiazine neuroleptics. A therapeutic window is a range of concentrations of a drug measured in the blood that are associated with a good therapeutic response. Plasma concentrations outside this range are either too low to ensure a therapeutic response or so high that they induce toxic side effects. Despite the numerous studies of the relationship between the plasma concentration and the therapeutic response for a number of "standard" neuroleptics, it would appear that such correlations rarely account for more than 25% of the variance in clinical response to treatment. The existence of a therapeutic window for neuroleptics would therefore appear to be unproven. However, there could be ranges of plasma concentrations associated with optimal antipsychotic action, but these must be defined separately for each drug. There is also evidence that some non-responders to treatment may improve when the plasma drug concentration is reduced rather than raised.

Besides the poor specificity of many of the assays used to determine plasma drug concentrations, another problem which has arisen from these studies has been the length of the "wash-out" period necessary before the patient is given the neuroleptic under investigation. As a result of the prolonged duration of blockade of dopamine receptors in the brain by conventional neuroleptics and their metabolites, it is necessary to allow a wash-out period of several weeks before the patients are subject to a pharmacokinetic study. This raises serious ethical questions. Perhaps with the advent of new imaging techniques it may be possible in the near future actually to determine the rate of disappearance of neuroleptics from the brain of the patient. This may enable the relationship between plasma concentration and clinical response to be accurately determined.

Relationship between plasma antidepressant concentrations and the therapeutic response

Over the past 20 years there has been widespread interest in monitoring plasma antidepressant, particularly tricyclic, levels to optimize the response to treatment. One aspect of this research that is universally agreed upon concerns the extensive interindividual variability among patients, but it is still uncertain whether a knowledge of the plasma drug concentration is of clinical value.

For the tricyclic antidepressants (TCAs) the two major oxidative pathways that occur in the liver are desmethylation and hydroxylation, the latter pathway being the main rate-limiting step that governs the renal excretion of these drugs. *First-pass metabolism*, whereby the drug passes via the portal system directly to the liver, is much greater following oral rather than intravenous administration of such drugs. For the major TCAs, first-pass metabolism accounts for approximately 50% or more of the drug concentration which enters the portal circulation. Such extensive first-pass metabolism probably occurs with the newer antidepressants that also undergo oxidation and desmethylation in the liver. It seems possible that the presence of high concentrations of the therapeutically inactive hydroxylated metabolites of the TCAs in the brain could result in a reduction in the therapeutic activity of the parent compound. The presence of desmethylated metabolites of the tertiary antidepressants such as norchlorimipramine and desipramine undoubtedly contribute to the antidepressant effects of the parent compound. Whereas the tertiary precursors show some selectivity for inhibiting the uptake of 5-hydroxytryptamine (5-HT) into the nerve terminal, the desmethylated metabolites show selectivity as noradrenaline uptake inhibitors. Thus no TCA can be considered to be selective in inhibiting the uptake of either of these biogenic amines. In the case of TCA overdose, the normal oxidative pathways in the liver are probably saturated, which leads to a disproportionately high concentration of the desmethylated metabolite.

The practical consequence of this finding is that toxic plasma concentrations of a TCA are very likely to occur if the dose of the drug is increased in those patients who fail to respond to normal therapeutic doses of the drug. Such a transition to toxic doses could occur suddenly.

There is good evidence that *genetic differences* in hepatic metabolism are responsible for the large interindividual variation in the metabolism of TCAs, including maprotiline and the monoamine oxidase inhibitors. Such genetic factors have been investigated using pharmacogenetic probes. Drugs such as antipyrine (phenazone) and debrisoquine have been investigated in patients treated with TCAs to see if the clearance of such drugs correlates with the metabolism of the antidepressants. It has been found that the clearance of antipyrine correlated well with the metabolism of the benzodiazepines but not with all of the TCAs. Those individuals who showed a deficient hydroxylation of debrisoquine also differed from the normal population in their metabolism of TCAs. However, at the present level of knowledge, it would appear that despite overall similarities in the metabolic pathways for most antidepressants, specific drugs are subject to specific metabolic processes that limit the application of pharmacokinetic phenotyping compounds such as debrisoquine. If the pharmacokinetic properties of an antidepressant in an individual patient need to be known, a test dose of the drug should be given. However, to date there is no convincing evidence that such information improves the frequency of the therapeutic response!

It may be concluded that, so far, a pharmacokinetic analysis of antidepressants is of limited clinical value because of:

1. Large interindividual variability in plasma concentrations which reflect genetically determined metabolic differences.
2. The effects of variables such as age, sex, race and drug interactions on the pharmacokinetics of the antidepressant.
3. The presence of therapeutically active metabolites that may contribute to the pharmacodynamic and toxic effects.

In contrast to the limited value of pharmacokinetics to the use of antidepressants, knowledge of the kinetics of *lithium* has been important in defining the therapeutic and toxic range in unipolar or bipolar manic patients. Prediction of the dose required by the individual patient by giving a single dose of the drug and measuring the erythrocyte/plasma lithium ratio has been shown to be useful, and non-compliance of a patient can be readily detected. The pharmacokinetic profiles of the various types of normal- and slow-release preparations now enable adjustment of the dosage to the needs of the individual patient. Such knowledge has also led to the clinical practice of maintaining the patient on the lowest plasma concentration of lithium for long periods of time, thereby prolonging the remission of both manic and depressive symptoms.

Pharmacokinetic aspects of TCAs

All TCAs are fairly well absorbed following oral administration. Although it is recommended that TCAs are administered in divided doses initially, their relatively long half-lives (12–20 hours) and relatively wide dose range (50–300 mg) mean that a once daily dose at night is often preferred. However, it must be remembered that, due to the structure of the drugs, the higher therapeutic doses have potent anticholinergic effects which lead to a reduction in gastrointestinal tract activity and gastric emptying. As a consequence, the absorption of the antidepressant is impeded, as is that of any drug given concurrently. The plasma concentration of most TCAs reaches a peak 2–8 hours after oral administration and once absorbed the drugs are widely distributed. As these drugs are highly protein bound, and also bind to tissue proteins, they have a high apparent volume of distribution. This implies that plasma drug monitoring to ensure optimal therapeutic response is of questionable value, even though it is often recommended that the most satisfactory antidepressant response occurs in the plasma concentration range of 50–300 ng/ml, toxic effects becoming apparent when the drug concentration reaches $0.5–1.0 \mu g/ml$.

The metabolism and elimination of TCAs takes several days to occur, the elimination half-life ranging from 20 hours for amitriptyline to 80 hours for protriptyline. The half-life values for the desmethylated metabolites such as desmethylimipramine and nortriptyline are approximately twice those of the parent compounds imipramine and amitriptyline. It is also well established that the half-life values of the TCAs are considerably greater in the elderly, which predisposes such patients to a greater possibility of severe side effects.

Pharmacokinetic aspects of MAOIs

All the commonly used MAOIs (monoamine oxidase inhibitors), exemplified by phenelzine, isocarboxazid and pargyline, are irreversible inhibitors of both forms of the enzyme, forming covalent bonds with the active sites on the enzyme surface. This is the reason why the effects of these drugs last for many days even though their blood concentrations are undetectable. This can result in an accumulation of the drugs following their long-term use as they can also inhibit their own metabolism. These drugs are metabolized in the liver largely by a process of acetylation. Because of the relevance of the genetic status of the patient to the rate of metabolism of many drugs that are acetylated (the half-life of a drug that is acetylated rapidly being shorter and therefore less likely to accumulate than one that is slowly acetylated), it was hypothesized that the acetylator status of patients being treated with the older type of MAOIs may be an important determinant of their therapeutic effects. Recent clinical studies, however, have failed to show that the acetylator status is an important determinant of the therapeutic action of the phenelzine type of drug.

Because the long duration of action of the older irreversible inhibitors of MAO could be responsible for unnecessary drug and dietary interactions, different types of MAOIs have been synthesized which are reversible inhibitors of the enzyme. Such compounds have the advantage that their action on the enzyme can be terminated by the presence of the high concentration of a natural substrate. Thus, should a patient on such a reversible inhibitor inadvertently take a tyramine-rich food, the tyramine would overcome the inhibitory effect of the drug on the MAO in the gastrointestinal wall and be metabolized. The tyramine would not then be absorbed and lead to the chance of a hypertensive episode. However, the MAO activity in other tissues, including the brain, would remain inhibited by the drug so that the therapeutic benefits would be maintained. In addition to the advantage of being less likely to interact with dietary amines, reversible MAOIs have a shorter duration of action than the irreversible inhibitors. Brofaromine, for example, has a half-life of 12 hours in the brain, in contrast to several days in the case of the phenelzine type of MAOI. A further advantage of the reversible and selective inhibitors lies in their effects on brain amines. Initially an irreversible inhibitor such as clorgyline may show selectivity, but will lose this following chronic treatment due to its long duration of action and possible accumulation. Such an effect is less likely to occur with the reversible MAOIs, which will be metabolized more readily, will not accumulate and will therefore be less likely to inhibit the non-preferred isoenzyme. Several selective MAO-A type inhibitors have now been synthesized (e.g. brofaromine, cimoxatone, moclobemide and tolox-atone) which have proven to be clinically effective antidepressants. There is evidence that some of these inhibitors, for example moclobemide, act as pro-drugs in that they form active metabolites *in vivo* which have a greater affinity for MAO-A than the parent compound. Of the selective and reversible MAO-B inhibitors, caroxazone and Ro 16-6491 are currently undergoing development.

Relationship between plasma anxiolytic concentrations and the therapeutic response

While the individual drugs in the benzodiazepine group differ in potency, all benzodiazepines in common use have anxiolytic, sedative-hypnotic, anticonvulsant and muscle-relaxant activity in ascending order of dose. The main clinical difference between the individual drugs lies in the time of onset of their therapeutic effect, and the intensity and duration of their clinical activity.

All benzodiazepines are derived from weak organic acids and some, such as midazolam, form water-soluble salts at a low pH. However, at normal physiological pHs, all benzodiazepines are lipophilic, the lipid solubility varying from highly lipophilic in the case of drugs like midazolam, flurazepam, diazepam and triazolam to slightly lipophilic for drugs such as clonazepam, bromazepam and lormetazepam. The benzodiazepines are also highly protein bound, so that at the plasma pH the proportion of the drug in the free form will vary from only 2% in the case of diazepam to about 30% with alprazolam. However, for most benzodiazepines the percentage of the drug in the pharmacologically active free form is independent of the total plasma concentration over a wide therapeutic range.

Transport of the benzodiazepines into the brain is rapid, the rate of uptake being determined by the physicochemical properties of the drug. Absorption from the gastrointestinal tract, or from an injection site, is the rate-limiting step governing the speed of onset of the therapeutic response. Oral absorption is more rapid when the drug is taken on an empty stomach.

The activity of benzodiazepines may be terminated when the drug is removed from the benzodiazepine receptor site and diffuses into peripheral adipose tissue sites and then metabolized in the liver, or when there is a decrease in the sensitivity of the benzodiazepine receptors following chronic exposure to the drug (termed *acute tolerance*). The rate of development of acute tolerance appears to vary with the different benzodiazepines, making it difficult to relate the changes in therapeutic response to the changes in plasma concentration.

Pharmacokinetic factors do play a role in terminating the pharmacological effects of these drugs however. It would appear that the distribution of the drug rather than its clearance is the most important factor governing the termination of action. The extent of peripheral distribution of a benzodiazepine increases according to the lipophilicity of the drug. This phase is usually rapid and leads to the termination of the therapeutic effects of the drug; the apparent elimination $t_{1/2}$ of the drug is usually much slower and is not necessarily related to the time course of the pharmacological effects. This means that drugs with apparently long half-lives may have very short durations of action due to their extensive distribution throughout the body, whereas those drugs that are less lipophilic have a smaller V_d and therefore a longer duration of action, particularly after a single dose. Midazolam is an unusual benzodiazepine in that it is very lipophilic, has a large V_d and is rapidly metabolized and excreted. Both clearance and distribution therefore contribute to the cessation of its therapeutic effect.

The extent of accumulation of an anxiolytic will depend on the elimination half-life in relation to the dosing interval. Thus drugs with long half-lives will have cumulative sedative effects, and may impair cognition, following repeated administration. However, despite increasing blood and presumably brain concentrations of the drug, central depression does not increase in parallel because of the development of tolerance to the non-specific depressant actions of the drug. Long half-life anxiolytics are slowly eliminated whereas short half-life drugs tend to be eliminated rapidly. This means that the dose of the latter type of drug must be tapered slowly to avoid withdrawal effects at the end of a period of treatment.

Oxidation and *conjugation* are the principal mechanisms whereby the benzodiazepines are metabolized. Nitroreduction is an additional pathway that is involved in the metabolism of nitrazepam, flunitrazepam and clonazepam. Aliphatic hydroxylation and *N*-dealkylation are the main oxidative routes and often lead to active metabolites (e.g. diazepam gives rise to desmethyldiazepam, oxazepam and temazepam as active metabolites). The second main mechanism is hepatic conjugation to glucuronic acid. Drugs such as oxazepam, lorazepam, temazepam and lormetazepam are inactivated in this way. The main oxidative pathways are influenced by physiological factors such as age, by pathological factors such as hepatitis and by drugs such as the oestrogens and cimetidine which affect hepatic oxidative metabolism.

The relative contribution of the active metabolites of the benzodiazepines to the overall therapeutic effect of the parent compound will depend on the concentration of the metabolite formed, its agonist potency at central benzodiazepine receptors and its lipophilicity. For example, after the chronic administration of diazepam, desmethyldiazepam accumulates in the brain. As this metabolite has potency at the benzodiazepine receptors equal to diazepam, the metabolite probably plays an important part in the overall action of diazepam. In the case of clobazam, however, even though the active metabolite desmethylclobazam is present in higher concentrations than the parent compound after chronic administration, it has a lower potency than clobazam and therefore is of less importance than the parent compound with regard to the anxiolytic effect.

Of the *non-benzodiazepines* that have been introduced recently for the treatment of anxiety and insomnia, buspirone and zopiclone have been the most extensively investigated so far. The pharmacokinetic characteristics of zopiclone have been studied in healthy subjects, in the elderly and in patients with renal and hepatic malfunction. It would appear that the kinetics of this drug only alter appreciably in patients in the terminal stages of renal or hepatic disease; in the elderly only a slight increase in the half-life of the drug was observed. Zopiclone is a short (approximately 5 hours) half-life hypnotic which is converted to another short half-life active metabolite, zopiclone N-oxide. The kinetics of the drug are not apparently altered by repeated daily dosing. Buspirone and its close analogue gepirone form the active metabolite 1-piperazine (1-PP). There is also extensive metabolism of the parent compound by hydroxylation and oxidation. The 1-PP metabolite is lipophilic and rapidly enters the brain, where it has an apparent $t_{1/2}$ of about 2.5 hours. This metabolite also accumulates in the brain after chronic dosing, thereby suggesting that it contributes to the anxiolytic action of the parent compound.

The importance of drug pharmacokinetics to drug interactions

Genetic polymorphism

In pharmacokinetics, genetic polymorphism refers to differences between individuals' ability to metabolize drugs. More than 25 years ago it was shown that the steady-state plasma concentration of the TCA nortriptyline was related to the genetic characteristics of the patient. Thus homozygous, but not heterozygous, twins had similar blood nortriptyline concentrations. Since that time it has become clear that many of the liver enzymes concerned with drug metabolism exhibit genetic polymorphism. This may be particularly important when depressed patients receiving antidepressant therapy are also given other drugs which compete for the same hepatic enzyme.

Each cytochrome P450 isoenzyme is the product of a separate gene, and so far more than 200 such genes have been identified. Furthermore, a number of cytochrome P450 genes have been shown to have different alleles which have resulted from mutation. Where such a mutation exists in more than 1% of the population, the term "genetic polymorphism" is applied. Many of the polymorphic forms of the cytochrome P450 enzyme appear to be of minor significance in drug metabolism. Substrates and inhibitors of these isoenzymes are presented in Table 3.1.

In some individuals an isoenzyme may be absent. This is an inherited trait which can vary in incidence according to racial background. Depending on whether the isoenzyme is absent or present, individuals are classified as extensive or poor metabolizers of the reference compound.

The clinical importance of genetic polymorphism depends on factors such as the health status of the patient and the concomitant administration of any drugs which might act as a substrate or inhibitor of a particular isoenzyme. For example, a depressed patient who metabolizes an SSRI (selective serotonin reuptake inhibitor) slowly will have higher plasma concentrations of that drug than another patient who metabolizes the drug at the normal rate. However, this is unlikely to be clinically significant given the high therapeutic index of the SSRIs. In contrast, TCAs have a low therapeutic

Table 3.1.   Characteristics, substrates and inhibitors of some cytochrome P450 isoenzymes

Isoenzyme	Polymorphism	Substrate	Inhibitor
1A2	Probably not, but very wide interpatient variability	Warfarin, propranolol, phenacetin, clozapine, theophylline, TCAs (desmethylation)	Fluvoxamine
2C	2–3% of Caucasians 15–25% of Orientals	Diazepam, tolbutamide, phenytoin, TCAs (desmethylation)	Fluvoxamine, fluoxetine, sertraline
2D6	5–8% of Caucasians Lower in other races	Codeine, dextromethorphan, such as haloperidol, thioridazine, perphenazine, nortriptyline, desipramine, fluoxetine, norfluoxetine, TCAs (hydroxylation), beta-blockers such as timolol and metoprolol, type 1C antiarrhythmics encainide, flecainide	Fluoxetine, paroxetine, sertraline, fluphenazine
3A4	Unknown	TCAs (desmethylation), triazolam, alprazolam, midazolam, carbamazepine, terfenadine, quinidine, lidocaine, erythromycin, cyclosporin	Very likely all SSRIs (norfluoxetine particularly), nefazodone, ketoconazole

index and the active metabolites of amitriptyline (nortriptyline) and imipramine (desimipramine) are usually hydroxylated via the cytochrome P450 2D6 pathway. Slow metabolizers of desmethylated TCAs will experience TCA accumulation, which may result in potentially toxic cardiovascular effects. Conversely, patients who are fast metabolizers may experience subtherapeutic plasma drug concentrations.

Another factor which should be considered is the relative importance of the defective metabolic pathway in the overall metabolism of a drug. For example, paroxetine is metabolized by at least two pathways and the suboptimal activity of one enzyme has a relatively minor effect on the elimination of the drug. For the other SSRIs, the hepatic enzymes responsible for oxidization have not been clearly identified. However, these agents have a high affinity for the cytochrome P450 system and drug–drug interactions may be important under certain circumstances.

Drug–drug interactions

Drugs may interact on a pharmacodynamic or pharmacokinetic basis. Pharmacodynamic drug–drug interactions arise with agents which act on the same receptors, sites of action or physiological systems. Pharmacokinetic interactions involve the interference of one drug with the absorption, transport, distribution, metabolism or elimination of another.

The SSRIs bind to and inhibit some forms of cytochrome P450 that are involved in oxidative metabolism. These enzymes are principally found in the liver, where most oxidative drug metabolism occurs, and to a lesser extent in tissues such as the gut wall, kidneys and brain. The propensity for interactions between SSRIs and other agents is not all-inclusive. Indeed, not all drugs undergo oxidative metabolism, and many are efficiently eliminated without undergoing extensive metabolism.

In the liver, the *cytochrome P450* isoenzyme system (CYP450) catalyses the oxidation of many endogenous substances (such as lipids and steroids) and a variety of lipophobic drugs. CYP450 comprises a group of isoenzymes located in the endoplasmic reticulum. There are four cytochrome P450 isoenzymes of theoretical importance in the metabolism of antidepressant drugs: 1A2, 2C, 2D6 and 3A4. While the metabolism of many therapeutically useful drugs has been attributed to specific cytochrome P450 isoenzyme(s), the isoenzymes involved in the metabolism of most drugs remain elusive.

When the affinity of a drug for an enzyme is high (i.e. the pair bind tightly), there is less opportunity for additional molecules to bind and the enzyme can metabolize only a portion of the drug molecules available in the hepatic circulation at any one time. Thus, if an SSRI binds with high affinity to an isoenzyme, then the metabolism of any other drug which usually binds to this isoenzyme will be potently inhibited when SSRIs are given concomitantly. Conversely, drugs that bind to an isoenzyme with low affinity have a greater propensity for metabolic inhibition through higher-affinity binding of other compounds.

There are several possible drug–drug interactions due to the SSRIs acting as inhibitors of different cytochrome P450 isoenzymes (Table 3.1). For example, fluoxetine and its active metabolite norfluoxetine can inhibit the isoenzymes 2C, 2D6 and 3A4, which suggests that a drug–drug interaction could occur with phenytoin (2C isoenzyme), TCAs, antipsychotic agents, type 1C antiarrhythmics (2D6) and carbamazepine (3A4). Fluvoxamine may interact with theophylline, clozapine, TCAs (1A2 isoenzyme), carbamazepine, alprazolam and triazolam (3A4). The only clinically significant interaction, however, has been between particular SSRIs and some TCAs. Indeed, fluoxetine may cause plasma TCA levels to rise within the toxic range, but only in a few patients who receive therapeutic doses of both fluoxetine and desipramine. Sertraline has also occasionally been associated with such interactions.

When more than one drug is necessary for the treatment of the depressed patient, it is always prudent clinical practice to consider the possibility of pharmacodynamic or pharmacokinetic interactions. For example, if treatment with an SSRI is to continue, it may be necessary to reduce its dose should a potential inhibitor of one of the cytochrome P450 isoenzymes be given concomitantly. This is particularly important when a TCA is administered with an SSRI. Furthermore, it is important to recognize not only that competitive substrate inhibition may commence shortly after the administration of the first dose of the SSRI, but also that the full clinical consequences of such an interaction may not occur until the SSRI has reached its steady-state concentration. For most SSRIs (fluvoxamine, paroxetine, sertraline and citalopram) this will occur within 4–6 days of starting treatment, although for fluoxetine (and its metabolite norfluoxetine), which have longer elimination half-lives, it may take several weeks. Special care should always be taken in adding drugs which have a narrow therapeutic index (such as the TCAs and theophylline), and in such cases plasma drug monitoring is a useful precaution. In general, metabolic interactions should always be considered when an SSRI is started or stopped or the dosage changed.

The potential interaction between SSRIs and MAOIs or L-*tryptophan* can cause the *serotonergic syndrome*, which is characterized by excitation and tremor and is sometimes fatal. For this reason, therapy with an MAOI should not be initiated *within 5 weeks* of stopping fluoxetine treatment, or *within 2 weeks* of stopping treatment with any other SSRI.

Drug–protein interactions

In addition to metabolic interactions, consideration should be given to drug–protein binding interactions, although there is little clinical evidence to suggest that such interactions are of any consequence with the SSRIs. It must be stressed that many liver enzymes are non-specific for their substrates and that most drugs are metabolized by multiple pathways. Good therapeutic practice demands that drug interactions should be considered carefully, particularly in subpopulations of depressed patients such as the elderly or those with hepatic dysfunction or a history of alcoholism.

In SUMMARY, it would appear that a detailed knowledge of the pharmacokinetics of the main groups of psychotropic drugs is only of very limited clinical use. This is due to limitations in the methods for the detection of some drugs (e.g. the neuroleptics), the presence of active metabolites which make an important contribution to the therapeutic effect, particularly after chronic administration (e.g. many antidepressants, neuroleptics and anxiolytics), and the lack of a direct correlation between the plasma concentration of the drug and its therapeutic effect. Perhaps the only real advances will be made in this area with the development of brain imaging techniques whereby the concentrations of the active drug in the brain of the patient may be directly measured. Until such time as the kinetics of psychotropic drugs in the brain can be properly assessed, it can be concluded that the routine determination of plasma levels of psychotropic drugs is of very limited value.

Despite the limited value of measuring plasma psychotropic drug concentrations to assess clinical response, a knowledge of the pharmacokinetics of such a drug can be of value in predicting drug interactions.

4 Molecular Genetics and Psychopharmacology

In recent years the psychopharmacologist has paid increasing attention to the examination of brain proteins with which psychotropic drugs react, and also the molecular mechanisms that control the synthesis and cellular function of these proteins. For this reason, any understanding of psychopharmacology requires some knowledge of the basic techniques of molecular genetics.

Genes are composed of deoxyribonucleic acid (DNA) which is a long polymer composed of deoxyribonucleotides. Each deoxyribose nucleotide has one of the following purine or pyrimidine bases, namely adenosine, guanine, thymine or cystosine. A single gene may contain from a few thousand to several hundred thousand bases that are arranged in a specific sequence according to the information contained in the gene. It is this sequence of bases which determines the structure of the gene product which is a protein. In addition, the gene also contains information regarding the way in which the gene is expressed during development and in response to environmental stimuli.

The role of DNA in storing and transferring genetic material is dependent on the properties of the four bases. These *bases are complementary* in that guanine is always associated with cytosine, and adenosine with thymine. Watson and Crick, some 40 years ago, showed that the stability of DNA is due to the double helix structure of the molecule that protects it from major perturbations. Information is ultimately transferred by separating these strands which then act as templates for the synthesis of new nucleic acid molecules.

There are two ways in which DNA molecules may act as templates. Firstly, DNA is used as a template for replicating additional copies during cell division. This occurs by free deoxyribonucleotides binding to the complementary bases of the exposed DNA strand and then being linked by the enzyme DNA polymerase to form a new DNA double helix. Secondly, small sections of the DNA molecule are used as a template for the synthesis of *messenger ribonucleotides* (mRNAs) which are responsible for carrying the message for the synthesis of specific proteins. mRNAs differ from DNA in that they are much shorter (generally 7000 base pairs in length) and are single stranded. mRNAs contain the information necessary for the synthesis of a specific protein and also contain the pentose sugar moiety ribose instead of deoxyribose found in DNA. In addition, thymine is replaced by the pyrimadine base uracil which, like thymine, is complementary to adenine.

The human genome contains approximately 100 000 genes which are distributed with a total DNA sequence of 3 billion nucleotides. The DNA of the human genome is divided into 24 exceptionally large molecules each of which is a constituent of a particular chromosome of which 22 are autosomes and 2 are sex chromosomes (X and Y chromosomes).

Translation of the information encoded in DNA, expressed as a particular nucleotide sequence, into a protein, expressed as an amino acid sequence, depends on the genetic code. In this code, sequences of three nucleotides (termed a *codon*) represent one of the 20 amino acids that compose the protein molecule. Because there are 64 codons which can be constructed for the four different bases, and only 20 different amino acids that are coded for, several amino acids may be coded for by more than one codon. There are also three codons, called *stop codons*, that terminate the transfer of information. Furthermore, although all cells contain the same complement of genes, certain cells (for example, the neurons) have specialized genes that encode specific proteins for the synthesis of specific transmitters. The expression of such genes is under the control of regulatory proteins called transcription factors which control the transcription of mRNA from the genes they control.

The expression of enzymes that control neurotransmitter systems is controlled not only by factors operating during embryonic development, but also by the degree of neuronal activity. Thus the more active the nervous system, the greater the genetically controlled synthesis of the neurotransmitters which clearly play an important role in the behaviour of the organism. Regulation of the genes also determines the response of the brain to drugs, hence the importance of molecular genetics to psychopharmacology.

One of the most important areas of molecular genetics concerns the role of specific base sequences, called *regulatory sequences*, that surrounded the sections of the gene that encode the amino acid sequence of a protein. These regulatory sequences are activated or inactivated by specific transcription factors and it is the complex interaction of regulatory sequences and transcription factors that underlies the adaptation of brain function to the effects of some psychotropic drugs. For example, it is well known that the optimal response to an antidepressant or neuroleptic drug requires several weeks of treatment. Such adaptive changes are probably a reflection of the molecular genetics of neurotransmitter function and may help to explain the lack of success in developing antidepressants or neuroleptics that have a rapid therapeutic action.

How may genes be manipulated?

One of the main goals of molecular genetics is to determine the base sequence of the human genome. This is the purpose of the Human Genome Project, an international collaborative research programme aimed at providing a complete analysis of the human genome within the next decade. The first step in such an analysis is to isolate the small sequences of bases in DNA that are transcribed into mRNAs. The information contained in the mRNAs can be isolated and amplified by a technique called *cDNA cloning*. In this technique, mRNAs from brain tissue, for example, are purified and then treated with reverse transcriptase which converts mRNAs into single complementary strands of DNA. This is called *complementary DNA* (cDNA). The cDNA provides a template for producing a second strand that is complementary to the first. This double-stranded cDNA is then incubated with bacterial plasmids to produce *recombination DNA plasmids*. Plasmids may be considered as bacterial viruses that can reproduce themselves when inserted into the appropriate bacteria so that during the process of bacterial cell division multiple copies of the cDNA that had been inserted in the plasmid is formed. As each bacterium is likely to be infected with a plasmid, containing a different type of cDNA, the resulting medium will contain a mixed population of cDNAs from the original brain tissue. This is called a *cDNA library*.

The individual components of the cDNA library may be obtained by grouping individual bacteria on a culture medium so that they reproduce to form identical clones. This enables a large quantity of specific cDNAs to be produced in a pure form. The cDNA within these plasmid-containing bacteria can then be removed, and the precise nucleotide sequence determined by standard automated analytical procedures.

Since the brain expresses many mRNAs that are also found in non-nervous tissue and are therefore of little interest to the psychopharmacologist, it is necessary to isolate only those cDNAs that, for example, encode for a specific enzyme or receptor protein. Several techniques have been developed to achieve this. For example, a specific cDNA plasmid may be inserted into cultured mammalian cells such as fibroblasts that can express the specific receptor or enzyme. Once this has been expressed in the culture medium, the receptor or enzyme can be identified by adding a specific ligand or substrate. This enables those cells that expressed the specific macromolecule of interest to be identified and subsequently isolated. Once a particular cDNA has been isolated in this way it can be used to make unlimited quantities of the macromolecule whose sequence it encodes. As mammalian cells are generally used for this method of amplification, the amino acid sequence is the same as that used in the limbic brain. Furthermore, if, for example, the cDNA encodes a neurotransmitter receptor,

Brain mRNAs

 Reverse transcriptase transcribes these different mRNAs into
 single complementary strands of DNA

    ↓

Single-stranded brain cDNAs formed

 Single-stranded cDNAs form template for double-stranded DNA

    ↓

Double-stranded brain cDNAs formed

 Double-stranded cDNAs added to bacterial plasmids that insert
 the cDNA into the plasmid

    ↓

Recombinant DNA plasmid containing the brain DNA

 Recombinant DNA then inserted into bacteria which reproduce
 the brain DNA

    ↓

cDNA library formed with each bacterium multiplying the specific cDNA
it contains

    ↓

Individual bacteria isolated and cultured to produce clones that yield
specific cDNAs

 Specific cDNAs (for example a receptor) inserted in plasmid that
 transfects a mammalian cell (e.g. fibroblasts) in culture

    ↓

Mammalian cell containing the specific cDNA then exposed in a culture
medium to a toxin which destroys all non-transformed mammalian cells

 Add radioligand that identifies the receptor of the mammalian cell

    ↓

Identification and isolation of transformed cells which can then be cultured
to provide unlimited quantities of the receptor protein

Figure 4.1. Summary of principal methods used in molecular genetics

it is likely that it will be integrated into the plasma membrane of the cell
surface and therefore largely reflect the portion of the receptor in the neuron.
This enables such receptor-containing cells to be used for screening the
affinity of putative psychotropic drugs on receptors that were derived from
human brain. This method is now commonly used in the pharmaceutical
industry to screen numerous compounds for their potential therapeutic
application; for example, screening compounds for their affinity for the
human D_4 receptor as potential atypical neuroleptics.

 Another important application of cDNAs is to identify specific proteins in
a tissue homogenate or tissue section. Since cDNAs undergo complementary

base pairing, adding a radioactively labelled cDNA to a homogenate or tissue slice will bind it to the complementary sequence by a process of *hybridization*. Thus the amount of radioactive cDNA that hybridizes to the tissue or tissue extract is a measure of the amount of mRNA that is complementary to it. When this procedure is undertaken on slices of brain, it is known as *in situ hybridization*. In this way it is possible to determine the distribution of specific receptors in a tissue by accurately determining the distribution of mRNA that encodes for the receptor protein. This is a particularly valuable technique for the administration of psychotropic drugs.

A variety of techniques have now been developed to manipulate gene expression using cDNAs. For example, it is possible to introduce copies of a new gene (in the form of cDNAs) into a cultured cell line by a process of *transfection*. This is achieved by means of plasmids that transfect the human or mammalian cells in culture. Those cells that have had the DNA sequence integrated into their chromosomes can then be separated from those cells in which integration has not occurred by incubating the mixed cell population with a toxin to which the engineered cells are resistant whereas the normal cells are not. In this way clones of cells that contain the new genetic material can eventually be isolated.

A major advance in this technique has arisen through the development of *transgenic mice*. This technique involves injecting foreign DNA into the genome of the mouse embryo. As a consequence, the foreign DNA can give rise to a line of mice that contain the foreign DNA. Using this technique, mice have now been produced whose brains express the A4 protein – a marker for Alzheimer's disease. A variant of this technique is to replace a normal gene with a foreign gene in the chromosome, thereby giving rise to a progeny that lack both the normal gene and its function. Sibling mating then gives rise to offspring which have two defective genes. This method has so far largely been confined to mice which are termed "knockout" mice. This method could prove to be particularly useful for determining the physiological role of specific neurotransmitter receptors.

In CONCLUSION, molecular genetics is providing important tools that enable the physiological role of specific receptors and enzymes to be elucidated. *In situ* hybridization is a powerful technique for locating receptors in specific brain regions and in studying the influence of drug treatment on these receptors. The accuracy, specificity and sensitivity of such a technique is substantially greater than any other available technique. Transgenic mice and "knockout" mice are also providing valuable models of human disease that have not been obtained by other methods. With regard to psychiatric illnesses, molecular genetic techniques are being used in human genome screening which are designed to locate those genes that may be responsible for bipolar disorder and schizophrenia. By collecting cell lines from family pedigrees, it may be possible to determine the genes that contribute to alcoholism and Alzheimer's disease in addition to those involved in schizophrenia and the affective disorders. This may eventually lead to the identification of new methods for the pharmacotherapy of such conditions.

5 Psychotropic Drugs that Modify the Serotonergic System

Over a century ago, a substance was recognized in clotted blood which was found to cause vasoconstriction. This substance was still present following adrenalectomy therapy suggesting that it differed from adrenaline and noradrenaline. Eventually, Rapaport, Green and Page in 1947, purified the vasoconstrictor factor from serum and identified as serotonin ("serum tonic"). Independently of the American investigators, Erspamer and colleagues in Italy had identified a substance they termed "enteramine" from the intestine. "Enteramine" was subsequently found to be identical to serotonin and was subsequently synthesized by Hamlin and Fisher in 1951. Chemically, serotonin or enteramine is the indoleamine 5-hydroxytryptamine (5-HT).

Following the isolation and synthesis of serotonin in the early 1950s, there has been increasing interest in the physiological function of this amine. Initially, it was assumed that its main function was that of a peripheral hormone because of the relatively high concentrations that were found in the gastrointestinal tract and blood. Twarog and Page soon showed, however, that it was also present in the mammalian brain thereby suggesting that it may have a neurotransmitter role there. Interest in the physiological role of serotonin in the central nervous system has preoccupied neurobiologists since that time.

The detection of serotonin in nervous and non-nervous tissue was aided by the development of the Falck–Hillarp histochemical technique, a method whereby freeze-dried sections of tissue, when exposed to formaldehyde vapour causes indoleamines to emit a yellow fluorescence. Dahlstrom and Fuxe used this technique to show that the highest concentration of serotonin in the brain is located in the raphé nuclei, projections from these cell bodies ascending to the forebrain via the medial forebrain bundle. Descending fibres were also shown to project to the dorsal and lateral horns and the intermediolateral column of the spinal cord. Detailed observation of the distribution of the serotonergic system in the brain became possible with the development of specific antibodies to the amine and the introduction of autoradiographic methods for both the human and rodent brain.

For serotonin to be considered as a neurotransmitter, it was essential to establish that it produced its physiological effects by activating specific receptors located on the intestinal wall, platelet membrane or on nerve cells. A major development occurred in 1957 when Gaddum and Picarelli showed that the action of serotonin on the guinea-pig ileum could be blocked by either phenoxybenzamine (dibenzyline) or morphine. These investigators termed the two types of serotonin receptors on the intestinal wall "D" (for dibenzyline) or "M" (morphine) receptors, the "M" type receptors being associated with the nerves supplying the intestine that produced contraction of the smooth muscle by facilitating acetylcholine release, while the "D" receptors were located on the smooth muscle wall. More recently, it has been realized that the "D" receptors are widely distributed in the body and coincide with 5-HT_2 receptors which, when activated by selective agonists, contract smooth muscle and aggregate platelets. They also occur in synaptosomal membranes where they are possibly associated with postsynaptic membrane structures. By contrast, the "M" receptor has not been unequivocally identified in neuronal membranes. However, increasing evidence now suggests that the peripheral "M" receptor is identical to the $5\text{-}HT_3$ receptor in the brain. Thus in a period of some 20 years, the distribution of serotonin in both nervous and non-nervous tissue has been determined, many of its physiological properties explained and the types of receptors upon which it acts to produce its diverse physiological effects evaluated.

5-HT receptor subtypes

Current knowledge of 5-HT receptors has been derived from advances in medicinal chemistry, from the synthesis of ligands that show considerable specificity for subpopulations of 5-HT receptors. The application of such ligands to our understanding of the distribution of the 5-HT receptor subtypes has been largely due to quantitative *in vitro* autoradiographic techniques and the application of such imaging techniques as positron emission tomography. Functional studies undoubtedly lag behind but the development of sophisticated electrophysiological techniques and studies of changes in secondary messenger systems which respond to the binding of selective ligands to the 5-HT receptor subtypes have opened up the probability that the physiological importance of the numerous receptor subtypes will soon be clarified.

As a consequence of the application of these various techniques, the International Union of Pharmacological Societies (IUPHAR) Commission on serotonin nomenclature has published two major reports which attempt to classify the various receptor subtypes according to their ligand binding properties and secondary messenger systems. The first report classified 5-HT receptors into 5-HT_1-like (comprising $5\text{-HT}_{1A,\ 1B,\ 1C}$ and $_{1D}$) 5-HT_2 (formerly the 5-HT-D receptor) and 5-HT_3 (formerly the 5-HT-M receptor). The detection of a novel 5-HT receptor, that could not be classified as 5-HT_1, 5-HT_2, or 5-HT_3, in both the peripheral and central nervous systems, extended the receptor types to 5-HT_4. The application of molecular biology techniques has led to the cloning and sequencing of at least six different 5-HT receptors namely 5-HT_{1A}, 5-HT_{1B}, 5-HT_{1C}, 5-HT_{1D}, 5-HT_2 and 5-HT_3. Further studies of the second messenger systems to which these receptor subtypes are attached have shown that the 5-HT_1-like, 5-HT_2 and 5-HT_4 receptors belong to the G protein coupled receptor superfamily, whereas the 5-HT_3 receptor belongs to the same family as the nicotinic, gamma-aminobutyric acid-A (GABA-A) and glycine receptors which are ion gated channel receptors.

The most recent publication of the IUPHAR Commission has redefined the 5-HT receptor subtypes according to their second messenger associations and thereby helped to stress the functional role of the receptor subtypes rather than relying primarily on the specificities of ligands that bind to them. This approach has led to the classification of 5-HT receptors into those linked to adenylate cyclase (5-HT_{1A}, 5-HT_{1B}, 5-HT_{1D}, 5-HT_4), those linked to the phosphatidyl inositol system (5-HT_{2A}, 5-HT_{2B} and 5-HT_{2C}), and those linked directly to ion channels (5-HT_3). Table 5.1 summarizes the accepted classification of the 5-HT receptor subtypes, all of which occur in the brain, together with the most specific agonists and antagonists which have been developed.

More recently, the family of 5-HT receptors has been dramatically increased to include 5-HT_4, 5-HT_{5A} and 5-HT_{5B}, 5-HT_6 and 5-HT_7. The 5-HT_6 and 5-HT_7 receptors are positively linked to adenylate cyclase. Of these, only the 5-HT_4 receptor has so far not been cloned. Of these newly discovered receptors, only the 5-HT_4 receptor has been investigated in some detail. This receptor is quite widely distributed in the brain and peripheral tissues where they are positively coupled to adenylate cyclase. In the brain, the 5-HT_4 receptors facilitate acetylcholine release and may play a role in peristalsis. It has been hypothesized that in the brain 5-HT_4 receptors may also play a role in facilitating cholinergic transmission and thereby have a potential role to play in presenting cognitive deficits which are associated with cortical cholinergic malfunction. The possible clinical significance of 5-HT_4 receptors must await the development of specific agonists and antagonists. So far, such compounds have not been developed.

Despite the dramatic advances which have taken place in the identification and characterization of 5-HT receptor subtypes, it is evident that many of the ligands used to characterize these receptor subtypes are not completely selective. It must also be emphasized that receptors are the products of genes and are therefore subject to genetic changes and, as a consequence, variability in physiological and pharmacological responsiveness. Thus affinity, potency and intrinsic activity of a drug at one receptor may vary depending on the time, species and receptor-effector coupling. It is already

Table 5.1.   Distribution and selectivity of drugs for 5-HT receptor subtypes

---

$5\text{-}HT_{1A}$ *receptors*
  Hippocampus, septum, amygdala, cortical limbic area
  Agonists: buspirone, gepirone, ipsapirone, flesinoxan
  Antagonists: WAY 100135: BMY 7378; NAN-190
  Possible clinical use of agonists: anxiolytics, antidepressants
$5\text{-}HT_{1B}$ *receptors*
  Substantia nigra, globus pallidus, dorsal subiculum, superior colliculi
  Non-selective: pinodol, propanolol
  ? selective partial agonists: CP-93, 129
  Possible clinical use of antagonists: antidepressants
$5\text{-}HT_{1D}$ *receptors*
  Caudate nucleus but widely distributed in human dry and GP brain, similar to
  $5\text{-}HT_{1B}$ of rat brain
  Non-selective: rauwolscine, yohimbine
  ? selective: L-694, 247
  Possible clinical use of antagonists: antidepressants
$5\text{-}HT_{1E}$ *receptor*
  In mammalian brain
  Possible clinical use: ?
$5\text{-}HT_{2A}$
  Neocortex but widely distributed in the mammalian brain
  Agonists: DOI, DOB
  Non-selective antagonists: ketanserin, ritanserin
  Possible clinical use of antagonists: antidepressants, anxiolytics, ? neuroleptics
$5\text{-}HT_{2B}$
  In mammalian brain
  Possible clinical use: ?
$5\text{-}HT_{2C}$
  Choroid plexus
  Non-selective antagonists: spiperone, amperozide, pimozide
  Possible clinical use of antagonists: neuroleptics
$5\text{-}HT_3$
  Area postrema, entorhinal and frontal cortex, hippocampus
  Agonists: ondansetron, granisetron, zacopride
  Possible clinical use of antagonists: antiemetics, anxiolytics, ? antidementia
$5\text{-}HT_4$
  Collicular and hippocampal neurons
  Antagonists SC-205-557, SC-53606
  Agonist: SC-49518
  Possible clinical use: ?

8-OHDPAT	= Dipropylamino-8-hydroxy-1,2,3,4-tetrahydronaphthylene
RU-24969	= 5-methoxy-3-(1,2,3,6-tetrahydropyridin-4-yl) 1H indol
mCPP	= 1-(3 chlorophenyl) piperazine
TFMPP	= 1-(m-trifluoromethylphenyl) piperazine
DOI	= 1-(2,5-dimethoxy-1-iodophenyl) 2-aminopropane
MDL 73005	= 8,2 (2,3-dihydro-1,4-benzodioxin-2yl) methylamino-ethyl-8-azaspirol (4,5) decan -7,9-dione
NAN 190	= 1-(2-methoxyphenyl) 4-(4(2-phthalimido)entyl-piperazine
5-CT	= 5-carboxamidotryptamine
ICI 169369	= (2-(2-dimethylamino-ethylthio-3-phenylquinoline))
ICS 205-930	= (3-tropanyl)-IH-indole-2-carboxylic acid ester
DOM	= 2,5,dimethoxy-4-diemethylbenzene ethamine

Table 5.2. Serotonin receptor subtypes and disease states

Physiological or pathological condition	Serotonin receptor subtype implicated
Feeding behaviour	5-HT_{1A} agonists enhance food consumption in experimental animals
	$5\text{-HT}_{1B}/5\text{-HT}_{2C}$ agonists decrease food consumption in experimental animals
Thermoregulation	5-HT_{1A} agonists cause hypothermia in experimental animals
	5-HT_{1B} and 5-HT_2 agonists cause hyperthermia in experimental animals
Sexual behaviour	5-HT_{1A} agonists both facilitate and inhibit sexual behaviour in male rats
	5-HT_{1B} agonists inhibit sexual behaviour in the male but facilitate the behaviour in the female rat
Cardiovascular system	5-HT_1, 5-HT_2 and 5-HT_3 receptors may be involved in the complex action of serotonin on blood pressure
	5-HT_2 agonists appear to be hypertensive agents whereas the antagonists are hypotensives
Sleep	5-HT_{1A} agonists delay the onset of REM sleep
	5-HT_2 antagonists suppress REM sleep
Hallucinogenic activity	Most "classical" hallucinogens such as LSD and mescaline are antagonists at 5-HT_2 receptors
Antipsychotic activity	Many atypical neuroleptics (e.g. amperozide and risperidone) are 5-HT_2 receptor antagonists. In animals, 5-HT_3 antagonists have profiles similar to chronically active neuroleptics
Anxiolytic activity	Several novel anxiolytics (e.g. buspirone, ipsapirone) are 5-HT_{1A} partial agonists.
	5-HT_2 and 5-HT_3 antagonists have anxiolytic properties
Depression	5-HT_{1A} receptors are functionally sensitized by chronic antidepressant treatments in rats
	5-HT_2 receptor numbers are increased and activity decreased, in depression; return to control values in response to treatment.

known, for example, that ipsapirone, buspirone, spiroxatrine and lysergic acid diethylamide (LSD) may behave either as agonists or antagonists depending on the functional model being used to assess their activity. A similar problem arises with intrinsic activity which is usually assumed to be a direct reflection of the pharmacological properties of the drug. It seems possible that the affinity can also be influenced by the nature of the genetically determined receptor-effector coupling and is therefore tissue (and species) dependent. Such factors may help to explain why the identification and subclassification of 5-HT receptor subtypes is complex and often confusing.

This dilemma can be illustrated by the attempts being made to identify the functional role of 5-HT receptor subtypes using ligands which are believed to be specific in their binding properties. Such ligands may prove to be non-selective, more selective for an as yet unidentified 5-HT receptor subtype or more selective for a non-5-HT receptor site. Conversely several non-5-HT ligands are known to bind to 5-HT receptors with a high affinity. For example, the alpha$_1$ adrenoceptor antagonist WB4101, and the beta adrenoceptor antagonist pindolol, have a high affinity to 5-HT$_{1A}$ receptors. Nevertheless, despite these cautions, there is a growing body of information which implicates different 5-HT receptor subtypes in a variety of physiological and pharmacological responses and these will be briefly reviewed (see Table 5.2).

Serotonin and sleep

It has been known for some years that the functional activity of 5-HT neurons in the brain changes dramatically during the sleep–wake arousal cycle. Thus from a stable, slow and regular discharge pattern during quiet wakening, neuronal activity gradually declines as the animal becomes drowsy and enters slow-wave sleep. During rapid eye movement (REM) sleep, 5-HT activity is totally suppressed but in anticipation of awakening the neuronal activity returns to its basal level several seconds before the end of the REM episode. During arousal or wakening, the 5-HT neuronal discharge pattern increases considerably above the quiet waking state.

Koella has reviewed the evidence implicating the involvement of serotonin in the sleep–wake cycle but the involvement of specific serotonin receptor subtypes in sleep mechanisms is unclear. Experimental evidence suggests that 5-HT$_{1A}$ agonists delay the onset of REM sleep while 5-HT$_2$ antagonists suppress REM and have variable effects on non-REM sleep.

It must be emphasized that most studies of the relationship between the serotonergic system and sleep have been conducted in rats and therefore the relevance of such findings to man remains unproven. From such experimental studies, it has been shown that blockade of 5-HT$_2$ receptors increases the proportion of slow-wave sleep and decreases the quantity of REM sleep. Whether this effect of 5-HT$_2$ antagonists can be ascribed to a specific effect on slow-wave sleep is however, a matter of conjecture as any increase in time spent in one stage of sleep will be reflected in a decrease in the time spent in other stages of sleep. However, experimental evidence suggests that most drugs that alter serotonergic transmission reduce REM sleep. There is evidence that the 5-HT$_2$ antagonist ritanserin improves sleep quality in those suffering from "jet lag" which suggests that the 5-HT$_2$ receptors may be involved in adjusting the sleep–wake cycle to the photoperiod. Furthermore, experimental data suggest that activation of 5-HT$_2$ receptors may vary according to the sleep–wake cycle. Such findings suggest that 5-HT$_2$ receptors are involved in the regulation of circadian rhythms and the sleep–wake cycle. With regard to the overall role of 5-HT in sleep, Koella has postulated that serotonin may produce its various effects on sleep architecture by influencing cognition and vigilance.

Details of the effects of psychotropic drugs on the sleep profile are discussed in Chapter 9.

Serotonin and hallucinogenic activity

There is abundant experimental evidence to show that serotonin plays a major role in the mechanism of action of hallucinogens, but it is presently unclear whether the actions of hallucinogens can be explained by their agonistic or antagonistic actions. LSD, for example, may behave either as an agonist or antagonist depending on the particular tissue, concentration and experimental condition, whereas the tryptamine type of hallucinogens usually act as agonists. Experimental evidence nevertheless suggests that the behavioural effects of a number of indole alkylamine (e.g. LSD-like) and phenylalkylamine (e.g. mescaline-like) hallucinogens can be attenuated by 5-HT$_{2A}$ antagonists and that the potency of these classes of hallucinogens at 5-HT$_{2A}$ (and possibly 5-HT$_{2C}$) sites correlate with their hallucinogenic potency in man. It seems unlikely however that all hallucinogens owe their activity to their potency in stimulating 5-HT$_{2A}$ receptors; LSD and 5-methoxydimethyltryptamine for example interact with 5-HT$_{2C}$ sites, while phenyclidine may owe its hallucinogenic potency to an action on N-methyl-D-aspartate (NMDA) and a subclass of sigma receptors. Nevertheless, the balance of evidence suggest that most "classical" hallucinogens such as LSD, mescaline and psilocybin act as partial agonists on 5-HT$_{2A}$ receptors.

Details of the pharmacological properties of hallucinogenic drugs are discussed in Chapter 14.

Serotonin and drugs of abuse

The role of 5-HT in the control of alcohol intake has received considerable attention following the discovery that 5-HT reuptake inhibitors reduce alcohol intake in alcohol dependent rats. Similar effects have been found for intracerebroventricularly administered 5-HT or its precursor 5-HTP. Regarding the type of 5-HT receptor involved, there is experimental evidence that the 5-HT$_{1A}$ partial agonists buspirone and gepirone are effective. Differences were found between the effects of the 5-HT$_3$ antagonist ondansetron and the $5\text{-}HT_{2A}/5\text{-}HT_{2C}$ antagonist ritanserin. Thus the $5\text{-}HT_3$ antagonist ondansetron reduces alcohol intake without affecting the alcohol preference of rats, while ritanserin reduces both the alcohol preference and intake. This suggests that, at least in rats, different populations of 5-HT receptors may be involved in alcohol intake and preference.

Regarding other types of drugs of abuse, the $5\text{-}HT_3$ antagonist MDL 72222 has been shown to block place preference conditioning induced in rodents by morphine or nicotine without affecting the preference for amphetamine. It is possible that these effects of $5\text{-}HT_3$ antagonists are associated with the reduction in dopamine release as it is well established that the rewarding effects of many drugs of abuse are due to increased dopaminergic activity in limbic regions. On the strength of the experimental findings, it has been proposed that $5\text{-}HT_3$ antagonists might be useful in treating drug abuse in man. Only appropriate placebo-controlled studies of $5\text{-}HT_3$ antagonists will clarify the therapeutic value of such agents in different types of drug abuse.

A further discussion of the pharmacological properties of alcohol and other drugs of abuse is given in Chapter 14.

Serotonin and the antipsychotic activity of neuroleptics

Given the complexity of the serotonergic system and its interaction with multiple neurotransmitter systems in the mammalian brain, it is not surprising to find that 5-HT plays a role in the aetiology of schizophrenia. Meltzer has suggested that in schizophrenia a malfunction of the mechanism whereby 5-HT modulates the release of dopamine (for example, due to the decreased inhibition by 5-HT of the release of dopamine in the mesencephalon and frontal cortex) might contribute to the enhanced neocortical dopaminergic function which probably forms the biochemical basis of the disease. The antipsychotic activity of atypical neuroleptics such as clozapine and risperidone may therefore lie in the normalization of the relationship between the malfunctioning 5-HT and dopaminergic systems.

The novel antipsychotic drug clozapine has a very complicated neurochemical profile in that it has a high affinity for $5\text{-}HT_{2A}$, $5\text{-}HT_{2C}$, $5\text{-}HT_3$, $5\text{-}HT_6$ and $5\text{-}HT_7$ receptors in addition to its action on D_4 and D_3 receptors. Risperidone likewise has a high affinity for $5\text{-}HT_{2A}$ receptors as well as acting as an antagonist of D_2 receptors. Such drugs have received attention recently because of their reduced propensity to cause extrapyramidal side effects and for their efficacy in treating the negative symptoms of schizophrenia. These properties may partly reside in the antagonistic actions of the atypical neuroleptics on the various sub-populations of 5-HT receptors of which the $5\text{-}HT_{2A}$ receptor may be of primary importance.

In experimental studies, many clinically effective neuroleptics have been shown to act as 5-HT$_{2A}$ receptor antagonists. Studies on post-mortem brain from schizophrenic patients have shown that the decrease in the number of 5-HT$_{2A}$ receptors in the prefrontal cortex might be related to the disease process. It therefore seems unlikely that the antipsychotic activity of neuroleptics can be explained solely in terms of their action on 5-HT$_{2A}$ receptors. Furthermore, no correlation exists between the average therapeutic doses of a neuroleptic and its affinity for 5-HT$_{2A}$ receptors. It does seem possible, however, that several atypical neuroleptics such as amperozide, risperidone and possibly ritanserin do owe at least part of the pharmacological profile to their ability to inhibit 5-HT$_{2A}$ receptors.

Following the discovery that selective 5-HT$_3$ antagonists reduce the behavioural effects of the infusion of dopamine into the nucleus accumbens, there has been considerable interest in the possible role of 5-HT$_3$ receptor antagonists as potential neuroleptic agents. While there is a growing body of evidence to suggest that 5-HT$_3$ antagonists may be therapeutically valuable for the treatment of disorders of the gastrointestinal tract, as antiemetics and possibly anxiolytic agents, there is currently little evidence to suggest that such drugs are effective in the treatment of schizophrenia. However, experimental studies of the 5-HT$_3$ antagonists on dopamine autoreceptors may eventually offer new leads to the development of novel antipsychotic drugs.

A more detailed discussion of the pharmacological properties of typical and atypical neuroleptics is given in Chapter 10.

Serotonin and anxiolytic activity

Although the benzodiazepine anxiolytics primarily interact with the GABA receptor complex, there is ample experimental evidence to show that secondary changes occur in the turnover, release and firing of 5-HT neurons as a consequence of the activation of the GABA-benzodiazepine receptor. Similar changes are observed in the raphé nuclei where a high density of 5-HT$_{1A}$ receptors occurs. Such findings suggest that 5-HT may play a key role in anxiety disorders.

Undoubtedly one of the most important advances implicating serotonin in anxiety has been the development of the azaspirodecanone derivatives buspirone, gepirone and ipsapirone as novel anxiolytics. All three agents produce a common metabolite, namely 1-(2-pyrimidinyl) piperazine or 1-PP, which may contribute to the anxiolytic activity of the parent compounds. It soon became apparent that these anxiolytic agents do not act via the benzodiazepine or GABA receptors but show a relatively high affinity for the 5-HT$_{1A}$ sites; the 1-PP metabolite however only possesses a very low affinity for the $5\text{-}HT_{1A}$ site although it may contribute to the anxiolytic effect of the parent compound by acting as an $alpha_2$ adrenoceptor agonist. In experimental studies, these atypical anxiolytics have mixed actions, behaving as agonists in some situations and antagonists in others. For this reason they are considered to be partial agonists at $5\text{-}HT_{1A}$ receptors, acting either as agonists on presynaptic $5\text{-}HT_{1A}$ receptors or antagonists on postsynaptic $5\text{-}HT_{1A}$ receptors.

In animal models of anxiety, $5\text{-}HT_2$ receptor antagonists have been shown to be active. Ritanserin appears to exhibit both anxiolytic and anxiogenic activity in different animal models. Nevertheless, in man, preliminary evidence suggests that ritanserin is an effective anxiolytic agent, although a placebo-controlled trial of the $5\text{-}HT_2$ antagonist ritanserin, has shown no differences in the Hamilton Anxiety and the Clinical Global Impression scales between the drug-treated and placebo-treated patients.

The anxiolytic properties of $5\text{-}HT_3$ receptor antagonists have been demonstrated in several animal models of anxiety. In these models, the $5\text{-}HT_3$ antagonists mimic the anxiolytic effects of the benzodiazepines but differ from the latter in their lack of sedative, muscle relaxant and anticonvulsant action. These compounds appear to be extremely potent (acting in the $ng\text{-}\mu g/kg$ range) and, providing the initial clinical finding of their anxiolytic activity is substantiated, this group of drugs could provide a valuable addition to the non-benzodiazepine anxiolytics. Thus experimental and clinical evidence suggest that $5\text{-}HT_{1A}$ receptor partial agonists, $5\text{-}HT_2$ and $5\text{-}HT_3$ antagonists may be useful and novel anxiolytic agents.

Serotonin and aggression, panic attack and related disorders

The possible overlap between anxiety, depression, panic attack, aggression and obsessive–compulsive disorders, and the involvement of serotonin in the symptoms of these disorders, has recently led to the investigation of various selective serotonin reuptake inhibitors (SSRIs) and selective 5-HT receptor agonists/antagonists in the treatment of these conditions. In experimental studies, there is evidence that drugs such as eltoprazine, which binds with high affinity to $5\text{-}HT_{1A}$, $5\text{-}HT_{1B}$ and $5\text{-}HT_{2C}$ sites, are active antiaggressive agents, whereas selective $5\text{-}HT_{1A}$ agonists, and $5\text{-}HT_2$ and $5\text{-}HT_3$ antagonists are inactive. There is also preliminary evidence to suggest that SSRIs such as fluoxetine reduce impulsive behaviour which may contribute to their therapeutic action in the treatment of obsessive–compulsive disorders and possibly in reducing suicidal attempts.

Zohar and Insel have suggested that the symptoms of obsessive–compulsive disorder are due to supersensitive $5\text{-}HT_1$ type receptors and that the function of SSRIs such as clomipramine, fluoxetine and the non-selective 5-HT antagonist metergoline owe their efficacy to their ability to reduce the activity of these receptors.

It now seems generally accepted that the effects of anti-obsessional drugs may be mediated by serotonergic mechanisms. The apparent hypersensitivity of obsessive–compulsive patients to the trazodone metabolite m-chlorophenyl piperazine (mCPP, a non-selective 5-HT_{1B}, 5-HT_{2C} and 5-HT_2 agonist) suggests that a diverse group of 5-HT_1 and 5-HT_2 receptors are involved. The efficacy of buspirone, a partial agonist of 5-HT_{1A} receptors in attenuating the obsessional symptoms further suggests that 5-HT_{1A} receptors are also involved. As the 5-HT reuptake inhibitors such as fluoxetine and fluvoxamine are particularly effective in attenuating the obsessive symptoms following several weeks of administration, it may be argued that the therapeutic effect of such drugs lies in their ability to desensitize the supersensitive 5-HT_1-type receptors. Which of the 5-HT_1 receptors is specifically involved is unclear, but neuroimaging studies on patients with obsessive–compulsive disorder implicates the striatum as the major brain region which is defective. The 5-HT receptors in the striatum are 5-HT_{1D} and 5-HT_2 in man which may implicate these receptor subtypes specifically in the aetiology of the condition.

With regard to generalized anxiety disorder, it has been postulated that an overactivity of the stimulatory 5-HT pathways occurs. Drugs such as buspirone and ipsapirone are effective in such conditions because they stimulate the inhibitory 5-HT_{1A} autoreceptors on the raphé nuclei and thereby reduce serotonergic function. It is noteworthy that the SSRIs often worsen anxiety initially because they temporarily enhance serotonergic function. Adaptive changes in the pre- and postsynaptic 5-HT receptors then occur leading to a reduction in the anxiety state.

A further discussion of the pharmacological properties of the anxiolytic drugs is given in Chapter 8.

Serotonin and its role in depression

Serotonin is believed to play a multifunctional role in depression which is to be anticipated from its involvement in the physiological processes of sleep, mood, vigilance, feeding and possibly sexual behaviour and learning, all of which are deranged to varying extents in severe depression. However, the involvement of precise serotonin receptor subtypes in depression, and in the action of antidepressants, is still far from clear. One approach to unravelling the changes in serotonin receptors in depression has been to study the effects of chronically administered antidepressants on serotonin receptor subtypes in rat brain. While there is evidence that most antidepressants show only a low affinity for the 5-HT_1 sites, there is experimental evidence to show that

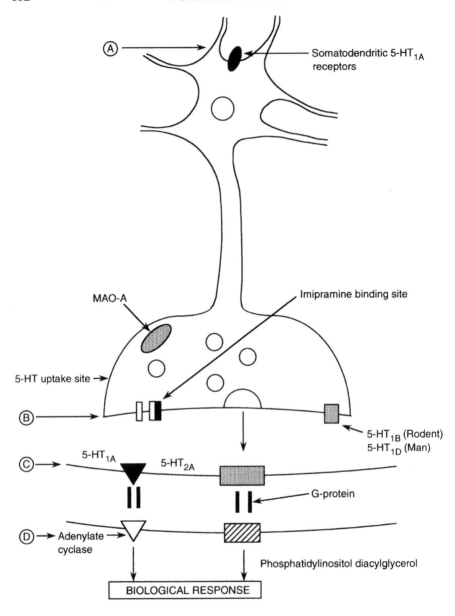

Figure 5.1. Changes that occur following the chronic administration of anti-depressants. Ⓐ SSRIs and MAOIs desensitize the inhibitory 5-HT$_{1A}$ somato dendritic receptors. Ⓑ SSRIs and MAOIs desensitize the inhibitory 5-HT$_{1B}$/5-HT$_{1D}$ inhibitory auto receptor on the presynaptic terminal. After acute administration, the TCAs and the SSRIs inhibit the uptake of 5-HT into the nerve terminal by binding to the

chronic antidepressant treatment results in a hypersensitivity of postsynaptic and a hyposensitivity of presynaptic 5-HT$_{1A}$ receptors. In contrast to the 5-HT$_{1A}$ receptors, many antidepressants from various chemical classes have a moderate affinity for 5-HT$_2$ receptors although there is no apparent correlation between the 5-HT$_2$ receptor affinity and the antidepressant potency.

Regarding the changes that occur in rat cortical 5-HT$_2$ receptor density following chronic antidepressant and lithium treatment, there is unequivocal evidence that the number of receptors increases in response to chronic drug treatment although it must be emphasized that chronic electroconvulsive shock results in a decrease in the receptor number. Similarly, in untreated depressed and panic patients, the density of 5-HT$_2$ receptors on the platelet membrane has been shown to be increased. The number of receptors normalizes on effective, but not ineffective, treatment. Using the serotonin-induced platelet aggregation response as a measure of the functional activity of 5-HT$_2$ receptors, it has been consistently shown that the 5-HT$_2$ receptor responsiveness is reduced in the untreated depressive but returns to control values following effective treatment irrespective of the nature of treatment. Thus changes in 5-HT$_2$ receptor density and function appear to be disturbed in the depressed patient and return to control values only following effective treatment. The increase in the receptor number, and decrease in their responsiveness to serotonin, in the untreated depressed patient may suggest an abnormality in the coupling mechanism between the receptor site and the phosphatidylinositol second messenger system that brings about the platelet shape change underlying aggregation.

It has been hypothesized that depression could arise from a pathological enhancement of 5-HT$_2$ receptor function. This view would concur with the

---

Figure 5.1. (*continued*) imipramine binding site (or its equivalent). 5-HT transport sites are also found on the cell body and axonal projection but their precise role in serotonergic transmission is unclear. Presumably the change in 5-HT is in the vicinity of the receptors. 5-HT$_{1B}$ and $_{1D}$ receptors appear to have a similar function but are structurally slightly different according to the species in which they are found. © TCAs, ECT and most non-SSRIs second generation antidepressants sensitize the postsynaptic 5-HT$_{1A}$ receptors thereby increasing serotonergic function. The density of 5-HT$_{2A}$ receptors is decreased by TCAs and SSRIs in rat brain following chronic treatment; in the depressed patient however the number of 5-HT$_{2A}$ receptors is increased and normalizes following effective treatment. ⒟ There is experimental evidence that the activity of the second messenger system associated with the 5-HT$_{2A}$ receptor is decreased following chronic antidepressant treatment. There is also circumstantial evidence that the G protein coupling mechanism between the 5-HT$_{2A}$ receptor and its second messenger is hypofunctional in depressed patients but normalizes following effective treatment. This suggests that some antidepressants may improve the receptor–second messenger G protein coupling mechanism.

observations that the functional activity of 5-HT_2 receptors on the platelet membrane is enhanced in depression and the increase in the density of 5-HT_2 receptors in the frontal cortex of brains from suicide victims. It is possible that enhanced 5-HT_2 receptor function is associated primarily with anxiety, a common feature of depression, and that the increased activity of the 5-HT_2 receptors results in an attenuation of the functioning of 5-HT_1 receptors thereby resulting in the symptoms of depression. Whether this change in the activity of 5-HT_1 receptors is due to direct effects of the altered 5-HT_2 receptor function is uncertain. There is evidence that hypercortisolaemia, which is a characteristic feature of depression, reduces the activity of these receptors probably through central glucocorticoid type 2 receptors. Clearly further research is needed to determine the precise interaction between the 5-HT_2 and 5-HT_1 receptor types.

More recently, it has been speculated that the $5\text{-HT}_{1B/1D}$ receptors may have a role to play in depression and in the mode of action of antidepressants. These receptors appear to be located presynaptically where they control the release of 5-HT; in experimental studies the non-selective 5-HT_1 antagonist methiotherpin has antidepressant properties. Thus it may be speculated that the $5\text{-HT}_{1B/1D}$ receptors are supersensitive in depression, thereby leading to a reduced intersynaptic concentration of 5-HT with a consequent increase in the number of postsynaptic 5-HT_2 receptor sites. However, only the development of highly selective $5\text{-HT}_{1B/1D}$ antagonists will enable this hypothesis to be tested.

Although the precise mechanism whereby antidepressants produce their therapeutic effects is incompletely understood, there is a growing body of evidence to suggest that serotonin receptors, particularly of the 5-HT_{1A} and 5-HT_2 subtype, play a role in their actions. Only the 5-HT_{2A} receptor has, so far, been convincingly demonstrated to be malfunctional in depression and to be normalized following effective treatment. A further consideration of the pharmacological properties of the different classes of antidepressants is considered in Chapter 6. Figure 5.1 summarizes some of the proposed sites of action of different classes of antidepressants that modulate central serotonergic transmission.

In SUMMARY, it is evident that serotonin is involved in a variety of physiological processes and that disturbances of serotonergic function may be of importance in the aetiology of many gastrointestinal, cardiovascular and central nervous system diseases. The existence of subtypes of serotonin receptors and the impetus that this has given to the development of drugs with selective actions on these receptor subtypes is already leading to the development of new therapeutic agents. Evaluation of the functional status of serotonin receptor subtypes in psychiatric and neurological diseases may be of future importance in the diagnosis and assessment of treatment response in such patients. In this regard, the development of serotonin receptor probes coupled with such techniques as positron emission tomography may be of considerable importance in diagnosis in the future.

To date, at least four major subtypes of serotonin receptor have been described in detail and a major advance has been made with the isolation of genomic clones for these receptor subtypes. We now await the further development of selective ligands for all the serotonin receptor subtypes which may ultimately lead to a better understanding of the functional significance and clinical relevance of serotonin receptors in health and disease. Hopefully such a development will also result in the availability of more effective drugs to treat neurological and psychiatric diseases.

6 Drug Treatment of Depression

Introduction

The *Oxford Dictionary* defines depression as a state of "low spirits or vitality". Clearly, this state has been experienced by most people at some stage during their lives. However, the psychiatrist is seldom concerned with such a mood change unless it persists for such a long time that it incapacitates the individual. Should the depressed mood be associated with feelings of guilt, suicidal tendencies and disturbed bodily functions (such as weight loss, anorexia, loss of libido or a disturbed sleep pattern characterized by early morning wakening) and persist for weeks or even months, often with no initiatory cause, then psychiatric assistance is usually required. It is not proposed to discuss the various types of depression that have been identified because the drug treatment is essentially similar irrespective of whether or not there appears to be an initiatory cause. For example, bereavement is often associated with a severe depressive episode, particularly in the elderly, and while counselling may be of considerable assistance in enabling the patient to adjust to the changed circumstances the use of an antidepressant is often advisable.

Many psychiatrists still divide depression into the endogenous (i.e. no apparent external cause) and reactive (i.e. an identifiable external cause) types and, while such a division may be of some value regarding ancillary treatment, there is presently no evidence to suggest that the biochemical changes that may be causally linked to the illness differ nor is there any evidence that the way in which the patient should be assisted by drugs differs substantially. Other international classifications of depression are based on the mono- and bipolar dichotomy, a system of classification that separates those patients with depressive symptoms only from those that fluctuate between depression and mania (i.e. manic-depression) or have only manic symptoms. In such cases treatment strategies differ as specific and antimanic drugs such as lithium or the neuroleptics would be used to abort an acute attack of mania, while antidepressants are the drugs of choice to treat the depressive episodes and anxiety associated with depression. Readers are referred to the various classification manuals, such as the *Diagnostic and Statistical Manual of Mental Disorders* of the American

Psychiatric Association (DSM-IV) or the *International Classification of Diseases*, 10th Revision (ICD10), for further details.

Historical development of antidepressants

The use of cocaine, extracted in a crude form from the leaves of the Andean coca plant, has been used for centuries in South America to alleviate fatigue and elevate the mood. It was only relatively recently, however, that the same pharmacological effect was discovered when the amphetamines were introduced into Western medicine as anorexiants with stimulant properties. Opiates, generally as a galenical mixture, were also widely used for centuries for their mood-elevating effects throughout the world. It is not without interest that while such drugs would never now be used as antidepressants, there is evidence that most antidepressants do modulate the pain threshold, possibly via the enkephalins and endorphins. This may help to explain the use of antidepressants in the treatment of atypical pain syndromes and as an adjunct to the treatment of terminal cancer pain. Finally, alcohol in its various forms has been used to alleviate anguish and sorrow since antiquity. Whilst the opiates, alcohol and the stimulants offer some temporary relief to the patient, their long-term use inevitably leads to dependence and even to an exacerbation of the symptoms they were designed to cure.

The development of specific drugs for the treatment of depression only occurred in the early 1950s with the accidental discovery of the monoamine oxidase inhibitors (MAOIs) and the tricyclic antidepressants (TCAs). This period marked the beginning of the era of pharmacopsychiatry.

Although the iminodibenzyl structure, which forms the chemical basis of the TCA series, was first synthesized in 1889, its biological activity was only evaluated in the early 1950s following the accidental discovery that the tricyclic compound chlorpromazine had antipsychotic properties. Imipramine is also chemically similar in structure to chlorpromazine, but was found to lack its antipsychotic effects. It was largely due to the persistence of the Swiss psychiatrist Kuhn that imipramine was not discarded and was shown to have specific antidepressant effects. It is not without interest that the first report of the antidepressant effects of imipramine was presented to an audience of 12 as part of the proceedings of the Second World Congress of Psychiatry in Zurich in 1957!

The introduction of the first MAOI in the early 1950s was equally inauspicious. Iproniazid had been developed as an effective hydrazide antitubercular drug, but was subsequently found to exhibit mood-elevating effects. This was shown to be due to its ability to inhibit MAO activity and was unconnected with its antitubercular action. Thus by the late 1950s, psychiatrists had at their disposal two effective treatments for depression, a

TCA and an MAOI. But it was only in attempting to discover how these drugs may work, together with the evidence that the recently introduced antipsychotic drug resperine caused depression in a small number of patients, that the hypothesis was developed that depression was due to a relative deficit of biogenic amine neurotransmitters in the synaptic cleft and that antidepressants reversed this deficit by preventing their inactivation. While this hypothesis has been drastically revised in the light of research into the biochemical nature of depression, at that time it had the advantage of unifying a number of disparate clinical and experimental observations and in laying the basis for subsequent drug development.

Aspects of the biochemical basis of depression

Research into the chemical pathology of depression has mainly concentrated on four major areas:

1. Changes in biogenic amine neurotransmitters in post-mortem brains from suicide victims.
2. Changes in cerebrospinal fluid (CSF) concentrations of amine metabolites from patients with depression.
3. Endocrine disturbances which appear to be coincidentally related to the onset of the illness.
4. Changes in neurotransmitter receptor function and density on platelets and lymphocytes from patients before and following effective treatment.

Changes in "classical" neurotransmitters in post-mortem brain

There are major problems in interpreting the data obtained from post-mortem studies, despite the obvious advantage which such an approach may have in allowing the researcher direct access to human brain material. Such problems arise from the fact that post-mortem changes inevitably affect the metabolism of the transmitters. It is seldom possible to fix the brain tissue in less than 12 hours from death and many transmitter changes can be caused by the anoxia that inevitably arises. In addition, many suicide victims have been taking psychotropic medication at the time of death and this could profoundly affect amine metabolism. Alcohol, frequently associated with an overdose of the antidepressant prescribed to treat the patient, is often used as a means of suicide. Such drugs have a profound effect on the concentrations and metabolism of the transmitters, thereby leading to erroneous conclusions regarding the relationship between suicide and the associated biochemical changes. Furthermore, the precise clinical diagnosis of the victim at the time of death is by no means certain in many cases. It has been variously estimated that only 40% of suicides have a primary diagnosis of depression, the majority suffering from alcoholism, mania, schizophrenia or some other major psychiatric illness. In the light of these difficulties perhaps it is not surprising to find that the evidence for an abnormality in the concentrations of the biogenic amine transmitters noradrenaline and 5-HT is inconclusive. A brief review of the evidence over the last 20 years shows that a consistent decrease in 5-HT and its metabolite 5-hydroxyindoleacetic acid (5-HIAA) is largely restricted to those studies reported before 1976, later studies which tended to use more sensitive and accurate means of analysis such as high performance liquid chromatography (HPLC) having provided only inconclusive evidence for such a change. There are no consistent reports that the catecholamines noradrenaline and dopamine are altered in the suicide brain.

More recent studies have concentrated on the changes in neurotransmitter receptors, as there is experimental evidence that such receptors are not so vulnerable to post-mortem changes as the transmitters that act upon them. From such studies it would appear that there is an increase in the density of 5-HT_2 receptors in the limbic regions of the suicide brain, a finding which would accord with the observation that these receptors are also increased on the platelet membranes of untreated depressed patients. However, not all investigators have been able to replicate these post-mortem findings.

An increase in the density of muscarinic receptors has been found, which may implicate the involvement of the cholinergic system in the aetiology of depression and help to explain why central cholinomimetic drugs can produce a dysphoric mood in depressed patients. Support for the hypothesis that the cholinergic system is hyperfunctional in the depressed patient comes from the observation that the endocrine response to the reversible anticholinesterase pyridostigmine is increased in depressed patients. Perhaps more attention should be directed to a possible disturbance in central cholinergic transmission as a causative factor in depression.

In view of the well-established experimental and clinical evidence that the beta adrenoceptor density is increased in the untreated depressed patient, it is noteworthy that in several studies the density of these receptors appears to be unchanged in the cortical regions of the suicide brain.

Some attention has also been directed to the 5-HT transport sites in the suicide brain. There would appear to be some evidence that the imipramine binding sites are decreased, which concurs with the finding that these sites are also decreased on the platelet membranes of untreated depressed patients. More recently it has been shown that [^{3}H] paroxetine is a more specific ligand for the 5-HT transport site, but preliminary studies show that the density of this site is unchanged in the suicide brain.

Thus it may be concluded that there is evidence of an abnormality in both the serotonergic and cholinergic systems in the brains of suicide victims.

Changes in CSF and urinary amine concentrations

Changes in the concentrations of the main 5-HT and dopamine metabolites, 5-HIAA and homovanillic acid (HVA), have been reported to occur in the CSF of untreated depressed patients. Åsberg and her coworkers at the Karolinska Institute in Stockholm reported that the 5-HIAA concentrations in a group of depressives showed a bimodal distribution, one subgroup having an unchanged level while another subgroup had a low concentration of this metabolite. The clinical history of the latter group showed that the patients had attempted suicide by dramatic, physical means (e.g. cutting the throat). Subsequently other investigators have suggested that a very low functional activity of the serotonergic system may be associated with impulsivity.

The introduction of probenecid to block the efflux of acid metabolites from the CSF has enabled investigators to assess the turnover of 5-HT in the conscious patient. The use of this technique is based upon the assumption that the efflux is equal to the rate of clearance of 5-HIAA, and studies have shown that the rate of accumulation of this metabolite is reduced in the untreated depressive and returns to normal following clinical improvement in approximately 50% of the patients. Those failing to show a normalization of the 5-HIAA accumulation on clinical recovery may be prone to subsequent episodes of the illness.

Several studies have attempted to define the relationship between the CSF metabolite levels and the response of the depressed patient to antidepressants that show specificity in inhibiting the reuptake of either noradrenaline (e.g. maprotiline) or 5-HT (e.g. zimelidine or fluoxetine). The CSF 5-HIAA, 3-methoxy-4-hydroxyphenylglycol (MHPG) and HVA concentrations enable an assessment to be made of the effects of these drugs on the serotonergic, noradrenergic and dopaminergic systems, respectively, both before and after antidepressant treatment. Despite the attractive hypothesis that selective antidepressants are particularly beneficial to those patients with specific neurotransmitter defects – for example those with a major defect in 5-HT or noradrenaline would be expected to respond best to a selective 5-HT or noradrenergic uptake inhibitor – there is no convincing evidence that this is the case. One must conclude from these studies that irrespective of the presumed specificity of antidepressants on the various neurotransmitters in the brain, in practice they modulate the activity of a number of different transmitters whose functions are inter-related.

Despite the findings that changes in CSF 5-HIAA may be related to the depressed state, there have been a number of criticisms of the use of this metabolite as a marker of central 5-HT activity. There is evidence, for example, that much of the 5-HIAA in the CSF comes from the spinal cord, not the brain. The ventricular 5-HIAA concentration would appear to be unchanged in the depressed patient, while the lumbar CSF concentration may reflect the general activity of the patient rather than the mood state. A similar argument can be made regarding the relevance of the decreased HVA levels frequently reported in depressed patients. These could also reflect the degree of motor retardation commonly seen in depressed patients and therefore not be of relevance to the mental state.

Since there is evidence that, under carefully controlled conditions of diet, exercise and time of day at which the body fluid is collected, there is an equilibrium in the distribution of MHPG between the CSF, blood and urine; studies on central noradrenergic function have been largely restricted to an analysis of urinary MHPG. Despite numerous studies during the 1970s on the concentration of this metabolite in the urine of uni- and bipolar patients with depression, there is so far little evidence that this metabolite is altered.

Thus it may be concluded that, although there is some evidence to suggest that serotonergic function is abnormal in some groups of depressives, as shown by CSF studies, it is by no means certain that such changes are a reflection of the mood states. Evidence for changes in the noradrenergic and dopaminergic systems in depression is equivocal.

Neuroendocrine correlates of depression

There is physiological evidence that the control of anterior pituitary hormone releasing factors by the hypothalamus is largely under the influence of the biogenic amine neurotransmitters. It would therefore seem a reasonable assumption to predict that any change in the activity of these transmitters that may be causally associated with depression would also be reflected in an abnormality of hormone release from the pituitary. It has long been known that depressed patients show an abnormality in the circadian fluctuations of most hormones, while the hypersecretion of cortisol which is not readily amenable to suppression by the glucocorticoid dexamethasone has been widely advocated as a biological marker of depression. A hypersecretion of cortisol is also found in patients with Cushing's disease, and since such patients frequently show evidence of depression it can be speculated that changes in the function of glucocorticoid receptors in the brain may play some role in the aetiology of the illness. Largely as a result of the seminal studies of Carroll and colleagues in the United States, the dexamethasone suppression test has been shown to be of predictive value for the diagnosis of further episodes of endogenous (or melancholic) depression in up to 95% of patients. However, it is now apparent that positive tests can occur in patients with senile dementia, alcoholism, anorexia nervosa and malnutrition, and in those subject to inadequate renal dialysis. Whether the changes in cortisol secretion in such patients are attributable to secondary symptoms of depression still awaits elucidation.

Recently there has been considerable interest in the possible modulatory role of glucocorticoid receptors on central neurotransmission. It is well established that there is a high density of steroid receptors in the limbic regions of the brain. Hypercortisolaemia occurs frequently in patients with depression, and the insensitivity of hypothalamic glucocorticoid receptors to the inhibitory effects of administered synthetic glucocorticoids such as dexamethasone forms the basis of the dexamethasone suppression test for depression. Failure of dexamethasone to suppress the hypersecretion of cortisol suggests that central glucocorticoid receptors are hypersensitive. Interest in the possible association of central glucocorticoid receptors with altered neurotransmitter function arose from the observation that these receptors occur in the nuclei of catecholamine- and serotonin-containing cell bodies in the brain. It has been shown that glucocorticoid receptors function as DNA binding proteins that can modify gene transcription, and that long-term imipramine treatment causes an increase in glucocorticoid receptor immunoreactivity in rat brain, particularly in the noradrenergic and serotonergic cell body regions. Such findings lend support to the hypothesis that the changes in central neurotransmission that occur in depression reflect the effects of chronic glucocorticoid hypersecretion on the transcription of proteins, which play a crucial role in neuronal structure and function. It has been postulated that antidepressants normalize both cortisol secretion and, indirectly, noradrenergic and serotonergic neuro-transmission, upregulating the desensitized central glucocorticoid receptors and thereby restoring their sensitivity to inhibitory feedback regulation. It therefore follows that if the pituitary–adrenal axis plays such an important role in the control of central aminergic neurotransmission, glucocorticoid synthesis inhibitors such as metapyrone or ketoconazole could restore central amine function by decreasing the elevated peripheral cortisol levels, and thereby upregulate central glucocorticoid receptors in a manner similar to that occurring after long-term antidepressant administration. Preliminary clinical data showing that metapyrone has antidepressant effects lend credibility to this view.

The link between glucocorticoid receptors, corticotropin-releasing factor, the interleukins (particularly interleukin-2 and interleukin-6), prostaglandin E_2 (PGE_2) and the biogenic amine neurotransmitters has also been the subject of recent attention. There is experimental evidence to show that long-term antidepressant treatment results in a reduction in brain concentrations of interleukins and PGE_2. There is evidence that plasma PGE_2 levels are increased in depressed patients and that presynaptic release of the biogenic amines is reduced by PGE_2. Therefore it has been hypothesized that antidepressants may normalize central neurotransmission by reducing brain levels of both the interleukins and PGE_2 by reducing central macrophage activity (e.g. the microglia, which release interleukins and thereby precipitate a cytokine cascade) and by inhibiting brain cyclo-oxygenase activity. These changes, together with those in glucocorticoid receptor function, may therefore incrementally bring about the normalization of defective central neuro-transmission during antidepressant treatment. This subject is discussed further in Chapter 17.

There is good evidence that growth hormone secretion is also disrupted in depression, which may reflect an abnormality in the postsynaptic alpha$_2$ adrenoceptor activity. Thus the incremental rise in growth hormone following an acute challenge with either desipramine or clonidine is diminished in depressed patients. Whether such changes are a direct consequence of hypoactivity of the postsynaptic alpha$_2$ receptors or an indirect result of changes in central 5-HT or gamma-aminobutyric acid (GABA) function is presently unclear.

A reduction in the responsiveness of the anterior pituitary gland to the stimulant effects of thyrotrophin-releasing hormone has been reported to occur in depressed patients. At present, however, there would not appear to be any consensus regarding the value of such challenge tests to the diagnosis of depression. There is clinical evidence that the efficacy of some types of antidepressant can be enhanced by the concurrent administration of a small dose of a thyroid hormone. From such studies it may be concluded that thyroid function could play a role in the response of the depressed patient to antidepressant treatment and also, due to the possible involvement of thyroid hormones in sensitizing peripheral and central adrenoceptors, in predisposing the patient to a depressive episode.

Most of the neuroendocrine challenge tests have been used to assess noradrenergic function in the depressed patient and have indicated that this function is suppressed. It is well established that the control of prolactin secretion is at least partly under central serotonergic control. The prolactin response to an intraveneous tryptophan challenge has been found to be decreased in depressed patients and to normalize following effective antidepressant treatment. The prolactin response to the 5-HT-releasing agent D-fenfluramine has also been shown to be blunted in the depressed patient. The precise cause of the blunted response is uncertain, but it presumably reflects a decrease in the activity of one of the populations of 5-HT receptors.

To date there has been little emphasis on the use of neuroendocrine challenge tests to investigate changes in the dopaminergic system. Preliminary evidence suggests that electroconvulsive shock treatment results in an enhancement of the inhibitory effect of bromocriptine on prolactin release, which suggests that the antidepressant effect of this treatment is associated with a sensitization of postsynaptic D$_2$ receptors.

In SUMMARY, the results of the neuroendocrine challenge tests imply that the noradrenergic and serotonergic postsynaptic receptors are functionally hypoactive in the depressed patient. There is some evidence that the responsiveness of these receptors normalizes after effective treatment.

Peripheral markers for the study of depression

The need for researchers to obtain a peripheral model of the nerve terminal in order that changes in transmitter receptor function and transport may be investigated in patients has led to an interest in the platelet as a possible model. Structurally, both the nerve terminal and the platelet contain mitochondria and dense core vesicles that store 5-HT or other amines. MAO activity is associated with the mitochondrial fraction of both nerve endings and platelets, the major difference being that in the platelet only one type of MAO, MAO-B, occurs, whereas in the nerve terminal both MAO-A and B occur, the subtype of enzyme depending on the function of the terminal. The storage vesicles in the platelet contain only 5-HT but, like in the nerve terminal, the release of this amine is a calcium-dependent process. Unlike nerve terminals, platelets cannot synthesize 5-HT, but this role is taken over by the closely associated amine precursor uptake and decarboxylation cells (APUD) cells, which are of the same embryonic origin as the nerve terminals and platelets, all of which contain the unique neuron-specific enolases. The APUD cells and platelets may therefore be considered to represent a paraneuronal system.

There are, however, a number of important differences between the platelet and the nerve terminal. Platelets store glycogen, whereas nerve terminals do not. Structurally, platelets are not directly connected with any other cells or with the nervous system, whereas neurons are directly and indirectly connected with hundreds of other nerve cells via their axonal and dendritic processes. It may therefore be concluded that, although platelets may be considered to be a useful model of the serotonergic nerve terminal, and that the shape changes which may be induced by selective alpha and 5-HT$_2$ agonists can give some degree of insight into the changes in receptor function which may occur in psychiatric illness, their relevance to other types of nerve terminal is necessarily limited. Figure 6.1 gives a diagrammatic representation of the inter-relationship between the structure and the function of the platelet.

Changes in peripheral receptors in depression

One method that has been used to monitor postsynaptic adrenoceptor changes in the depressed patient *in vivo* involves measuring the pressor response to intravenously administered alpha agonists such as phenyleph-rine or noradrenaline, or the indirectly acting amine tyramine. An enhanced pressor response has been reported to occur in untreated patients, which suggests that the postsynaptic alpha receptors are hyperactive. Other studies

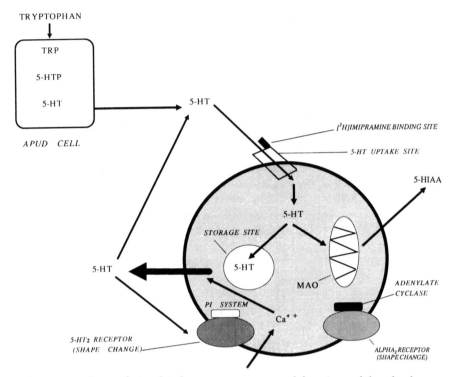

Figure 6.1. Inter-relationship between structure and functions of the platelet.

have concentrated on changes in the density and aggregating function of the alpha$_2$ receptors on the platelet membrane. While there would appear to be little evidence that the functional activity of these receptors is altered, there is conflicting evidence regarding the density of these receptors, with some investigators reporting an increase, others a decrease and yet others no change. A major problem in evaluating these studies stems from the nature of the ligand used to detect the receptors and the relative specificity of the ligand for the alpha receptors. Studies with the highly specific ligand [^{3}H] rauwolscine consistently show that the density of these receptors is unchanged.

Studies on the density and function of beta adrenoceptors on the lymphocyte membrane have also yielded equivocal results. Some of the changes reported are undoubtedly due to the heterogeneity of the patients studied, lack of control for age, different periods being allowed for the wash-out of any psychotropic medication being taken by the patients and the specificity of the ligand for the beta receptors. The most consistent studies in which attempts have been made to control for some of these factors show that the beta receptor density is raised in the untreated patient and returns to control values in those patients responding to treatment. Thus the beta receptor density would appear to be a useful state marker of depression. Regarding the beta receptor function, there is some evidence that the receptor-linked cyclase activity is decreased. Thus it may be surmized that there is a deficit in the link between the beta receptor and the secondary messenger system which may be causally related to depression.

While there has been widespread interest in possible changes in adrenoceptor activity that may be linked to depression, less attention seems to have been paid to serotonin receptor function. There is evidence that 5-HT-induced platelet aggregation is significantly reduced in the untreated depressed patients but normalizes on effective treatment irrespective of the nature of that treatment. This provides clinical evidence for the view that 5-HT receptor function is augmented following effective treatment and that the time of onset of the clinical response coincides with the improvement.

Circadian changes in neurotransmitter function in depression

Both clinical and experimental studies have shown that a number of transmitter receptors and amine transport processes show circadian changes. It is well established that depression is associated with a disruption of the circadian rhythm as shown by changes in a number of behavioural, autonomic and neuroendocrine aspects. One of the main consequences of effective treatment is a return of the circadian rhythm to normality. For example, it has been shown that the 5-HT uptake into the platelets of depressed patients is largely unchanged between 0600 and 1200, whereas the 5-HT transport in control subjects shows a significant decrease over this period. The normal rhythm in 5-HT transport is only re-established when the depressed patient responds to treatment. Thus it may be hypothesized that the mood of action of antidepressants is to normalize disrupted circadian rhythms. Only when the circadian rhythm has returned to normal can full clinical recovery be established.

Chronobiological studies have shown that circadian rhythms occur in the responsivity of animals to light, dark and psychotropic drugs. This implies that the timing of drug administration so that the drug reaches the target organ at its optimum sensitivity could help to improve its therapeutic efficiency. The results of experimental studies suggest that most anti-depressants delay the circadian phase and lengthen the circadian period. These changes could be due to the drugs acting on the circadian pacemaker in the superchiasmatic nucleus. However, other brain regions could also be responsible together with antidepressant-induced changes in the retina which would lead to a modification of the processing of light stimuli; the lateral geniculate nucleus may also have a role to play. Seasonal affective disorder (SAD) generally consists of recurrent depressive episodes in autumn and winter that alternate with euthmia or hypomania in spring and summer. The seasonal rhythms of mood, sleep and weight change seen in SAD patients resemble hibernation seen in animals. This led to the hypothesis that extension of the photoperiod in winter could counteract the depressive symptoms. Exposure to bright light had indeed been shown to be efficacious. Clinical studies show that carbohydrate craving, a common feature of SAD, is possibly linked to a decreased serotonin turnover. Such a hypothesis is supported by the fact that the serotonin releasing agent D-fenfluramine is effective in treating SAD. Chronobiology is clearly an important area of research for the psychopharmacologist which needs more attention.

Drugs used in the treatment of depression

It is generally accepted that the high affinity, energy-dependent mechanism whereby the biogenic amines noradrenaline, dopamine and 5-HT are transported into the presynaptic neuron in the brain is of primary importance in terminating the physiological action of these transmitters on their receptor sites. From this it follows that a drug that inhibits the reuptake mechanism would not only prolong the physiological action of the transmitter, but also produce behavioural changes. *Cocaine* is an example of a psychotropic drug that selectively inhibits the uptake of noradrenaline and dopamine and its psychostimulant properties are partly attributable to this effect. The *amphetamines*, such as D-amphetamine and methamphetamine, also impede the reuptake of catecholamines, but in addition they enhance the release of these amines, an action which underlies their marked euphoriant, stimulant and anorexiant properties. Nevertheless, despite the actions of these drugs in prolonging the intersynaptic activity of the catecholamines, there is no evidence that they have antidepressant properties. From this evidence it must be concluded that the ability of a drug to inhibit the reuptake process of a neurotransmitter is not in itself indicative of antidepressant potential!

The *tricyclic antidepressants* (TCAs), as exemplified by amitriptyline, imipramine and clomipramine, and most of the more recently introduced antidepressants such as fluoxetine, maprotiline and fluvoxamine, are potent inhibitors of noradrenaline and/or 5-HT reuptake both *in vitro* and *in vivo*. Even allowing for the fact that many of these drugs produce pharmacologically active metabolites *in vivo* (e.g. desipramine from imipramine, and norfluoxetine from fluoxetine), there is no evidence to suggest that the

Table 6.1. Effect of different classes of antidepressants on the uptake of [³H]5-HT, noradrenaline and dopamine into nerve ending fractions from rat brain

Type of antidepressant	Uptake (μM)		
	5-HT	Noradrenaline	Dopamine
Tricyclics			
Imipramine	0.50	0.20	8.7
Desipramine	0.20	0.03	50.0
Amitriptyline	0.49	0.05	4.0
Nortriptyline	1.60	1.30	5.5
Clomipramine	0.04	0.30	12.0
Lofepramine			
Non-tricyclics			
Nomifensine	12.00	0.03	0.14
Maprotiline	30.00	0.08	–
Citalopram	0.014	32.00	–
Fluoxetine	0.06	10.00	–
Zimelidine	0.24	2.70	12.0
Mianserin	8.00	0.30	–

Values expressed are the 50% inhibitory concentration following *in vitro* addition of the antidepressants to the nerve ending fractions. Thus the lower the value, the more potent the antidepressant is in inhibiting the transport of the amine. – implies that values are not available.

potency or specificity of action of the drug in inhibiting amine reuptake is in any way related to its therapeutic effect. Perhaps this is not surprising when it is realized that the transport of 5-HT, and possibly other amine transmitters, is defective in the depressed patient and therefore it would seem contradictory for an antidepressant to correct the symptoms of depression by further impeding the mechanism which is already defective in the untreated patient. Furthermore, it has long been known that the effects on amine uptake occur acutely, whereas it takes many days, and sometimes weeks, before the antidepressant effects of the drugs become apparent. As has already been discussed elsewhere in this volume, such findings suggest that antidepressants ameliorate the symptoms of the disease by re-adapting the abnormal neurotransmitter transport and receptors that are defective in the depressed patient. Such a process probably takes many days, or weeks, and appears to correlate with the onset of the clinical response.

The effects of a number of commonly available tricyclic and non-tricyclic antidepressants on the reuptake of the biogenic amines are summarized in Table 6.1. Figure 6.2 gives a measure of the potency of a number of typical and atypical antidepressants in inhibiting noradrenaline or 5-HT uptake *in vitro*.

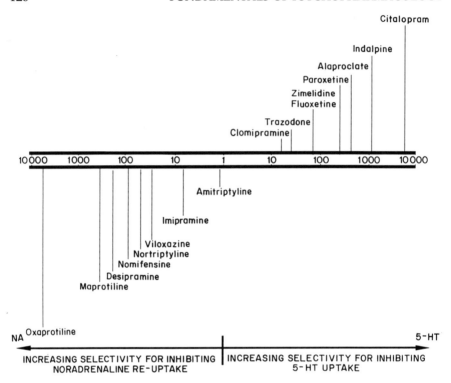

Figure 6.2. Selectivity of antidepressants in inhibiting the uptake of [³H] noradrenaline (NA) or [³H]5-HT into synaptosomes from rat brain *in vitro*. It should be noted that the potency of an antidepressant in inhibiting amine uptake *in vitro* may differ from its inhibitory potency following acute administration *in vivo*. Furthermore, there appears to be no direct relationship between the potency of the antidepressant *in vitro* and the therapeutic dose.

The selectivity of antidepressants in inhibiting noradrenaline or 5-HT uptake has led to the introduction of a large number of drugs that lack the dibenzazepine structure found in many TCAs. However, there is no evidence that any of the newer antidepressants in current use are therapeutically more effective than imipramine. Their main advantage lies in their lower cardiotoxicity, safety in overdose and fewer adverse side effects at therapeutic doses.

Second generation antidepressants

A summary of the different classes of second generation antidepressants is given in Table 6.2.

Table 6.2.   Some second generation antidepressants

Drug class	Examples
Selective MOA-A inhibitors	Brofaromine, cimoxatone, moclobemide
Alpha$_2$ adrenoceptor antagonists	Idazoxan*, mianserin, mirtazapine (mepirzapin)
Selective serotonin (5-hydroxytryptamine; 5-HT) reuptake inhibitors	Citalopram, fluoxetine, fluvoxamine, paroxetine, sertraline, zimelidine**
Noradrenaline (norepinephrine) reuptake inhibitors	Levoprotiline*, nomifensine**, oxaprotiline
Serotonin reuptake enhancer	Tianeptine
5-HT$_{1A}$ partial agonists	Gepirone*, ispapirone*
Benzodiazepine analogues	Alprazolam, adinazolam, zometapine*
Drugs modulating dopaminergic function	Amfebutamone (bupropion)
Gamma-aminobutyric acid (GABA-mimetics)	Fengabine, progabide*
Non-tricyclic antidepressants	Lofepramine

*Clinical efficacy uncertain; **drugs withdrawn because of serious adverse effects.

The frequency of adverse effects associated with first generation antidepressants, and the lack of patient compliance that arise from such effects, has led to the development of a number of second generation antidepressants. These include such chemically diverse drugs as the new TCAs (e.g. lofepramine), the tetracyclic compound mianserin, various bi- and tricyclic antidepressants (e.g. trazodone, viloxazine and amfebutamone), and a series of selective serotonin reuptake inhibitors (SSRIs) (e.g. fluoxetine, fluvoxamine, paroxetine and sertraline). These drugs are sometimes called atypical antidepressants.

Despite the initial enthusiasm that greeted the introduction of the second generation antidepressants, these drugs have not provided the ideal solution to safe and effective antidepressant therapy. Most of the second generation drugs have the distinct advantages over first generation drugs of reduced toxicity, improved patient compliance and lower toxicity in overdose. However, like the TCAs their therapeutic effect only becomes manifest after several weeks of treatment. In addition, up to 30% of depressed patients treated with an effective dose of any of the currently available antidepressants fail to improve following several weeks of drug therapy.

It has been estimated that there are currently 125 antidepressants in varying states of development. All appear to be based on the traditional concepts of enhancing the availability of biogenic amine neurotransmitters. There appears to be little likelihood that the overall antidepressant efficacy or the speed of onset in therapeutic response will improve following the introduction of such chemically novel entities. It is hoped that the third generation of antidepressants, when it appears, will combine the increased speed of onset with greater efficacy and a further reduction in the adverse effect profile to that shown by the second generation drugs.

Novel TCAs

With the exception of lofepramine, all of the more recently introduced TCAs (such as dothiepin, doxepin, maprotiline and amoxapine) are at least as toxic as the predecessors such as amitriptyline and imipramine. Lofepramine is a unique TCA, probably because of the phenyl piperazine substitution in its side chain. This moiety prevents the attachment of the side chain nitrogens to the muscarinic receptor site. It largely lacks the anticholinergic, antihistaminic and cardiotoxic properties of the traditional TCAs.

Safety in overdose and an improved adverse effect profile makes lofepramine a particularly useful TCA. It is especially useful for the treatment of elderly depressed patients who have compromised cardiac function, or any patient likely to attempt suicide.

Selective monoamine oxidase inhibitors

Factors contributing to the decline in the use of the first generation of MAOIs included the need for dietary restrictions, the toxicity of some MAOIs when taken in overdose, and the unfavourable report regarding the relative lack of efficacy of phenelzine when compared to imipramine and ECT in the treatment of depression. These factors led to the use of MAO inhibitors being limited to atypical depression and, more recently, panic attacks.

The discovery that MAO exists in two isoenzymic forms led to the development of MAOIs that show selectivity for one or the other form. Under physiological conditions, MAO-A primarily deaminates noradrenaline and serotonin, while MAO-B deaminates dopamine. The MAO-B isoenzyme predominates in the brain and platelets, while MAO-A predominates in the gastrointestinal tract. Selective MAOIs have been introduced for the treatment of depression (MAO-A inhibitors, such as moclobemide) and as an adjunct to levodopa in the treatment of Parkinson's disease (MAO-B inhibitors, exemplified by selegiline).

Whereas the older MAOIs are irreversible inhibitors of MAO, the new MAO-A inhibitors such as moclobemide, toloxatone (Figure 6.3) and brofaromine are reversible inhibitors of MAO-A. The potential advantage of the reversible over the irreversible inhibitors is that the tyramine-potentiating effects of reversible inhibitors of monoamine oxidase (RIMAs) is much reduced compared with the older MAOIs.

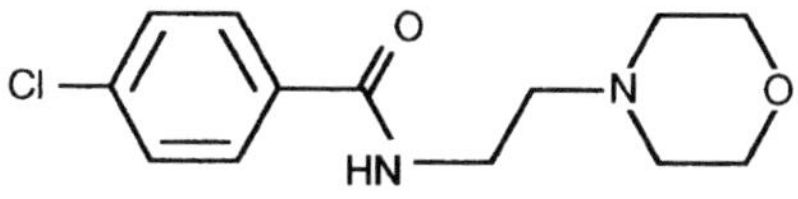

Moclobemide

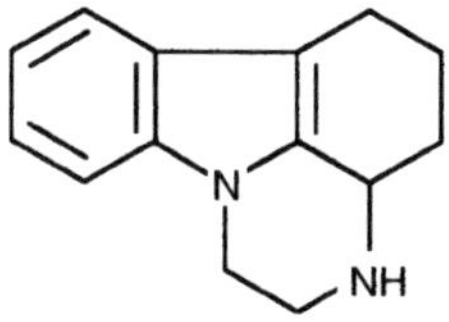

Pirlindole

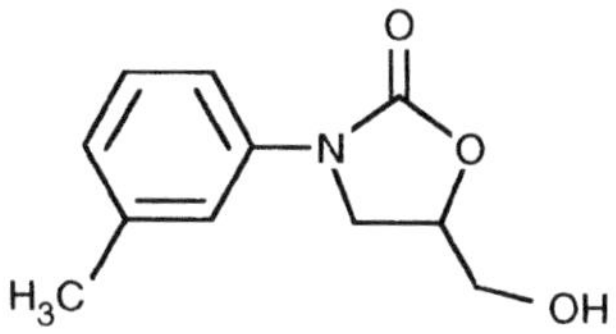

Toloxatone

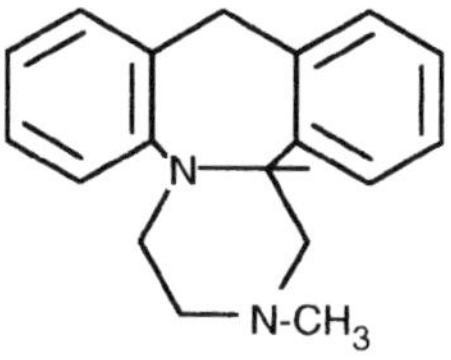

S-Mirtazapine

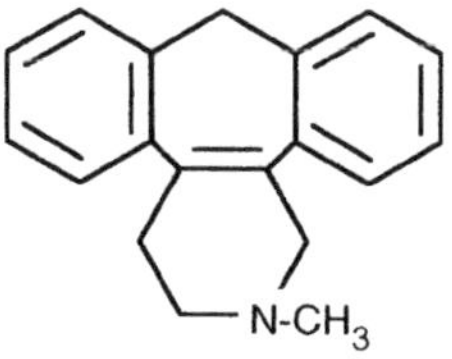

Setiptiline (teciptiline)

Figure 6.3. Structural formulae of some monoamine oxidase inhibitors (moclobemide, pirlindole and toloxatone) and alpha$_2$ adrenoceptor antagonists [S-mirtazapine and setiptiline (teciptiline)].

It is still unclear whether RIMAs are as effective as TCAs and second generation antidepressants in the treatment of all types of depression. However, there is evidence that moclobemide is effective in the treatment of both endogenous depression and atypical depression, and does not apparently interact with dietary tyramine when the amine is consumed in usual amounts.

Novel MAO-A inhibitors have been developed that are irreversible in their action, but which do not apparently interact with dietary tyramine. Both experimental and clinical studies have shown that an enantiomer of the pro-drug MDL-72394 is decarboxylated by brain *l*-aromatic amino acid decarboxylase to form an irreversible MAO-A inhibitor. When combined with a peripheral levodopa decarboxylase inhibitor, MAO-A activity in the periphery is largely unaffected. Whether this compound will eventually be marketed as an antidepressant will depend on the success of placebo-controlled trials against such comparators as amitriptyline.

The use of MAO-B inhibitors has been largely restricted to adjunctive therapy for Parkinson's disease. There have been some controlled clinical trials in depressed patients, in which high doses of selegiline have been shown to have antidepressant properties. At the doses required to show antidepressant activity, however, it appears that selegiline loses its selectivity of action on MAO-B and also inhibits MAO-A. Thus, it seem unlikely that MAO-B inhibitors will be developed for the treatment of depression in the future.

Alpha$_2$ adrenoceptor antagonists

More than 15 years ago, it was discovered that clonidine reduced blood pressure by activating alpha$_2$ adrenoceptors in the vasomotor area of the brain. This was important in defining the physiological role of alpha$_2$ adrenoceptors in controlling the release of noradrenaline.

More recently, it has been discovered that alpha$_2$ adrenoceptors may be classified into several subtypes, namely alpha$_{2A}$, alpha$_{2B}$ and alpha$_{2C}$. The alpha$_{2A}$ subtype predominates in the cortex of the rat. The precise physiological role of the different subtypes of alpha$_2$ adrenoceptors still remains an enigma. Nevertheless there is evidence that presynaptically located alpha$_2$ adrenoceptors function as inhibitory receptors to control the release of noradrenaline.

Mianserin was the first truly atypical antidepressant to be discovered that largely lacked an inhibitory effect on the reuptake of biogenic amines and had no MAOI properties. Mianserin was shown to facilitate the release of noradrenaline from brain slices *in vitro* and to antagonize the action of clonidine *in vivo*. In addition, mianserin has an antagonistic effect on postsynaptic 5-HT$_2$ receptors in the rat brain. The adverse effects of this antidepressant, namely postural hypotension and sedation, have been attributed to its antagonistic action on alpha$_1$ adrenoceptors and histamine H$_1$ receptors, respectively.

The unique effect of mianserin as an alpha$_2$ adrenoceptor (probably alpha$_{2B}$) antagonist has led to the development of numerous selective alpha$_2$ adrenoceptor antagonists as putative antidepressants. To date, over 35 alpha$_2$ adrenoceptor antagonists have been patented as putative antidepressants. However, only two other tetracyclic compounds have been shown to be clinically effective antidepressants, namely mirtazapine, the aza derivative of mianserin, and setiptiline (teciptiline) (Figure 6.3).

Mirtazapine and setiptiline are both potent alpha$_2$ adrenoceptor (predominantly alpha$_{2B}$) specific antagonists, which have little effect on noradrenaline reuptake. However, it seems unlikely that the clinical efficacy of mirtazapine is limited to an antagonistic action on alpha$_2$ adrenoceptors. There are experimental studies to show that this drug, probably by its action on alpha$_2$ heteroreceptors located on serotonergic terminals, also facilitates serotonergic transmission.

The affinity of mianserin, mirtazapine and setiptiline for several neurotransmitter receptor sites restricts any conclusions being drawn regarding the precise role of alpha$_2$ adrenoceptor antagonism as the antidepressant mode of action.

A further complication relates to the recently discovered imidazoline receptors in the mammalian brain. These receptors have been shown to be functionally involved in drug-induced modulation of electrically stimulated noradrenaline release from rat vascular tissue. It is possible that such receptors are also involved in the control of noradrenaline release in the brain. At present, there appears to be little published evidence regarding the action of the novel TCAs on these receptors.

Idazoxan is the most widely researched non-tetracyclic, highly selective presynaptic alpha$_2$ adrenoceptor antagonist. Despite some initial evidence of antidepressant activity, its development has been discontinued recently because of its lack of efficacy in placebo-controlled, double-blind trials. One of the reasons for this lack of efficacy may lie in its partial agonist action at alpha$_2$ adrenoceptors.

Noradrenaline reuptake inhibitors

The antidepressant activity of classic TCAs, as exemplified by amitriptyline and imipramine, has been ascribed to their ability to impede the reuptake of noradrenaline and serotonin. However, it was soon established that their adverse effects (dry mouth, sedation, postural hypotension, etc.) were due to their antagonism of muscarinic, H$_1$ receptors and alpha$_1$ adrenergic receptors in the periphery.

Attention was therefore directed towards the development of drugs that showed a high degree of specificity for the noradrenaline and/or serotonin transport sites, but which had negligible effects on neurotransmitter receptors either in the brain or in the periphery.

Maprotiline was one of the first modified TCAs to be developed which showed a high selectivity for the noradrenaline transport site with little action on muscarinic or histamine receptors. Unfortunately, like the older TCAs, maprotiline was cardiotoxic in overdose. Furthermore, it was liable to precipitate seizures in those patients predisposed to epilepsy.

Close analogues of maprotiline, namely oxaprotiline (Figure 6.4) and levoprotiline, showed greater selectivity for the noradrenaline transporter than maprotiline, and had fewer adverse effects. Unfortunately, the clinical efficacy of these drugs is still uncertain and no comment can be made regarding their clinical usefulness.

Nomifensine was one of the first relatively selective catecholamine reuptake inhibitors with proven clinical efficacy and few adverse effects. While the parent compound is a selective inhibitor of both noradrenaline and dopamine reuptake, the main metabolite, 5-hydroxynomifensine, inhibits serotonin reuptake. Presumably, the enhanced noradrenergic and dopaminergic activity that results from the inhibition of catecholamine reuptake could account for the stimulant effect of the drug. Whether the serotonin reuptake inhibitory effect of the 4-hydroxy metabolite contributes to the antidepressant action of the drug is unknown.

A major advantage of nomifensine over other antidepressants lay in its lack of effect on the seizure threshold. It therefore had a special role to play in the treatment of depressed patients who also had epilepsy. However, this very useful antidepressant was withdrawn 10 years ago because of the rare occurrence of haemolytic anaemia.

Selective dopamine reuptake inhibitors have also been developed as putative antidepressants. To date, only amfebutamone (Figure 6.4) has been developed as an effective antidepressant that shows some selectivity for inhibiting the reuptake of dopamine in the rat brain. However, there is evidence that the major metabolite of amfebutamone in humans is a potent and selective inhibitor of noradrenaline reuptake. This metabolite may make a major contribution to the antidepressant properties of the agent.

The selective noradrenaline reuptake inhibitor viloxazine has been available for clinical use since 1974. The main adverse effects of this antidepressant are nausea, vomiting and occasionally migraine attacks. Furthermore, the clinical efficacy of viloxazine is in some doubt. A close analogue of viloxazine, reboxetine, has recently been developed. This is a potent inhibitor of noradrenaline reuptake and has little effect on other neurotransmitter receptors. Whether reboxetine will lack the adverse effects of viloxazine is presently unknown.

In recent years, several antidepressants have been developed that inhibit the reuptake of both noradrenaline and serotonin. Unlike the older TCAs,

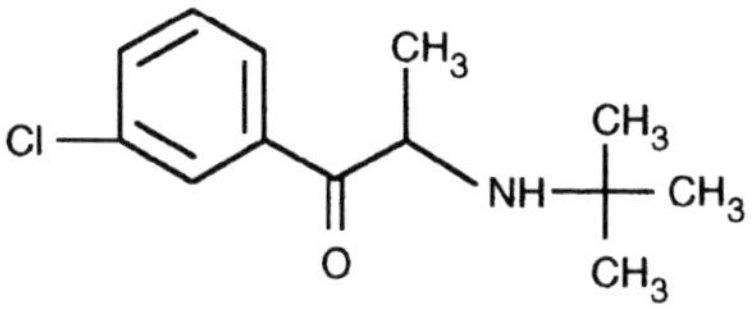

Amfebutamone (bupropion)

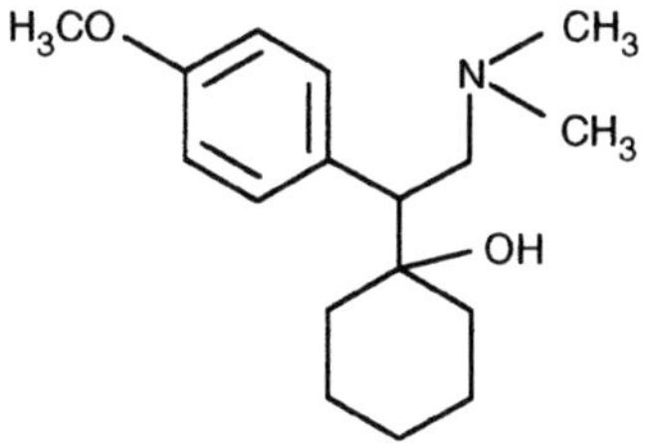

Venlafaxine

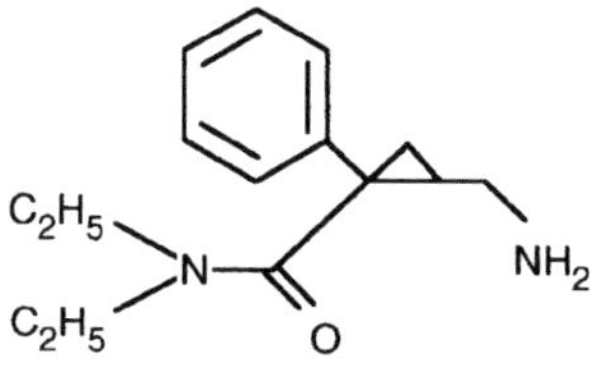

Milnacipran

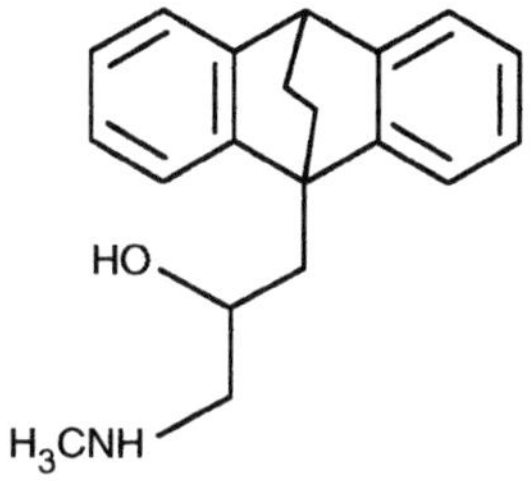

Oxaprotiline

Figure 6.4. Structural formulae of the noradrenaline (norepinephrine)/dopamine reuptake inhibitor amfebutamone (bupropion) and some nonselective noradrenaline and serotonin (5-hydroxytryptamine; 5-HT) reuptake inhibitors (venlafaxine, milnacipran and oxaprotiline).

these agents have little effect on muscarinic, histaminic and adrenergic receptors. Of the drugs in development, venlafaxine and milnacipran (Figure 6.4) have been shown to be effective antidepressants in clinical trials. However, it appears that these antidepressants do cause some nausea and anorexia.

Table 6.3.   Potency of some antidepressants in inhibiting the uptake of $[^3H]5\text{-}HT$ into rat brain

Antidepressants	Potency *in vitro* $(\mu M)\text{-}IC_{50}$	Potency *ex vivo* $(mg/kg)\text{-}ED_{50}$	Therapeutic dose mg/day
Paroxetine	0.01	1.9	20–50
Sertraline	0.06	2.9	50–200
Fluoxetine	0.27	7.0	20–40
Zimelidine	0.45	6.2	200
Fluvoxamine	0.54	7.4	100–200
Clomipramine	0.10	17.0	75–150
Imipramine	0.81	30.0	75–150
Amitriptyline	1.20	30.0	75–150

Selective serotonin reuptake inhibitors

During the last two decades there has been a major effort by the pharmaceutical industry to develop drugs that have a high degree of selectivity for the serotonin transport site in the brain. SSRIs are widely used for the treatment of depression, and are also used for panic attacks, obsessive–compulsive disorder, alcohol abuse and bulimia nervosa. The usefulness of these drugs in treating such a diverse group of psychiatric conditions reflects the primary role that serotonin plays in the physiological regulation of sleep, mood, impulsivity and feeding behaviour. The clinical pharmacology of SSRIs has been reviewed elsewhere.

The major biochemical difference between these SSRIs lies in their relative potencies for inhibiting the reuptake of serotonin *in vitro* and *in vivo*. A comparison of some of the most widely used SSRIs with regard to their ability to inhibit the reuptake of serotonin is shown in Table 6.3.

The dosage range of these drugs used to treat depression is also shown in Table 6.3. It can be seen that there is no apparent correlation between the potency of these drugs in inhibiting serotonin reuptake and the daily dosage. This suggests that inhibition of serotonin reuptake may be a necessary condition for the antidepressant activity of the SSRIs, but is not by itself a sufficient explanation.

The main clinically significant difference between the most widely available SSRIs lies in their duration of action. Only fluoxetine has an active metabolite, and the combined half-life of fluoxetine and its metabolite norfluoxetine exceeds 7 days. This may be of some therapeutic advantage should the depressed patient miss taking the drug for 1 or 2 days. However, it could be a disadvantage in a patient who fails to respond to fluoxetine and, therefore, requires an alternative antidepressant that may interact pharmaco-kinetically with the SSRI. For this reason, MAOIs should only be administered some 5 weeks after the withdrawal of fluoxetine.

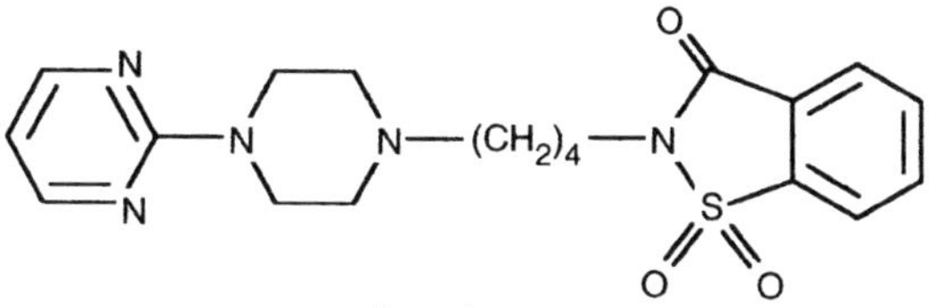

Ipsapirone

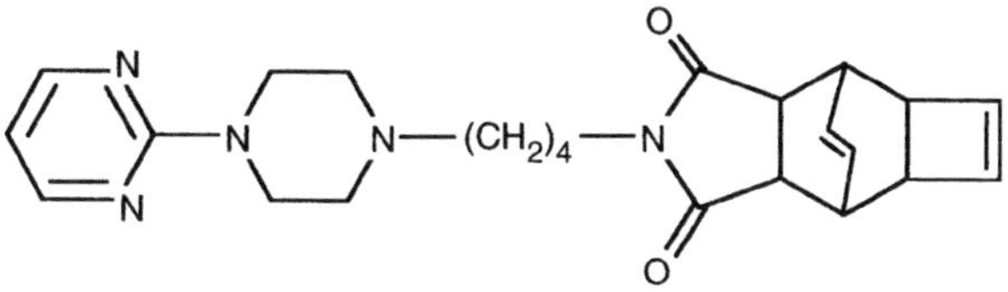

Zalospirone

Figure 6.5. Structural formulae of the 5-HT$_{1A}$ partial agonists ipsapirone and zalospirone.

All SSRIs produce qualitatively similar adverse effects that may largely be ascribed to an activation of different populations of serotonin receptors in the gastrointestinal tract (e.g. 5-HT$_3$ receptors) and brain. These adverse effects include nausea, diarrhoea or constipation, insomnia, tremor, dizziness and headache. Bodyweight gain, which is a major problem with the older TCAs, does not occur with the SSRIs. In general, the severity of adverse effects associated with the SSRIs is slight and, unlike the consequences of the adverse effects caused by the TCAs, compliance is generally good.

In addition, the behavioural toxicity of the SSRIs, as indicated by their effects on psychomotor functions, memory and sedation, is relatively low when compared with the older TCAs.

There is little experimental or clinical evidence to show that the clinical efficacy and adverse effect profiles of recently marketed (e.g. citalopram) or late-stage development (e.g. viqualine and cericlamine) SSRIs will differ appreciably from the SSRIs that are already well established.

Because of the clinical importance of the SSRIs in the treatment of mental illness, a detailed discussion of the role of serotonin is discussed further in Chapter 5. The structures of some SSRIs together with nefazodone are shown in Figure 6.6.

Nefazodone is a novel antidepressant which has recently been launched in North America and in many European countries. From its pharmacological properties it may be considered to be a modified SSRI. Thus it has an affinity for the serotonin transporter but, in addition, inhibits the postsynaptic 5-HT$_{2A}$ receptors. The action on the 5-HT$_2$ receptor may account for its anxiolytic activity which has enabled it to be licensed for mixed anxiety-depression.

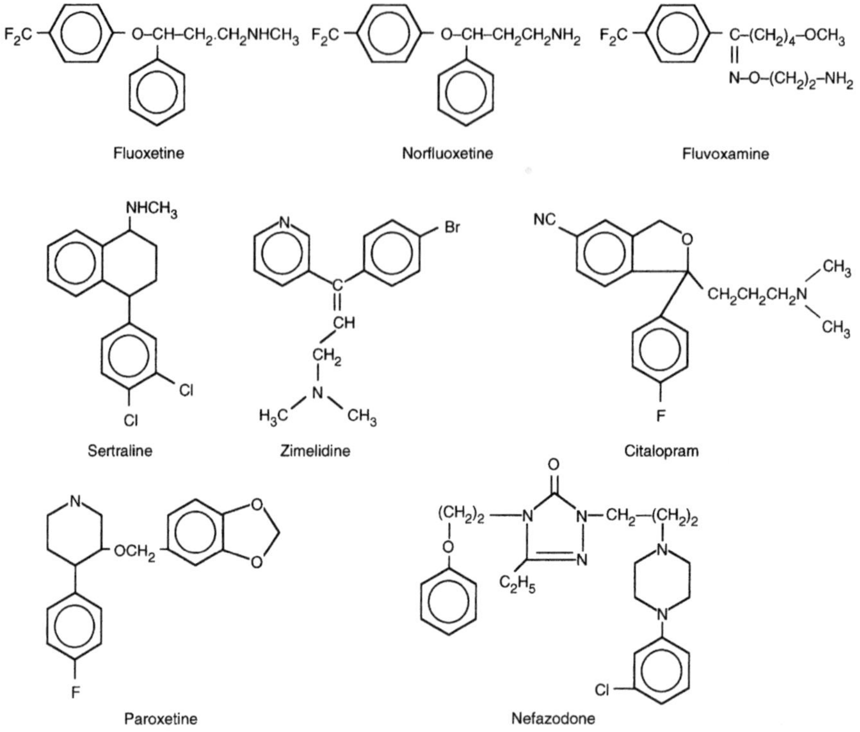

Figure 6.6. Chemical structure of some 5-HT uptake inhibitors. Zimelidine has been withdrawn due to serious adverse side effects. Norfluoxetine is an active metabolite of fluoxetine.

Perhaps the most unique feature of nefazodone lies in its ability to increase rapid eye movement (REM) sleep, an effect which might be associated with its action on 5-HT_{2A} receptors. Most classes of antidepressants have been shown to decrease REM sleep; as the sleep pattern of the depressed patient is grossly disturbed (both in terms of the slow-wave sleep and the REM sleep profile) this could be a significant advantage in using an antidepressant that improves the sleep profile particularly in the initial stages of treatment. The side effects of nefazodone are somewhat similar to those of the SSRIs.

It would appear that established antidepressants, together with the various putative antidepressants with diverse chemical structures and different acute effects on central neurotransmission, all have two things in common at the cellular level, namely an ability to decrease the functional activity of postsynaptic beta adrenoceptors and enhance the activity of 5-HT_2 receptors in the limbic regions of the brain. As there is evidence that the beta

Table 6.4. Common effects of antidepressants (ADs) and electroconvulsive shock treatment (ECT) on the function of neurotransmitter receptors; experimental studies

Alpha$_2$ adrenoceptors	Decreased
Alpha$_1$ adrenoceptors	Increased after AD
Beta adrenoceptors	Decreased
5-HT$_2$ receptors (postsynaptic)	Decreased (ECT increased)
5-HT$_1$ somatodendritic autoreceptors	Decreased
GABA$_B$ receptors	Increased
Dopamine autoreceptors	Decreased

GABA=gamma aminobutyric acid; 5-HT=5-hydroxytryptamine (serotonin).

receptors are increased in density in the depressed patient, while the 5-HT$_2$ receptors show a functional decrease in activity, it can be hypothesized that the action of antidepressants on these receptors provides the link between their cellular actions and their clinical effects. Only further research on the mechanism of action of such drugs on the adaptational changes in other transmitter systems (e.g. the GABAergic system, which also appears to be impaired in depression) will enable any conclusions to be drawn regarding the precise mechanism(s) of action of antidepressants.

Modification of the amine modulation hypothesis of antidepressant action

Experimental studies show that changes occur in adrenoceptors, serotonin receptors, GABA-B receptors, dopamine autoreceptors and muscarinic receptors in the rat cerebral cortex after long-term administration of most types of antidepressants (see Table 6.4). Because of the disparate changes in amine receptors that occur, it is unlikely that there is a common mechanism of action of antidepressants. Nevertheless, it is possible that these drugs could modulate excitatory amino acid receptors. Such changes in excitatory amino acid receptors occur slowly and therefore account for the adaptation of the various types of neurotransmitter receptors that have been found to occur after long-term antidepressant treatment.

Several groups of investigators have independently shown that antagonists of N-methyl-D-aspartate (NMDA) receptors exhibit activity in animal models that is predictive of antidepressant activity in man; these drugs include both tricyclic and nontricyclic antidepressants. Such NMDA receptor antagonists also reduce the density of cortical beta adrenoceptors in a qualitatively similar manner to that found after TCA administration. It has also been shown that after TCA and electroconvulsive shock treatment (ECT) the ligand binding properties of both glycine and glutamate to the specific sites on the NMDA receptor-complex are altered.

It is of course possible that the mechanisms whereby antidepressants indirectly modulate NMDA receptors ultimately lead to the changes in aminergic neurotransmission that, for more than two decades, have formed the basis of the amine hypothesis of depression and the explanation of the mode of action of antidepressants. However, other structural and functional changes within the mammalian brain occur after antidepressant adminis-tration. While these changes have not received the same degree of attention as the changes in biogenic amines, they have been the subject of recent reviews. In brief, after long, but not short-term, administration of TCAs and such second generation antidepressants as fluoxetine, there is an increase in the phosphorylation of the neuronal microtubule assembly, which results in a change in the signal transduction process distal to the neurotransmitter receptors. Thus, antidepressants may cause changes in the cytoskeletal structure of the neuron. Other investigators have shown that, in cell culture, amitriptyline inhibits neurite outgrowth from chick embryonic cerebral explants, a finding that lends further support to the view that anti-depressants facilitate structural changes in nerve cells.

Electroconvulsive Shock Treatment

One of the pioneers in the application of electroconvulsive shock treatment (ECT) was the Italian clinician Cerletti who stated that the ". . . electricity itself is of little importance . . . the important and fundamental factor is the epileptic-like seizure no matter how it is obtained". ECT is undoubtedly an effective treatment for a range of psychiatric diseases varying from severe depression and mania to some forms of schizophrenia. Despite the considerable use of ECT over the last 50 years, it still arouses intense emotional and scientific debate. While the opposition to the use of ECT has been more evident in some Continental European countries and the United States than in Britain or Ireland, it was a British study of the use of ECT which, following a survey of over 100 centres, found that many units were badly equipped and had poor facilities and staff training. This report resulted in a considerable improvement in the application of ECT, with the establishment of guidelines governing the management and use of the technique; somewhat similar guidelines were instituted by the American Psychiatric Association.

It is now generally agreed that ECT is singularly effective and useful. There has been controversy over the relative merits in using unilateral or bilateral ECT. In general, it would appear that unilateral ECT is effective in the treatment of most depressed patients, whereas manic patients appear to respond best to bilateral ECT. Following a course of treatment, twice weekly for several weeks, the success rate in treating depression is about 80%. This is more successful than using antidepressants (up to 70% for a single course of treatment). Seizure monitoring is essential to ensure an adequate response. The principal side effect of ECT is a temporary cognitive deficit, specifically memory loss. There is evidence that such impairment is reduced if unilateral ECT is applied to the non-dominant hemisphere. Brief pulse-current ECT machines are now favoured in Britain and the United States to ensure optimal efficacy and minimal side effects. As Cerletti hypothesized in 1938, chemically induced seizures are equally effective as ECT and at one time pentamethylenetetrazole or flurothyl were used to produce seizures. However, the safety and ease of application of ECT means that such methods have been largely replaced.

How does ECT work?

While there are various psychological, neurophysiological and neuroendocrine theories that have been developed to explain the beneficial effects of ECT, most attention has been given to the manner in which ECT causes changes in those neurotransmitters that have been implicated in psychiatric illness. It is known that the rise in the seizure threshold during the course of treatment, and the corresponding alteration in cerebral blood flow, may reflect profound changes in cerebral metabolism that could be of crucial importance regarding the action of ECT. Changes in the hypothalamo–pituitary–adrenal axis have also been reported, but most studies suggest that such changes are secondary to the clinical response. The major emphasis of research has therefore been in the functional changes in brain neurotransmission, but it must be emphasized that most detailed studies have been conducted in rodents and therefore their precise relevance to changes in the human brain are a matter of conjecture.

Experimental studies in rodents have largely centred on the changes in biogenic amine neurotransmitters following chronic ECT treatments. Under these conditions, noradrenaline and 5-HT have been shown to be increased; the number of presynaptic alpha$_2$ receptors and their functional activity has been shown to be decreased, as has the functional activity of the dopamine autoreceptors. Such changes have also been found following the chronic administration of antidepressant drugs. The most consistent changes reported have been those found in postsynaptic receptor function. The functional activity of the postsynaptic beta adrenoceptors is decreased, a change which is also found with antidepressants. The postsynaptic 5-HT$_2$ receptor sensitivity is enhanced by chronic ECT and antidepressant treatment. Thus there appears to be a consistency between the chronic effects of both ECT and antidepressants in enhancing 5-HT responsiveness and diminishing that of noradrenaline. Regarding the dopaminergic system, while there is speculation that changes in the activity of this system may be important in the action of novel antidepressants such as bupropion, the only consistent changes found following chronic application of ECT and antidepressants is a functional decrease in the dopamine autoreceptor activity. This would lead to a reduction in the release of this transmitter.

In contrast to the plethora of animal studies, few clinical studies have shown consistent changes in the biogenic amines. There is evidence that the urinary and CSF concentrations of the noradrenaline metabolites normeta-nephrine and MHPG are decreased, suggesting that the turnover of noradrenaline is decreased, the opposite to that found in animals. Neuroendocrine challenge tests that have been used as probes to assess central noradrenergic function (e.g. with clonidine) show no consistent changes in patients following chronic ECT. Consistent changes have been reported in serotonergic function, however, with enhanced prolactin release occurring in response to a thyroid-stimulating hormone challenge. This is in agreement with the view that chronic ECT sensitizes postsynaptic 5-HT$_2$ receptors. Furthermore, platelet imipramine binding, which according to the results of some studies is increased in the untreated depressed patient, is attenuated by both antidepressant and ECT treatments, although it must be emphasized that not all investigators can replicate these findings. The transport of [^{3}H]5-HT into the platelets of depressed patients is also normalized following ECT and chronic antidepressant treatments. There is no evidence of any change in the dopaminergic system in depressed patients following ECT.

The central cholinergic system has been implicated in the pathogenesis of affective disorder and in memory function, which is frequently found to be malfunctioning in depressed patients. The memory deficit elicited by chronic ECT in both patients and animals may be related to the decreased density and function of central muscarinic receptors, but it should be emphasized that the changes reported in cholinergic function are small and their relevance to the clinical situation remains to be established.

Brain GABA is closely associated with the induction of seizures. In animals, chronic ECT decreases GABA synthesis in the limbic regions. While consistent changes in GABA-A receptor activity have not been reported, it would appear that GABA-B receptor density increases in the limbic regions following chronic ECT. This is qualitatively similar to the changes that have been reported following antidepressant treatment. The recent interest in the involvement of GABA in the aetiology of depression and in the mode of action of antidepressants is based on the hypothesis that GABA plays a key role not only in the induction of seizures but also in modulating the changes in the serotonergic system that are induced by both antidepressants and ECT.

Due to the ubiquitous distribution of peptides as cotransmitters and neuromodulators in the brain, it is not surprising to find that ECT produces changes in their concentrations and in their possible functional activity. Increased metenkephalin concentrations have been reported following chronic ECT. Such changes may be due to increased opioid receptor binding sites. Opioid-mediated behavioural changes such as catalepsy and reduced pain responses are increased following ECT in animals. Whether such changes are relevant to the effects of ECT and antidepressants in depressed patients is still unknown.

Other possibilities that have been suggested as a cause of the antidepressant action of ECT include an enhanced adenosine$_1$ receptor density in the cortex; agonists at these receptor sites are known to have anticonvulsant properties, while antagonists such as caffeine can cause convulsions, at least in high doses. Thyroid-stimulating hormone activity has also been shown to be enhanced. This peptide may exert antidepressant effects in its own right, but may also act by modulating both serotonergic and dopaminergic activity.

In SUMMARY, it would appear that ECT produces a number of changes in central neurotransmission that are common to antidepressants. These include a decrease in the functional activity of beta adrenoceptors and an enhanced activity of 5-HT$_2$ and possibly GABA-B receptors. The functional defect in central muscarinic receptors may be associated with the memory deficits caused by ECT treatment. It must be emphasized that the changes reported have largely been derived from animal experiments and their precise relevance to the mode of action of ECT in man is still a matter of conjecture.

Adverse effects of drug treatment for depression

TCAs

Significant side effects have been estimated to occur in about 5% of patients on TCAs, most of these effects being attributed to their antimuscarinic properties, for example, blurred vision, dry mouth, tachycardia and disturbed gastrointestinal and urinary tract function. Orthostatic hypotension due to the block of alpha$_1$ adrenoceptors and sedation resulting from antihistaminic activity frequently occur at therapeutic doses, particularly in the elderly. Excessive sweating is also a fairly common phenomenon, but its precise mechanism is uncertain. In the elderly patient, the precipitation of prostatic hypertrophy and glaucoma by the TCAs is also a frequent cause of concern.

Adverse effects of the TCAs on the brain include confusion, impaired memory and cognition and occasionally delirium; some of these effects have been reported to occur in up to 30% of patients over the age of 50. These effects may occasionally be confused with a recurrence of the symptoms of depression and are probably due to the central antimuscarinic activity of these drugs. Tremor also occurs frequently, particularly in the elderly, and may be controlled by the concurrent administration of propanolol. Neuroleptics are normally not recommended to be used in combination with TCAs as they are liable to accentuate the side effects of the latter drugs. The risk of seizures, and the switch from depression to mania in bipolar patients has also been reported following TCA administration.

Weight gain is a frequent side effect and is of considerable concern, particularly in the female patient, an effect probably associated with increased appetite. Other less common side effects include jaundice (particularly with imipramine), agranulocytosis and skin rashes.

Acute poisoning

This occurs all too frequently with the TCAs and can be life threatening. Death has been reported with doses of 2000 mg of imipramine, or the equivalent quantity of other TCAs, which approximates to 10 daily doses or less! Severe intoxication has been reported at doses of 1000 mg. Because of the toxicity of these drugs and the nature of the illness, in which suicidal thoughts are a common feature, it is generally recommended that no more than a 1 week's supply should be given at any one time to an acutely depressed patient.

The symptoms of overdose are to some extent predictable from the antimuscarinic and adrenolytic activity of these drugs. Excitement and restlessness, sometimes associated with seizures, and rapidly followed by coma, depressed respiration, hypoxia, hypotension and hypothermia are clear signs of TCA overdose. Tachycardia and arrhythmias lead to diminished cardiac function and thus to reduced cerebral perfusion, which exacerbates the central toxic effects. It is generally accepted that dialysis and forced diuresis are useless in counteracting the toxicity, but activated charcoal may reduce the absorption of any unabsorbed drug. The risk of cardiac arrhythmias may extend for several days after the patient has recovered from a TCA overdose.

It is partly due to the toxicity of the TCAs that the newer non-tricyclic drugs have been developed. All the evidence suggests that the non-tricyclics are much safer in overdose. Table 6.5 gives a survey of the relative toxicity of the older and newer antidepressants in overdose.

Drug interactions

Another area of concern regarding the use of the TCAs is their interaction with other drugs which may be given concurrently. Such interactions may

Table 6.5. Relative toxicity of antidepressants in overdose (UK data for period 1985–1990)

Drug	Deaths per million prescriptions
Tricyclics	
Amitriptyline	46.5
Dothiepin	50.0
Nortriptyline	39.2
Doxepin	31.3
Imipramine	28.4
Clomipramine	11.1
Maprotiline	37.6
Lofepramine	0.0*
Non-tricyclics	
Nomifensine	2.5
Trazodone	13.6
Mianserin	5.6
Viloxazine	9.4
Fluoxetine	0.0
Fluvoxamine	6.4
MAOIs	
Tranylcypromine	58.1
Phenelzine	22.8
Isocarboxazid	12.9

Mortality data obtained from Office of Population and Statistics of England and Wales and Registrar-General of Scotland. Data for single drug or single drug+alcohol.
*Since above data were reported, six cases of mortality following overdose have been identified in which lofepramine may be the causative agent.

arise due to the drugs competing for the plasma protein binding sites (e.g. phenytoin, aspirin and the phenothiazines) or for the liver microsomal enzyme system responsible for the common metabolism of the drugs (e.g. steroids, including the oral contraceptives, sedatives, apart from the benzodiazepines, and the neuroleptics). All of the TCAs potentiate the sedative effects of alcohol and any other psychotropic drug with sedative properties given concurrently. Smoking potentiates the metabolism of the TCAs. There is a well-established interaction between the TCAs and the adrenergic neuron blocking antihypertensives (e.g. bethanidine and guanethidine) which results from the TCA impeding the uptake of the neuron blocker into the sympathetic nerve terminal, thereby preventing it from exerting its pharmacological effects.

There is also a rare, but occasionally fatal, interaction between TCAs and MAOIs in which hyperpyrexia, convulsions and coma can occur. The precise mechanism by which this is brought about is unclear, but it may be associated with a sudden release of 5-HT.

Following prolonged TCA administration, abrupt withdrawal of the drug can lead to generalized somatic or gastrointestinal distress, which may be associated with anxiety, agitation, sleep disturbance, movement disorders and even mania. Such symptoms may be associated with central and peripheral cholinergic hyperactivity that is a consequence of the prolonged muscarinic receptor blockade caused by the TCAs.

MAOIs

The toxic effects of these drugs may arise shortly after an overdose, the effects including agitation, hallucinations, hyperreflexia and convulsions. Somewhat surprisingly, both hypo- and hypertension may occur, the former symptoms arising due to the accumulation of the inhibitory transmitter dopamine in the sympathetic ganglia leading to a marked reduction in ganglionic transmission, while hypertension can result from a dramatic release of noradrenaline from both central and peripheral sources. Such toxic effects are liable to be prolonged, particularly when the older irreversible inhibitors such as phenelzine and tranylcypromine are used. Treatment of such adverse effects should be aimed at controlling the temperature, respiration and blood pressure.

The toxic effects of the MAOIs are more varied and potentially more serious than those of the other classes of antidepressants in common use. Hepatotoxicity has been reported to occur with the older hydrazine type of MAOIs and led to the early demise of iproniazid; the hepatotoxicity does not appear to be related to the dose or duration of the drug administered.

Excessive central stimulation, usually exhibited as tremors, insomnia and hyperhidrosis, can occur following therapeutic doses of the MAOIs, as can agitation and hypomanic episodes. Peripheral neuropathy, which is largely restricted to the hydrazine type of MAOI, is rare and has been attributed to a drug-induced pyridoxine deficiency. Such side effects as dizziness and vertigo (presumably associated with hypotension), headache, inhibition of ejaculation (which is often also a problem with the TCAs), fatigue, dry mouth and constipation have also been reported. These side effects appear to be more frequently associated with phenelzine use. They are not associated with any antimuscarinic properties of the drug but presumably arise from the enhanced peripheral sympathetic activity which the MAOIs cause.

Drug interactions

Predictable interactions occur between the MAOIs and any amine precursors, or directly or indirectly acting sympathomimetic amines (e.g. the amphetamines, phenylephrine and tyramine). Such interactions can cause pronounced hypertension and, in extreme cases, stroke.

MAOIs interfere with the metabolism of many different classes of drugs that may be given concurrently. They potentiate the actions of general anaesthetics, sedatives, including alcohol, antihistamines, centrally acting analgesics (particularly pethidine due to an enhanced release of 5-HT) and anticholinergic drugs. They also potentiate the actions of TCAs, which may provide an explanation for the use of such a combination in the treatment of therapy-resistant depression.

The *"cheese effect"* is a well-established phenomenon whereby an amine-rich food is consumed while the patient is being treated with an irreversible MAOI. Foods which cause such an effect include cheeses, pickled fish, yeast products (red wines and beers, including non-alcoholic varieties), chocolate and pulses such as broad beans (which contain dopa). It appears that foods containing more than 10 mg of tyramine must be consumed in order to produce a significant rise in blood pressure. Furthermore, it is now apparent that there is considerable variation in the tyramine content of many of these foods even when they are produced by the same manufacturer. Therefore it is essential that all patients on MAOIs should be provided with a list of foods and drinks that should be avoided.

Changing a patient from one MAOI to another, or to a TCA, requires a "wash-out" period of at least 2 weeks to avoid the possibility of a drug interaction. There is evidence to suggest that a combination of an MAOI with clomipramine is more likely to produce serious adverse effects than occurs with other TCAs. Regarding the newer non-tricyclic antidepressants, it is recommended that a "wash-out" period of at least 5 weeks be given before a patient on fluoxetine is given an MAOI; this is due to the very long half-life of the main fluoxetine metabolite norfluoxetine.

Although it is widely acknowledged that the older MAOIs have the potential to produce serious adverse effects, the actual reported incidence is surprisingly low. Tranylcypromine was one of the most widely used drugs, involving several million patients by the mid 1970s, and yet only 50 patients were reported to have severe cerebrovascular accidents and, of these, only 15 deaths occurred. Nevertheless, it is generally recommended that this drug should not be given to elderly patients or to other patients with hypertension or cardiovascular disease.

The newer non-tricyclic antidepressants

With the possible exception of maprotiline, which is chemically a modified TCA with all the side effects attributable to such a molecule, all of the newer non-tricyclic drugs have fewer anticholinergic effects and are a less cardiotoxic than the older tricyclics. *Lofepramine* is an example of a modified tricyclic that, due to the absence of a free NH_2 group in the side chain, is relatively devoid of anticholinergic side effects. Thus by slightly modifying the structure of the side chain it is possible to retain the efficacy while reducing the cardiotoxicity.

Of the plethora of new 5-HT *uptake inhibitor antidepressants* (e.g. zimelidine, indalpine, fluoxetine, fluvoxamine, citalopram, sertraline and paroxetine), the most frequently mentioned side effects following therapeutic administration are mild gastrointestinal discomfort, which rarely leads to nausea and vomiting, occasional diarrhoea and headache. Such changes may be attributable to increased peripheral serotonergic function. Some severe idiosyncratic and hypersensitivity reactions such as the Gullain–Barré syndrome and blood dyscrasias have led to the early withdrawal of zimelidine and indalpine. For the well-established antidepressants such as fluoxetine, the side effects appear to be mild and infrequent, although akathisia and agitation have been reported and may be more pronounced in elderly patients.

Nomifensine, viloxazine, bupropion and oxaprotiline are examples of non-tricyclic antidepressants that facilitate *catecholaminergic function*. These drugs have the advantage over the TCAs of being non-sedative in therapeutic doses. The rare, although fatal, occurrence of haemolytic anaemia and pyrexia following therapeutic administration of nomifensine led to its withdrawal from the market a few years ago. Bupropion was also temporarily withdrawn from clinical use following evidence of seizure induction, but it has now returned to the market in the United States; viloxazine has also been reported to precipitate seizures and cause nausea in some patients at therapeutic doses. Idiosyncratic reactions have been reported to occur with the tetracyclic antidepressant *mianserin*, several cases of agranulocytosis have been reported in different countries. Elderly patients would appear to be most at risk from such adverse effects. Whether such side effects are a peculiarity of the mianserin structure or will also be found with the 6-aza derivative, mirtazepine, is unknown. Other frequent side effects associated with therapeutic doses of mianserin are sedation and orthostatic hypotension.

Clearly the major advantage of all the recently introduced antidepressants lies in their relative safety in overdosage and reduced side effects. These factors are particularly important when considering the need for optimal patient compliance and in the treatment of the elderly depressed patient who is more likely to experience severe side effects from antidepressants.

Treatment-resistant depression

It has been estimated that at least 30% of patients with major depression fail to respond to a 6-week course of TCA medication. Besides ECT, various strategies have been adopted to treat such non-responsive patients. These include a combination of a TCA with an MAOI or with lithium. Other approaches have involved combining lithium with an MAOI or with a combination of tryptophan and the 5-HT uptake inhibitor clomipramine. It must be emphasized that such drug combinations are not without risk or serious side effects! Nevertheless, it would appear that the effect of such combinations is to facilitate central serotonergic transmission, which suggests that the failure of a patient to respond to the usual course of antidepressant treatment may be related to a primary deficit in this particular system. A major problem for the investigator studying the biochemical and pharmacological aspects of therapy resistance, however, is the lack of an internationally recognized definition of resistant depression. Clearly such factors as patient compliance and the dose and duration of antidepressant used are key aspects that must be considered before treatment resistance can be established. There is also evidence that subgroups of patients with delusional depression, rapid-cycling affective disorders and post-stroke depression are more resistant to standard therapy and are therefore more likely to be termed therapy resistant.

In addition to those strategies already mentioned, there has been good clinical evidence to suggest that a combination of lithium with clomipramine or an SSRI (such as fluoxetine) is often successful. More recently, the discovery that pindolol can enhance serotonin release under experimental conditions has led to clinical studies in which pindolol in combination with an SSRI can not only treat resistant depression in some cases but also produce a more rapid therapeutic effect than the SSRI alone. There is some evidence that buspirone, the 5-HT$_{1A}$ partial agonist, in combination with an SSRI, may be useful in the treatment of resistant depression.

In CONCLUSION it appears that the chemically and pharmacologically diverse drugs that act as antidepressants have two properties in common. Firstly, they demonstrate approximately equal clinical efficacy and require several weeks' administration to produce an optimal therapeutic effect. Secondly, they all modulate a number of different types of mainly postsynaptic neurotransmitter receptors in animals and in depressed patients. Such effects occur irrespective of their specific effects on a particular neurotransmitter system that may arise after their short-term administration. Thus, the amine hypothesis of depression, in which it was postulated that depression arises from a deficiency in one or more of the biogenic amine neurotransmitters, which is corrected following effective antidepressant treatment, has now evolved into the "receptor sensitivity hypothesis". This hypothesis explains the delay in the therapeutic effects of antidepressant treatments as being due to time dependent adaptational changes in neurotransmitter receptors. Thus, depression may be related to an underlying abnormality in neurotransmitter receptor function. Whether this is sufficient to cause the abnormal affect state is still a matter of debate. It is possible, for example, that the changes in receptor function that ultimately produce the behavioural changes associated with depression are a consequence of changes in central glucocorticoid receptor activity that reflect the response of the patient to prolonged hypercortisolaemia.

Clearly, more research is needed to elucidate the precise mechanisms of action of antidepressants and the psychopathology of the condition. Only then may it be possible to develop antidepressants that show a clear therapeutic superiority over those available today.

7 Drug Treatment of Mania

Introduction

The term "bipolar disorder" originally referred to manic-depressive illnesses characterized by both manic and depressive episodes. In recent years, the concept of bipolar disorder has been broadened to include subtypes with similar clinical courses, phenomenology, family histories and treatment responses. These subtypes are thought to form a continuum of disorders that, while differing in severity, are related. Readers are referred to the *Diagnostic and Statisticial Manual of Mental Disorders* of the American Psychiatric Association (DSM–IV) for details of this classification.

The diagnosis of mania is made on the basis of clinical history. Key features of mania include elevated, expansive or irritable mood accompanied by hyperactivity, pressure of speech, flight of ideas, grandiosity, hyposomnia and distractibility. Such episodes may alternate with severe depression, hence the term "bipolar illness", which is clinically similar to that seen in patients with "unipolar depression". In such cases, the mood can range from sadness to profound melancholia with feelings of guilt, anxiety, apprehension and suicidal ideation accompanied by anhedonia (lack of interest in work, food, sex, etc.).

Mania, manic-depression and depression, which comprise the affective disorders, are relatively common; it has been estimated that there is an incidence of at least 2% in most societies throughout the world. There is good evidence to suggest that *genetic factors* play a considerable role in predisposing a patient to an affective disorder. In a seminal Danish twin register study, in which the incidence of affective disorders was determined in all twins of the same sex born in Denmark between 1870 and 1920, a total of 110 pairs of twins were identified in which one or both had manic-depression. The concordance rates, that is the rate of coexistence of the disorder in twin pairs, for all types of affective disorder were found to be 67% for the mono- and 20% for the dizygotic twins. Further analysis showed that the discrepancy in concordance rates for manic-depression was even greater between the mono- and the dizygotic pairs, being 79% for the former and 54% for the latter. There was no difference in the concordance rate for bipolar and unipolar affective disorders in the dizygotic twins, the values being 24% and 19%, respectively. Such findings strongly suggest that affective disorders are inherited. Nevertheless, despite the apparent differences in the genetic loading for monopolar and bipolar affective illness, there is increasing evidence that both types of illness can be associated with the same genetic make-up. Thus a substantial portion of unipolar patients have the same genetic and biological vulnerability as bipolar patients. What causes some patients to display mania or hypomania whereas others do not is unknown.

More recently attempts have been made to define the mode of genetic transmission of affective disorders. A study of single autosomal locus markers in such patients has concluded that there is a lack of evidence to indicate single locus transmission, and that a polygenic model is more consistent with the available data. Linkage markers (e.g. the link between the X chromosome and colour blindness), autosomal markers such as those associated with human leucocyte antigen (HLA), and restriction fragment length polymorphism (RFLP) have also been studied in populations of patients with affective disorders. There was much excitement generated by the discovery that the RFLP analysis of the manic patients in the unique Amish population in Pennsylvania showed a link between the disorder and the insulin-*ras*-1 oncogene on chromosome 11. Unfortunately, a more detailed analysis of the data has failed to confirm these initial findings. At present it must be concluded that, while the heritability of manic-depression is evident from clinical studies, the mode of transmission and the identity of the transmitted defect have not been demonstrated. Nevertheless, with the spectacular developments in molecular genetics now taking place, one may expect considerable advances in the identification of the locus of inheritance to be made in the coming decade.

Biochemical changes associated with mania

The various hypotheses that have been advanced regarding the biochemical cause of mania mainly centre on the idea that it is due to a relative excess of noradrenaline, and possibly dopamine, with deficits also arising in the availability of 5-hydroxytryptamine (5-HT) and acetylcholine. This simplistic view forms the basis of the *amine theory of affective disorders* which, in summary, states that depression arises as a consequence of biogenic amine deficit, while mania is due to an excess of these amines in central synapses. In mania, evidence in support of this hypothesis comes from the limited studies that have been undertaken on patients before and after effective treatment. An alternative approach has been to study drugs such as lithium that have been used to treat the condition.

Most studies of the changes in the urine concentration of the main central metabolite of noradrenaline, 3-methoxy-4-hydroxyphenylglycol (MHPG), have shown abnormalities in manic patients. However, there is a discrepancy in the literature regarding the duration and extent of the change. Urinary noradrenaline concentrations have, however, been found to be increased during the active phase of the illness and to return to normal following effective treatment; the increase is said to reflect a rise in the concentration of MHPG in the cerebrospinal fluid (CSF). The concentration of the main dopamine metabolite, homovanillic acid (HVA), is also reported to rise in mania, but whether such changes are causally related to the core symptoms of the illness is debatable as it would be anticipated that an increase in the sympathetic drive would be necessarily associated with the illness.

While there have been a number of studies of changes in the sympathetic system in mania, few studies have attempted to assess changes in the serotonergic system. Hypomania has been reported to occur in depressed patients being treated with 5-hydroxytryptophan, the precursor amino acid of 5-HT, in combination with the peripheral decarboxylase inhibitor carbidopa. Mania has also been reported to occur in depressed patients following treatment with tryptophan in combination with clomipramine, a 5-HT uptake inhibitor. Nevertheless, there are no reports of a 5-HT agonist exacerbating the symptoms of mania in patients who are hypomanic! This suggests that a serotonergic stimulus may trigger a manic episode but alone is not a sufficient cause. Regarding the changes in serotonergic function in mania, only one study to date has investigated $[^3H]$5-HT transport into the platelets of patients before and after effective treatment. Unlike depression, where the $[^3H]$5-HT uptake is reduced, in mania the uptake is enhanced before treatment and normalized on recovery.

Regarding the dopaminergic system, there is experimental evidence to show that dopaminomimetic agents such as amphetamine, piribedil, bromocriptine and L-dopa can initiate mania in predisposed patients during remission. Indeed, the behavioural excitation and hypomania following D-amphetamine withdrawal has been proposed as a model of mania. Other evidence implicating a change in the dopaminergic system has been derived from the efficacy of neuroleptics (dopamine antagonists), which effectively attenuate the symptoms of the illness.

Unlike the biogenic amines, the cholinergic system has received relatively little attention as a possible factor in mania. Experimental evidence shows that cholinomimetic drugs and anticholinesterases have antimanic properties, although their effects appear to be short-lived. Furthermore, their effects appear to be associated with a reduction in the affective core symptoms and locomotor components of the illness, but not in the grandiose thinking and expansiveness.

Which, if any, of these different types of neurotransmitters is causally involved in the illness is still a matter for conjecture.

Pharmacological treatment of mania

Lithium salts

Of the various types of psychotropic drugs which have been used to treat mania, lithium salts are universally acclaimed to be the most important and effective treatment of mania and manic-depression.

It can be argued that the introduction of lithium salts into the practice of psychiatry in 1949 heralded the beginning of psychopharmacology, as it predated the discovery of chlorpromazine, imipramine, monoamine oxidase inhibitors and resperine. Lithium came into clinical use serendipitously, the Australian psychiatrist Cade having by chance given it to a small group of manic patients and found that it had beneficial effects, whereas it appeared to lack activity when given to schizophrenics and depressives. However, lithium salts did not come into regular use in most industrialized countries until the early 1970s, partly because of the toxicity of the drug and partly because of the lack of commercial interest in a drug that could be dug out of the soil!

Lithium salts, generally in the form of the carbonate or bicarbonate, are rapidly absorbed from the gastrointestinal tract and reach a peak plasma concentration after 2–4 hours. Extreme fluctuations in blood lithium levels, which are associated with side effects such as nausea, diarrhoea and abdominal cramp, are reduced by using sustained release preparations. Lithium is not protein bound and therefore is widely distributed throughout the body water, which accounts for the adverse effects it has on most organ systems should it reach toxic levels. To avoid toxicity, and ensure optimal efficacy, it is essential to monitor the plasma levels at regular intervals to ensure that they lie between 0.6 and 1.2 mEq/litre; there is evidence that lower levels (0.4–0.6 mEq/litre) may be sufficient when lithium salts are used to prevent relapse in the case of patients with unipolar depression.

As lithium is an alkaline earth metal which readily exchanges with sodium and potassium, it is actively transported across cell membranes. The penetration of kidney cells is particularly rapid, while that of bone, liver and brain tissue is much slower. The plasma:CSF ratio in man has been calculated to be between 2:1 and 3:1, which is similar to that found for the plasma:red blood cell (RBC) ratio. This suggests that the plasma:RBC ratio might be a useful index of the brain concentration and may be predictive of the onset of side effects, as these appear to correlate well with the intracellular concentration of the drug.

Most of the lithium is eliminated in the urine, the first phase of the elimination being 6–8 hours after administration, followed by a slower phase which may last for 2 weeks. Sodium-depleting diuretics such as frusemide, ethacrynic acid and the thiazides increase lithium retention and therefore

Table 7.1. Main side effects of lithium

Gastrointestinal tract
Anorexia
Nausea
Vomiting
Diarrhoea
Thirst
Incontinence

Neuromuscular changes
General muscle weakness
Ataxia
Tremor
Fasciculation and twitching
Choreoathetoid movements
Hyperactive tendon reflexes*

Central nervous system
Slurred speech*
Blurring of vision
Dizziness
Vertigo
Epileptiform seizures
Somnolence
Confusion*
Restlessness*
Stupor*
Coma*

Cardiovascular system
Hypotension
Pulse irregularities
ECG changes
Circulatory collapse

Other effects
Polyuria
Glycosuria
General fatigue* and lethargy*
Dehydration

*Side effects usually associated with the toxic effects of lithium.

toxicity, while osmotic diuretics as exemplified by mannitol and urea enhance lithium excretion. The principal side effects of lithium are summarized in Table 7.1.

The *mode of action* of lithium is still the subject of debate! Because of its similarity to sodium it was initially believed that it acted by competing with sodium in the brain and other tissues. However, it is now known that lithium interacts equally well with potassium, calcium and magnesium ions, all of which are widely distributed and essential for the functioning of most biological processes. It seems likely that lithium displaces sodium and potassium from their intracellular compartments and thereby substitutes for them; calcium magnesium and phosphate concentrations are also altered. These effects of lithium on the electrolyte balance were once considered to be related to an action of the drug on sodium/potassium dependent adenosine triphosphatase ($Na^+K^+-ATPase$), an enzyme primarily involved in the repolarization of excitable membranes. Lithium appears to compete with a common binding site on the carrier, the site having a greater affinity for the lithium than the sodium ion. This could account for the ability of the drug to slow the speed of repolarization of nervous tissue. Other effects on brain function may be associated with an increase in the permeability of the blood–brain barrier resulting from an interaction of lithium with membrane phospholipids. The increased concentration of amino acids in the CSF may be a reflection of this.

It has long been apparent that the uptake, storage, release and metabolism (i.e. the turnover) of biogenic amines can be affected by both mono- and divalent cations. The effect on dopamine receptor sensitivity may be a particularly important action of lithium. It has been speculated that dopamine receptor hypersensitivity is closely associated with the onset of mania. Both acutely and chronically administered lithium can reduce the supersensitivity of both pre- and postsynaptic dopamine receptors, an effect which may help to explain its mood-stabilizing action but not its somewhat controversial ability to initiate tardive dyskinesia. Regarding the effects of lithium on noradrenergic function, it has long been known that it increases the reuptake of noradrenaline into neurons, increases the turnover of this amine in the brain without markedly affecting its turnover in the periphery, decreases its release and enhances its metabolism. The net effect of lithium is therefore to lead to a reduction in noradrenergic function which presumably is reflected in its antimanic properties.

At the postsynaptic level, lithium has been shown to reduce the function of beta adrenoceptors, presumably by affecting the coupling between the receptor and the secondary messenger system. This effect only becomes apparent following chronic treatment, which may help to explain the delay of several days, or even weeks, before an optimal beneficial effect is observed. All antidepressants are known to reduce the functional activity of postsynaptic beta receptors, which may explain why lithium has both an antimanic and an antidepressant effect in patients with manic-depression.

Relationship between the mode of action of lithium and its side effects

Many of the adverse effects of lithium can be ascribed to the action of lithium on adenylate cyclase, the key enzyme that links many hormones and neurotransmitters with their intracellular actions. Thus antidiuretic hormone and thyroid-stimulating-hormone-sensitive adenylate cyclases are inhibited by therapeutic concentrations of the drug, which frequently leads to enhanced diuresis, hypothyroidism and even goitre. Aldosterone synthesis is increased following chronic lithium treatment and is probably a secondary consequence of the enhanced diuresis caused by the inhibition of antidiuretic-hormone-sensitive adenylate cyclase in the kidney. There is also evidence that chronic lithium treatment causes an increase in serum parathyroid hormone levels and, with this, a rise in calcium and magnesium concentrations. A decrease in plasma phosphate and in bone mineralization can also be attributed to the effects of the drug on parathyroid activity. Whether these changes are of any clinical consequence is unclear.

Prolactin secretion, at least in experimental animals, is increased following chronic lithium treatment, probably as a consequence of the enhanced sensitivity of postsynaptic 5-HT receptors and the decreased sensitivity of dopamine receptors. In patients on therapeutic doses of the drug, however, the plasma prolactin levels would not appear to be markedly altered. There is little evidence that circulating gonadotrophin concentrations are affected by therapeutic doses of lithium.

One major side effect of lithium that causes great concern to patients is weight gain; this has been estimated to occur in up to 60% of patients according to some investigators. In addition to increased food intake, lithium also has an effect on the intermediary metabolism of carbohydrates. During the acute phase of lithium administration, insulin release is decreased leading to a raised plasma glucose; the insulin concentration then rises and increased fat synthesis could then occur. This appears to be due to an inhibition of several enzymes at the beginning of the glycolytic pathway, which could lead to enhanced lipid synthesis.

Recently research has focused on the action of lithium on serotonergic function. Lithium has been shown to facilitate the uptake and synthesis of 5-HT, to enhance its release and to increase the transport of tryptophan into the nerve terminal, an effect which probably contributes to the increased 5-HT synthesis. The net effect of these changes is to produce postsynaptic receptor events, which might explain why lithium, in combination with tryptophan and a monoamine oxidase inhibitor or a 5-HT uptake inhibitor, is often effective in therapy-resistant depression.

Drugs which enhance the activity of the central cholinergic system have been shown to have antimanic effects. Experimental studies have shown that lithium increases acetylcholine synthesis in the cortex, which is probably associated with an increase in the high affinity transport of choline into the neuron; the release of this transmitter is also increased. Whether these effects on the cholinergic system are relevant to its therapeutic action in manic patients remains to be proven.

So far attention has concentrated on the effects of lithium on excitatory transmitters. There is evidence that the drug can also facilitate inhibitory transmission, an effect that has been attributed to a desensitization of the presynaptic gamma-aminobutyric acid (GABA) receptors, which results in an increase in the release of this inhibitory transmitter. The increased conversion of glutamate to GABA may also contribute to this process. Thus it would appear that lithium has a varied and complex action on central neurotransmission, the net result being a diminution in the activity of excitatory transmitters and an increase in GABAergic function.

When receptors are directly linked to ion channels, fast excitatory or inhibitory postsynaptic potentials occur. However, it is well established that slow potential changes also occur and that such changes are due to the receptor being linked to the ion channel indirectly via a secondary messenger system. For example, the stimulation of beta adrenoceptors by noradrenaline results in the activation of adenylate cyclase. The antimanic and antidepressant effects of lithium are linked to a reduction in the functional activity of postsynaptic beta adrenoceptor-linked cyclase, combined with a reduction in the activity of the presynaptic noradrenergic neuron. The adverse effects of the drug on renal and thyroid function are due to the inhibition of the hormone-linked cyclases in these organs. Undoubtedly, transmitter receptor changes (e.g. serotonergic, noradrenergic, dopaminergic and GABAergic) play a major role in the therapeutic effects of lithium. Such changes may be related to the ability of the drug to re-synchronize disrupted circadian rhythms, which appear to be an essential feature of the affective disorders.

Other drug treatments for mania

The long-term toxic effects of lithium, such as nephrogenic diabetes insipidus, which has been calculated to occur in up to 5% of patients, and the rare possibility of lithium combined with neuroleptics being neurotoxic, has stimulated the research for other drug treatments. However, apart from the neuroleptics, these drugs have not been studied as extensively in the treatment of acute mania, but are worthy of consideration because of their reduced side effects.

Neuroleptics

Most psychotic and non-compliant patients are difficult to treat with lithium alone and need to be treated with neuroleptics. Haloperidol has been widely used alone to control the more florid symptoms of mania, but doubts have arisen concerning its toxic interactions with lithium. Such considerations are based on a report that such a combination caused neurotoxicity in a small group of manic patients, but it should be emphasized that a variety of other neuroleptics have also been rarely found to cause these effects. The symptoms of neurotoxicity include ataxia, confusion, hyperactive reflexes, chorea, slurred speech and even coma. It seems likely that some of these patients suffered from the malignant neuroleptic syndrome rather than enhanced lithium toxicity, but problems such as dehydration and over-sedation may have enhanced the drug interaction.

Tardive dyskinesia can occur in manic patients on neuroleptics alone, the frequency may be greater than in schizophrenics who are more likely to be on continuous medication. One possible explanation for this lies in the fact that neuroleptics are often administered to manic patients for short periods only, sufficient to abort the active episode, and then abruptly stopped. Thus high doses of neuroleptics are separated by drug-free periods, leading to a situation most likely to precipitate tardive dyskinesia. The recent increase in prescribing high potency neuroleptics such as haloperidol instead of low potency drugs such as chlorpromazine or thioridazine has undoubtedly increased the frequency of tardive dyskinesia.

Carbamazepine

This is a tricyclic compound somewhat similar to imipramine that is an anticonvulsant widely used in the treatment of temporal lobe epilepsy. Following its widespread use as an antiepileptic, it soon became evident that it had psychotropic effects. These included an improvement in mood, reduced aggressiveness and improved cognitive function. *Kindling* refers to the development of seizures after repeated delivery of a series to subthreshold stimuli to any region of the brain. This phenomenon can most readily be induced in limbic structures and, whereas conventional anticonvulsants such as phenytoin and phenobarbitone have little effect in attenuating kindled seizures, carbamazepine and the benzodiazepine anticonvulsants prevent such seizure development. It is now well established that carbamazepine is relatively selective in attenuating seizure activity in the hippocampus and amygdala, which suggests that it acts preferentially at limbic sites in the brain.

The mechanism of action of carbamazepine is complex, and is complicated by the fact that is has a long half-life metabolite, carbamazepine epoxide, which also has pronounced psychotropic properties.

The anticonvulsant properties of the drug would appear to be due to its ability to inhibit fast sodium channels, which may be unrelated to its psychotropic effects. Like lithium, it has been shown to decrease the release of noradrenaline and reduce noradrenaline-induced adenylate cyclase activity; unlike lithium, it seems to have little effect on tryptophan or 5-HT levels in patients at therapeutically relevant concentrations. It also reduces dopamine turnover in manic patients and increases acetylcholine synthesis in the cortex, an effect also seen with lithium. The effect of carbamazepine on GABAergic function appears to be related to its interaction with GABA-B type receptors, which may be relevant to its usefulness in the treatment of trigeminal neuralgia. There is no evidence that it changes GABA levels in the CSF of patients. Furthermore, while it would appear that the drug has no effect on central benzodiazepine receptors, there is evidence that it has a high affinity for the peripheral type of benzodiazepine receptor. These receptors are found in the mammalian brain but differ from the central receptors in that they are not linked to GABA receptors and therefore do not affect chloride ion flux. The main function of the peripheral type of benzodiazepine receptor would seem to be to control calcium channels. This may help to explain some of the psychotropic effects of carbamazepine, particularly as calcium channel antagonists such as *verapamil* have antimanic effects.

Changes in the activity of adenosine receptors have been implicated in the stimulant effects of drugs like caffeine. Carbamazepine exhibits mixed agonist–antagonist effects on adenosine receptors, and experimental evidence suggests that the reduced reuptake and release of noradrenaline caused by the drug are due to its interaction with these receptors. The precise relevance of these findings to its anticonvulsant and psychotropic effects is presently unclear.

Of the various peptides (e.g. the opioids, vasopressin, substance P and somatostatin) thought to be involved in the actions of carbamazepine, there is evidence that the reduction in the CSF concentration of somatostatin might be important in explaining its effects on cognition and also on the hypothalamo–pituitary–adrenal axis; somatostatin is a major inhibitory modulator of this axis and hypercortisolism frequently occurs in patients following carbamazepine administration.

There is still controversy regarding the general usefulness of carbamazepine as an alternative to lithium. It is apparent that the nature of the illness alters throughout the lifetime of the patient, so that pharmacological interventions may differ according to the stage of the illness. Preliminary clinical studies suggest that lithium may be particularly beneficial during the early and intermediate stages of the illness, whereas carbamazepine and related anticonvulsants may be more useful, either alone or in combination with lithium, at later stages, particularly, when the patient shows rapid, continuous cycling between mania and depression.

Other drugs

Other drugs that are reported to have beneficial effects but which have not undergone such extensive evaluation as the neuroleptics or carbamazepine include the *calcium channel antagonists* such as verapamil. A small open study has suggested that the alpha$_2$ adrenoceptor agonist *clonidine* may have some activity. More substantial studies have been conducted on the benzodiaze-pines *lorazepam* and *clonazepam*, and the anticonvulsant *sodium valproate*. All these drugs facilitate GABAergic function in some way, the first two by acting as agonists at benzodiazepine receptor sites and the latter by desensitizing the GABA autoreceptor and thereby enhancing the release of this inhibitory transmitter. Lastly, electroconvulsive shock treatment (ECT) has been claimed to be effective in attenuating the symptoms of an acute manic attack, but there is evidence that patients treated with ECT should not receive lithium concomitantly to reduce the possibility of neurotoxic side effects.

In CONCLUSION, lithium is universally accepted as a mood-stabilizing drug and an effective antimanic agent whose value is limited by its poor therapeutic index (i.e. its therapeutic to toxicity ratio). Neuroleptics are effective in attenuating the symptoms of acute mania but they too have serious adverse side effects. High potency neuroleptics appear to increase the likelihood of tardive dyskinesia. Of the less well-established treatments, carbamazepine would appear to have a role, particularly in the more advanced stages of the illness when lithium is less effective.

8 Anxiolytics and the Treatment of Anxiety Disorders

Introduction

Until the late 1960s, the symptoms of anxiety and insomnia were mainly treated with barbiturates. The barbiturates are known to cause dependence, and severe withdrawal effects were sometimes reported following the abrupt termination of their administration. Furthermore, their efficacy in the treatment of anxiety disorders was limited. The discovery of the benzodiazepine anxiolytic chlordiazepoxide some 30 years ago, and the subsequent development of numerous analogues with an essentially similar pharmacological profile, rapidly led to the replacement of the barbiturates with a group of drugs that have been widely used for the treatment of anxiety disorders, insomnia, muscle spasm and epilepsy and as a preoperative medication. The benzodiazepines have also been shown to have fewer side effects than the barbiturates, to be relatively safe in overdose and to be less liable to produce dependence than the barbiturates. They have now become the most widely used of all psychotropic drugs; during the last 25 years it has been estimated that over 500 million people worldwide have taken a course of benzodiazepine treatment.

In recent years there has been growing concern among members of the public and the medical profession regarding the problem of dependence and possible abuse of the benzodiazepines, and the recent decrease in the number of prescriptions of these drugs for the treatment of anxiety reflects this concern. And yet, despite the decline in the short-term use of benzodiazepine drugs to treat anxiety, their use as hypnotic sedatives is largely unchanged. Furthermore, their long-term use for the treatment of anxiety and/or insomnia continues. Thus in the UK approximately 1.5% of the adult population have taken benzodiazepines continuously for 1 year or more, while nearly half of these have taken the drugs for at least 7 years. It has been variously estimated that approximately 0.25 million people have taken benzodiazepines continuously for several years in the UK. The benzodiazepines commonly available are shown in Table 8.1.

The pharmacological properties of all these drugs are essentially similar, despite the fact that they may be prescribed for the treatment of anxiety or for insomnia. There is little objective evidence to suggest that the drugs listed

Table 8.1. Benzodiazepines on the "selected list" for the NHS

	Half-life (range in hours)	Accumulation
Drugs used for anxiety		
Chlordiazepoxide*	20–90	+++
Diazepam*	20–90	+++
Oxazepam	6–28	+
Lorazepam	8–24	±
Alprazolam	6–16	+
Drugs used for insomnia		
Nitrazepam	16–40	+++
Temazepam	6–10	+
Lormetazepam	8–12	+
Loprazolam	6–12	+
Triazolam	4–10	–

*Includes active metabolites.
+++=marked accumulation; +=some accumulation; ±=?some accumulation; –=no accumulation.

are more specific for the treatment of anxiety or of insomnia; an anxiolytic benzodiazepine given at night is likely to be an effective hypnotic, while a low dose of a hypnotic benzodiazepine given in the morning may be an effective anxiolytic. The reason for the similarity in the pharmacological profile of these drugs lies in the similarity of their mechanism of action and also in their metabolite inter-relationship (see Figure 8.1).

In essence, all of the older benzodiazepines that are structurally related to chlordiazepoxide and diazepam are termed 1,4-benzodiazepines. The chemical structure of some commonly used benzodiazepines is shown in Figure 8.2. They enhance the actions of the inhibitory neurotransmitter gamma-aminobutyric acid (GABA) in the brain. As a consequence, they affect the activities of the cerebellum (concerned with the balance and coordination), the limbic areas of the brain and the cerebral cortex (thought and decision making, fine movement control).

The half life of a benzodiazepine is not predictive either of its onset of action or of the therapeutic response of the patient. However, the rate of absorption and distribution within the body are important parameters in determining the pharmacodynamic response. The period for maximal response to treatment may be as long as 6 weeks, and there is no evidence that prolongation of the treatment, or increasing the dose of the drug, will lead to additional improvement in the response.

Chemical pathogenesis of anxiety

Although different authors have ascribed different meanings to the term "anxiety", and have often used the terms "fear" and "anxiety"

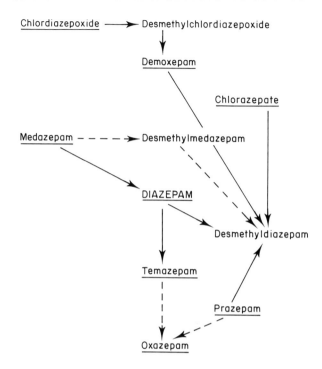

Figure 8.1. The metabolic pathways for the principal 1,4-benzodiazepines. The major pathway is shown with solid arrows and the minor pathway with broken arrows. Commercially available drugs are underlined.

interchangeably, it is generally accepted that anxiety is an unpleasant state accompanied by apprehension, worry, fear, nervousness and sometimes conflict. Arousal is usually heightened. An increase in the autonomic sympathetic nervous system is often associated with these psychological changes and may be manifest as an increase in blood pressure and heart rate, an erratic respiratory rate, decreased salivary flow leading to dryness in the mouth and throat, and gastrointestinal disturbances. Whilst "physiological" anxiety is usually short-lived, often with a rapid onset and abrupt cessation once the aversive event has terminated, "pathological" anxiety occurs when the response of the individual to an anxiety-provoking event becomes excessive and affects the ability of the individual to lead a normal life. It has been estimated that 2–4% of the population suffer from pathological anxiety and frequently no causative factor can be identified. The benzodiazepines, and non-benzodiazepine anxiolytics such as buspirone, may be useful in alleviating the symptoms of pathological anxiety. The three neurotransmitters that appear to be most directly involved in different aspects of anxiety are noradrenaline, 5-hydroxytryptamine (5-HT) and GABA.

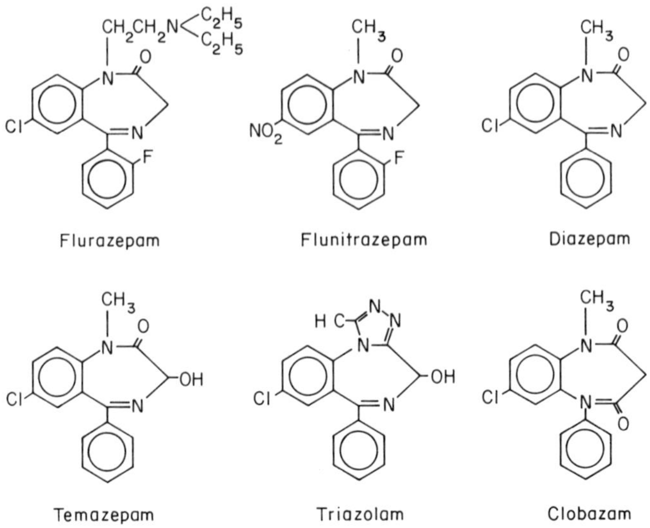

Figure 8.2. Chemical structure of some commonly used benzodiazepines. Clobazam differs from the other benzodiazepines shown, being a 1,5- rather than a 1,4-benzodiazepine.

Noradrenaline is the neurotransmitter most closely associated with the peripheral and central stress response. There is experimental evidence to show that drugs such as yohimbine that block the noradrenergic autoreceptors (e.g. on cell bodies and nerve terminals) and thereby enhance noradrenaline release cause fear and anxiety in both man and animals. Conversely, drugs that stimulate these autoreceptors (as exemplified by clonidine) diminish the anxiety state because they reduce the release of noradrenaline. Benzodiazepines have been shown to inhibit the fear-motivated increase in the functional activity of noradrenaline in experimental animals, but it is now widely believed that the action of the benzodiazepines on the central noradrenergic system is only short term and may contribute to the sedative effects which most conventional benzodiazepines produce, at least initially. Nevertheless, altered noradrenergic function may underlie certain forms of severe anxiety such as that seen in patients with panic attacks or anxiety states associated with major depression. Such forms of anxiety generally respond to treatment with antidepressants or benzodiazepines that also have some mild antidepressant properties (e.g. alprazolam).

Several experimental studies have suggested that a reduction in the activity of 5-HT in the brain results in anxiolysis, and therefore the anxiolytic effects of the benzodiazepines may be at least partly mediated by a reduction in central serotonergic neurotransmission. Other studies have shown that benzodiazepines inhibit the firing of serotonergic neurons in the midbrain raphé region, an area that contains serotonergic cell bodies which send projections to the limbic and cortical regions of the brain.

The link between the serotonergic pathways and the control of anxiety has been further strengthened by the introduction of non-benzodiazepine anxiolytics such as buspirone, ipsapirone and gepirone, which decrease central serotonergic function by stimulating a subclass of 5-HT receptors (5-HT$_{1A}$), leading to a decrease in serotonergic release. Despite the connection between the decreased functional activity of the serotonergic system and the anxiolytic effects of the benzodiazepines, it would appear that their effect on serotonergic transmission is indirect and probably mediated via a facilitation of the principal inhibitory neurotransmitter, GABA.

Unlike the biogenic amines, noradrenaline and 5-HT, GABA is one of the most widely distributed neurotransmitters in the mammalian brain, occupying some 40% of all synapses. Whereas noradrenaline and 5-HT are primarily excitatory in their actions, GABA is an inhibitory transmitter and therefore reduces the firing rate of excitatory neurons with which it is in contact. In various animal models of anxiety, the facilitation of GABAergic activity is associated with a reduction in anxiety. Conversely, drugs such as bicuculline, which specifically block GABA receptors, precipitate the symptoms of anxiety. There is also experimental evidence to show that the antianxiety effects of the benzodiazepines may be inhibited by GABA receptor antagonists or by drugs that reduce the synthesis of GABA. From such studies it may be concluded that the primary action of "classical" benzodiazepines such as diazepam is to facilitate central GABAergic transmission but, due to the modulatory effects of GABAergic neurons on other neurotransmitter systems in the brain, secondary changes occur in noradrenergic and serotonergic pathways which may contribute to their anxiolytic effects.

Pathophysiological basis of panic disorder and obsessive–compulsive disorder: Pharmacological treatment

A number of models of anxiety disorder have been proposed which help to explain differences in human behaviour in terms of their possible genetic and biological determinants. Of these models the one developed by Gray is particularly appealing to the neuroscientist in that it seeks to link three interdependent systems in the brain to specific behavioural functions. Thus one system is concerned with behavioural variations in response to signals of reward and non-punishment, a system concerned with impulsiveness. The second is located in the septo-hippocampal area and is concerned with behavioural inhibition; this is particularly relevant to the genesis of anxiety. The third system controls the escape and defensive–aggressive behaviour (the fight–flight response) and involves the amygdala-hypothalamus-midbrain regions. Thus the model of Gray regards anxiety disorders as arising from variations in the activities of several interdependent regions of the limbic system.

In recent years there has been considerable interest in the neurobiological basis of the anxiety disorders. It is generally accepted that the noradrenergic and serotonergic systems are causally involved in the pathogenesis of these disorders. Both the locus ceruleus and the dorsal raphé project to the septo-hippocampal circuit which, in turn, projects to the other regions of the limbic system that mediate anxiety. The hippocampus and the amygdala are of particular importance in that they are interconnected and also project to both subcortical and cortical nuclei. Their main neurophysiological function appears to involve the integration of external and internal sensory perception. It is well established that infusion of lactate in patients who are vulnerable to panic attack can initiate the full symptoms of the attack. Positron emission tomography (PET) imaging studies on such patients show that there is an abnormal hemispheric asymmetry in the parahippocampal gyrus blood flow and oxygen consumption together with an increase in glucose utilization in this area of the brain. Such studies help to locate the sites of the anxiety disorders in subcortical regions of the brain and also to provide a rational basis for defining the sites of action of the drugs that are used to treat them. They also suggest which of the numerous neurotransmitter systems found in these areas may be causally connected with the disorders.

Panic disorder is one of the most prevalent psychiatric disorders in industrialized countries. It is often associated with agoraphobia and has an estimated prevalence of between 1% and 6%. The use of imipramine in the treatment of anxiety by Klein and Fink, and the discovery by William Sargant that monoamine oxidase inhibitors (MAOIs) were effective in the treatment of "atypical depression" over 30 years ago led to the investigation of the efficacy of such treatments in patients with panic disorder. Since that time, such drugs have been shown to attenuate the symptoms of panic in addition to those of phobic avoidance and anticipatory anxiety. As both the tricyclic antidepressants (TCAs) and the non-specific MAOIs such as phenelzine affect both the noradrenergic and serotonergic systems it was unclear which of these neurotransmitters was causally related to the beneficial effects of antidepressant treatment. However, by determining the plasma concentrations of imipramine (which inhibits the reuptake of both noradrenaline and serotonin) and its major metabolite desipramine (which is selective in inhibiting noradrenaline reuptake) it has been shown that the antipanic action of imipramine is largely attributable to its effect on serotonergic function. This view has been strengthened in recent years by the widespread use of clomipramine, the most specific inhibitor of 5-HT reuptake of the conventional TCAs, in the treatment of panic disorder. However, there is convincing clinical evidence that other TCAs such as the "second generation" tricyclic lofepramine which inhibits both noradrenaline and 5-HT uptake, is equi-effective with clomipramine and has an advantage of fewer adverse effects.

Undoubtedly one of the major advances in the treatment of panic disorder in the last two decades has resulted from the introduction of the selective 5-HT reuptake inhibitors (the SSRIs). Detailed double-blind placebo controlled studies have shown that these drugs are effective in reducing the frequency of panic attacks, anxiety and the associated symptoms of the disorder. The importance of the serotonergic system in the therapeutic response to the SSRIs is indicated by studies in which fluvoxamine was compared with the selective noradrenaline reuptake inhibitor maprotiline. Whereas the number of panic attacks and the severity of anxiety significantly decreased following fluvoxamine, no such beneficial effects were seen following maprotiline treatment. Thus the SSRIs would appear to exhibit specific antipanic properties which are related to their chronic modulatory effects on serotonergic transmission. Generally all the SSRIs show a latency of several weeks before the optimal antipanic effect is established. This suggests that major changes in 5-HT receptor function must occur before the full clinical effect is manifest, a situation which is similar to that occurring when these drugs are used in the treatment of depression. In support of this hypothesis it has been found that a transient increase in anxiety frequently occurs when patients start treatment on an SSRI; this generally disappears as treatment proceeds and has been explained by an initial hypersensitivity of 5-HT$_1$ receptor subtypes which normalize following chronic drug treatment.

Despite the clear evidence that the serotonergic system is involved in the therapeutic efficacy of the antidepressants, it should be noted that the antipanic effect of the triazolobenzodiazepine alprazolam does not appear to be directly mediated by changes in the serotonergic system. This further emphasizes the complexity of the inter-relationships between the various biogenic amine and peptide (for example, cholecystokinin which has been implicated in the aetiology of panic disorder) neurotransmitters and also accounts for the diverse range of drugs that have been used in the treatment of the disorder.

According to the DSM-IV classification, anxiety as a disorder can be divided into panic disorder with or without agoraphobia, generalized anxiety disorder, obsessive–compulsive disorder (OCD) and social phobia. Patients with generalized anxiety disorder appear to respond best to anxiolytic benzodiazepines and the properties and adverse effects of these drugs has been discussed in detail elsewhere. In recent years there have been a number of largely "open" studies showing that the SSRIs and the reversible MAOI moclobemide are effective in the treatment of social phobia. However considerable attention has been paid recently to the pharmacological treatment of OCD, a condition which, until it was discovered that clomipramine could effectively attenuate some of the symptoms, was largely unaffected by drug treatment.

By using imaging methods it has been shown that blood flow rates were greater in parts of the cortex in OCD patients than in matched control subjects. Similarly PET imaging studies in which the uptake of fluorodeoxyglucose was used to determine the activity of different brain regions, showed that the activity of the inferior prefrontal cortex was significantly greater in untreated OCD patients. There is evidence that these abnormalities are reversed following effective treatment with clomipramine.

Despite the convincing evidence that the SSRIs are effective in the treatment of OCD, whereas antidepressants that lack an inhibitory effect on 5-HT reuptake (such as desipramine and nortriptyline) are largely ineffective, direct evidence implicating an abnormality in serotonergic function is limited. Thus there is evidence that the non-specific $5-HT_1$ receptor agonist m-chlorophenyl piperazine (mCPP) (a metabolite of trazodone and the new antidepressant nefazodone) can enhance the anxiety and obsessional state of some OCD patients but these changes are not associated with an increase in plasma cortisol and prolactin which would be indicative of $5-HT_1$ receptor hypersensitivity. Other clinical studies have shown that in patients responding to fluoxetine, there is no correlation between changes in $5-HT_{1A}$ receptor function and the reduction in the OCD symptoms. Thus it would appear that while the serotonergic system may be abnormal in OCD, and that drugs which selectively enhance serotonergic function are therapeutically effective in treating the condition, the nature of the abnormality in serotonergic function remains obscure. Nevertheless, there is now abundant clinical evidence that clomipramine and the SSRIs have made a major contribution to the pharmacological treatment of this disorder.

In CONCLUSION, the recognition of the high frequency of such anxiety states as panic disorder in the general population in recent years has led to the widespread interest in the aetiology and treatment of the condition. The introduction of the SSRIs has been important not only because of their proven efficacy in the treatment of panic disorder and OCD but also because of the light they have thrown on the possible abnormality in the serotonergic system which may underlie the cause of such anxiety disorders.

The benzodiazepine receptor and GABA function

Schmidt and colleagues in 1967 were the first to show that diazepam could potentiate the inhibitory effect of GABA on the cat spinal cord. Later it was shown that the effect of diazepam could be abolished if the endogenous GABA content was depleted, thus establishing that diazepam, and related benzodiazepines, did not act directly on GABA receptors but in some way modulated inhibitory transmission via GABA. It was subsequently demonstrated that the benzodiazepines bind with high affinity and specificity to neuronal elements in the mammalian brain and that there is an excellent correlation between their affinity for these specific binding sites and their pharmacological potencies in alleviating anxiety in both man and animals. The binding of a benzodiazepine to this receptor site is enhanced in the presence of GABA or a GABA agonist, thereby suggesting that a functional, but independent, relationship exists between the GABA receptor and the benzodiazepine receptor.

The *barbiturates*, and to some extent *alcohol*, also seem to produce their anxiolytic and sedative effects by facilitating GABAergic transmission. This action of chemically unrelated compounds can be explained by their ability to stimulate specific sites on the GABA receptor complex, the most marked effect being due to the benzodiazepines when they activate their specific receptor site. Thus benzodiazepines bind with high affinity to the benzodiazepine receptor and, as a result, change the structural conformation of the GABA receptor so that the action of GABA on its receptor is enhanced. This enables GABA to produce a stronger inhibition of the postsynaptic neuron than would occur in the absence of the benzodiazepine, the anxiolytic effect being produced by an allosteric enhancement of the action of GABA. The relationship between the various components of the GABA receptor and the GABA nerve terminal is shown in Figure 2.17 (see p. 57).

The inhibitory effect of GABA is mediated by chloride ion channels. When the GABA receptor is occupied by GABA, or by a drug acting as an agonist such as muscimol, the chloride channels open and chloride ions diffuse into the cell (see p. 57 for details). The chloride ion channel contains at least two binding sites. One of these sites is activated by barbiturates that have weak anxiolytic and hypnotic properties (e.g. pentobarbitone and phenobarbitone). Such drugs facilitate inhibitory transmission by increasing the duration of opening of the chloride ion channel. Another class of experimental anxiolytic agents that are not structurally related to the benzodiazepines (the pyrazolopyridines, of which etazolate is a clinically active example) also act at a specific site within the chloride ion channel and enhance GABAergic function by increasing the frequency of channel opening.

Thus it may be concluded that the "classical" benzodiazepines such as diazepam, and structurally related drugs, act as anxiolytics by activating a specific benzodiazepine receptor which facilitates inhibitory GABAergic transmission. Other drugs with anxiolytic properties, such as some of the barbiturates and alcohol, also facilitate GABAergic transmission by acting on sites associated more directly with the chloride ion channel.

Diversity of drugs acting on the benzodiazepine receptor

Until about 1980, it was widely accepted that the benzodiazepine structure was a prerequisite for the anxiolytic profile and for the recognition of and binding to the benzodiazepine receptor. More recently, however, a chemically unrelated drug, the *cyclopyrrolone* zopiclone, has been shown to be a useful sedative hypnotic with a benzodiazepine-like profile. Other chemical classes of drugs that are also structurally dissimilar to the benzodiazepines (e.g. triazolopyridazines) have also been developed and shown to have anxiolytic activity in man; these non-benzodiazepines also act via the benzodiazepine receptor. Thus the term *"benzodiazepine receptor ligand"* has been introduced to describe all drugs, irrespective of their chemical structure, that act on benzodiazepine receptors and thereby modulate inhibitory transmission in the brain.

Over the last decade there has been an increase in our knowledge of the relationship between the structure of benzodiazepine receptor ligands and their pharmacological properties. This has led to the development of potent receptor *agonists* that stimulate the receptor and produce pharmacological effects qualitatively similar to diazepam and related "classical" benzodiazepines, *antagonists*, which block the effects of the agonists without having any effects themselves, and a group of drugs that have a mixture of agonist and antagonist properties (so-called *partial agonists*). In addition, an intriguing group of compounds have been developed that have the opposite effect on the benzodiazepine receptor to the pure agonists. These are known as *inverse agonists*. The pharmacological properties of these different types of benzodiazepine receptor ligands are summarized in Figure 8.3.

At the molecular level, the differences between the agonist and antagonist benzodiazepines are ascribed to the ability of the drug to induce a conformational change in the fine structure of the receptor molecule that produces functional consequences in terms of cellular changes. The partial agonists have intrinsic activity that lies between the full agonists and the antagonists. When administered they have qualitatively similar effects to full agonists, but may not be quite as potent; when given with full agonists they reduce the potency of the full agonist. Some 7 years ago, the Danish investigators Braestup and Nielsen found that a group of non-benzodiazepine compounds, the beta-carbolines, not only antagonized the actions of the full agonists but also had intrinsic activity themselves. Such compounds were clearly not pure antagonists, which lack intrinsic activity, but were found to be inverse agonists because they had the exact opposite biological effects to the pure agonists, i.e. they caused anxiety, convulsions and facilitated memory function. Thus the benzodiazepine receptor is so far unique in that it has a bidirectional function. This discovery could be of major importance in designing drugs in which the adverse effects of the

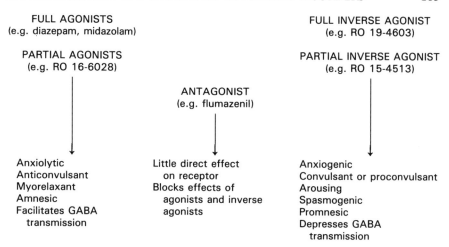

Figure 8.3. Properties of the various types of benzodiazepine receptor ligands.

"classical" benzodiazepines could be reduced but their beneficial effects maintained. The development of partial agonists may be particularly important in the production of anxiolytics that lack the sedative and amnestic properties of full agonists such as diazepam.

Are there natural ligands for the benzodiazepine receptor in the brain?

The presence of benzodiazepine receptors in the brain would suggest that there are natural ligands present which modulate these receptors. To date, a specific compound has not been unequivocally identified, but a number of candidates have been isolated that show agonist or inverse agonist activity. Some of these candidates are listed in Table 8.2.

Of the putative ligands for the benzodiazepine receptors that are listed in Table 8.2, diazepam-binding inhibitor (DBI), nephentin and tribulin appear to be particularly interesting. *DBI* is a polypeptide that has been isolated, and its structure elucidated, from mammalian and human brain. It is called "diazepam-binding inhibitor" because it can inhibit the binding of tritiated diazepam to the benzodiazepine receptor; recently it has also been shown to inhibit the binding of antagonists and inverse agonists to this receptor. Pharmacological studies show that DBI has anxiogenic properties and its concentration in the brain appears to be sufficiently high to block benzodiazepine receptors under appropriate conditions. It is only present in trace amounts in tissues other than the brain.

Tribulin is a relatively low molecular weight compound with acidic or neutral properties that has been isolated from human urine by Sandler and

Table 8.2. Putative endogenous ligands for the benzodiazepine receptor in the mammalian brain

---

Nicotinamide
Inosine and hypoxanthine
Ethyl-beta-carboline-3 carboxylate
Tribulin
Nephentin
Diazepam-displacing activity in human cerebrospinal fluid
Diazepam-binding inhibitor (DBI)

---

colleagues in the UK. The presence of this compound increases following stress and it has been found to inhibit the binding of benzodiazepines to their receptor site. In 1983 Sandler suggested that tribulin might be related to the endogenous anxiogenic factor and structurally related to the beta-carbolines. More recently it has been shown that tribulin is a mixture of at least three low molecular weight compounds.

Nephentin is also a large polypeptide that has been shown to have a relatively high affinity for the benzodiazepine receptor and does not have any effect upon other neurotransmitter receptors. Unlike DBI, however, the concentration of nephentin is much higher in non-nervous peripheral tissues such as the bile duct than it is in the brain. Furthermore, the distribution of nephentin in the brain does not coincide with that of the benzodiazepine receptors. It is possible, nevertheless, that nephentin is a precursor of a lower molecular weight peptide that can block the benzodiazepine receptor.

Less progress has been made in the detection of natural compounds that may act as agonists on the benzodiazepine receptor. Three non-peptides (nicotinamide, inosine and hypoxanthine) have been shown to have low affinities for the benzodiazepine receptor and there is some experimental evidence suggesting that they have mixed agonist–antagonist properties. Nevertheless, the consensus of opinion would appear to suggest that these substances are not the endogenous ligands for the benzodiazepine receptor. It is possible that purinergic mechanisms are activated by inosine and hypoxanthine and that the modulation of benzodiazepine receptor function is a secondary consequence of this.

There is some evidence to suggest that the benzodiazepines exist not only in plants such as the potato but also in the mammalian brain, including the brains of individuals who have never taken benzodiazepine anxiolytics or hypnotics. While such findings are still controversial, they do point to the possibility that the benzodiazepines are endogenous modulators of the GABA receptor and that a defect in their synthesis may have a role to play in the aetiology of anxiety disorders.

It may be concluded that there is some evidence to suggest that anxiety arises as a consequence either of a deficiency of an endogenous agonist or the presence of an endogenous inverse agonist acting on the benzodiazepine–GABA receptor complex. Thus one possible approach to drug design in the future may be the development of drugs that either facilitate the synthesis of endogenous agonists or reduce the synthesis of inverse agonists at the benzodiazepine receptor sites.

Changes in benzodiazepine receptor function following chronic administration of benzodiazepines

It is a well-established biological phenomenon that receptors adapt to the prolonged presence or absence of an agonist by changing their sensitivity, thereby attempting to return their function to normal levels. Thus prolonged blockade of dopamine receptors in the basal ganglia by neuroleptics such as chlorpromazine or haloperidol causes a *supersensitivity* of these receptors. Conversely, conditions in which the receptor is chronically stimulated by its endogenous neurotransmitter, or by an agonist drug, result in a decrease in the functioning of the postsynaptic receptors; this phenomenon is known as *subsensitivity*, an event which may be accompanied by a decrease in the number of receptors. Such changes, sometimes termed "up"- or "down"-regulation, may develop slowly or rapidly, the former being due to changes in the synthesis of the receptor while the latter probably reflects the movement of receptors into, or out of, the neuronal membrane.

Experimental studies in rodents have clearly demonstrated that high doses of "classical" benzodiazepines such as diazepam, lorazepam and flurazepam cause a decrease in benzodiazepine receptors in the cortex of the brain but the number of receptors rapidly returns to normal (after approximately 5 days) following the abrupt cessation of drug treatment. There is also electrophysiological evidence to show that the functional activity of the GABA receptors that are linked to the benzodiazepine receptors is also decreased following prolonged treatment with chlordiazepoxide, even though the actual number of GABA receptors is increased. *In vitro* evidence suggests that chronic benzodiazepine treatment results in an uncoupling of the benzodiazepine receptor from the GABA receptor complex.

Functional tolerance following chronic treatment with the benzodiazepines is well documented in animals and man and represents a pharmacodynamic rather than pharmacokinetic phenomenon. Tolerance appears to occur more rapidly with the sedative and anticonvulsant rather than the anxiolytic properties of the "classical" benzodiazepines. However, since clinically relevant tolerance develops with therapeutic doses, but changes in receptor tolerance only occur with very high doses of the drugs that are usually far in excess of those used clinically, little experimental evidence exists at present whereby the functional tolerance to benzodiazepines can be explained on the basis of benzodiazepine receptor desensitization. However, one must be cautious in extrapolating the results of animal experiments to the patient with an anxiety disorder who is being treated with a benzodiazepine. The benzodiazepine receptor complex shows marked plasticity in the animal brain, but relatively few changes have been noted in this receptor system in samples obtained from post-mortem human brain, even when the patients suffered from epilepsy at the time of death. This suggests that the regulation or plasticity of the benzodiazepine receptor in the human brain differs considerably from that in the brain of the experimental animal, although the molecular properties of the benzodiazepine receptor appear to be remarkably similar.

Adverse effects of benzodiazepines

The short-term effects are mainly those of sedation but following longer term use accumulation may occur, particularly in the case of drugs like diazepam and chlordiazepoxide that have long half-lives due to their active metabolites. After long-term administration (weeks to months) *tolerance* develops. While most patients rapidly become tolerant to the sedative side effects of these drugs, some patients, particularly the elderly, experience excessive sedation, poor memory and concentration, motor incoordination and muscle weakness. In extreme cases in the elderly, an acute confusional state may arise which simulates dementia. All sedatives, including the benzodiazepines, interact with alcohol and therefore these drugs should not be taken in combination.

In addition to the tolerance that occurs following the long-term treatment of a patient with a benzodiazepine, *dependence* also arises. Dependence is defined as a situation occurring as a consequence of the compensatory adaptive changes in the brain as a result of chronic drug administration. Evidence for *physical dependence* is obtained from the *withdrawal* effects that arise on discontinuation of the medication. *Rebound* effects are defined as an increase in the severity of the initial symptoms beyond that occurring in the patient before treatment started. Rebound insomnia following abrupt discontinuation of benzodiazepine hypnotics is well described, and rebound anxiety arises not uncommonly in those patients in whom an anxiolytic benzodiazepine has been suddenly terminated. Slowly tapering the dose of a benzodiazepine over a period of many days or weeks largely overcomes the problem of rebound effects.

Sudden withdrawal from a high chronic dose of benzodiazepine has long been known to provide a variety of side effects, including seizures and paranoid behaviour in extreme cases. Withdrawal symptoms include psychological changes such as anxiety, apprehension, irritability, insomnia and dysphoria, bodily symptoms such as palpitations, tremor, vertigo and sweating, and perceptual disturbances, including hypersensitivity to light, sound and pain, and depersonalization. The perceptual disturbances that occur on withdrawal are not generally seen in those patients exhibiting rebound effects and it therefore may be possible to distinguish between these two phenomena. It has been estimated that 15–30% of patients on benzodiazepines for longer than a year may encounter problems in trying to discontinue their medication.

Use of non-benzodiazepines in the treatment of anxiety disorders

The *barbiturates* and *meprobamate* have been entirely superseded by the benzodiazepines and because of their low benefit-to-risk ratio (dependence producing, lethality in overdose, potent sedative effects) they should never be used as anxiolytics. Despite their popularity as short-term sedatives, *antihistamines* are ineffective anxiolytics, while the use of *sedative antidepressants* such as amitriptyline should be limited to the treatment of patients with symptoms of both anxiety and depression due to their limited efficacy and the poor patient compliance associated with their adverse effects. However, patients with panic disorder do appear to show a beneficial response to antidepressants (see Chapter 5). A similar argument can be made regarding the use of low doses of *antipsychotics*, although drugs such as chlropromazine may have some value in treating severely anxious patients who had previously been dependent on sedatives. *Beta adrenoceptor antagonists* such as propranolol may have a place in the treatment of anxious patients with pronounced autonomic symptoms (palpitations, tremor and gastrointestinal upset).

The azaspirodecanedione anxiolytics

A series of non-benzodiazepine anxiolytics have recently been introduced which, unlike the benzodiazepines, do not facilitate GABAergic function but appear to act as agonists at $5\text{-}HT_{1A}$ receptors. *Buspirone* is an example of this novel class of anxiolytics, and is structurally similar to gepirone and ipsapirone. The latter compounds are reported to show both anxiolytic and antidepressant properties. The structure of these novel compounds is shown in Figure 8.4.

In vitro ligand binding studies have shown that buspirone binds with high affinity to $5\text{-}HT_{1A}$ and D_2 receptor sites. However, it is known that in vivo the main metabolite of buspirone and ipsapirone is 1-pyrimidylpiperazine (1-PP),

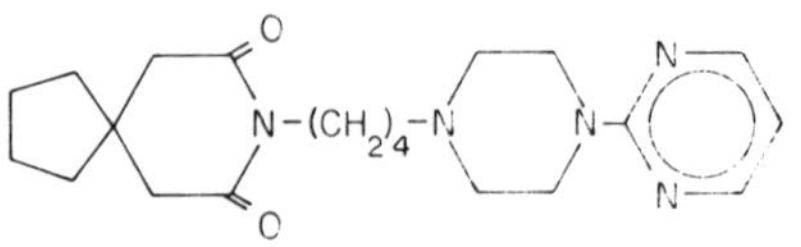

Buspirone

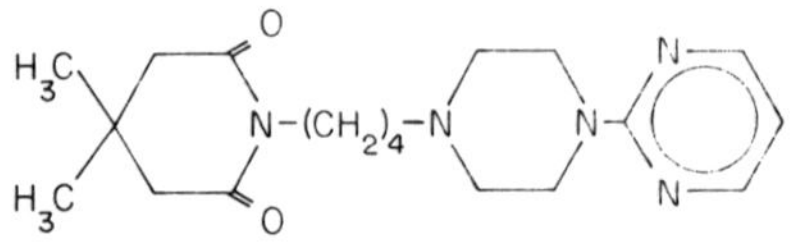

Gepirone

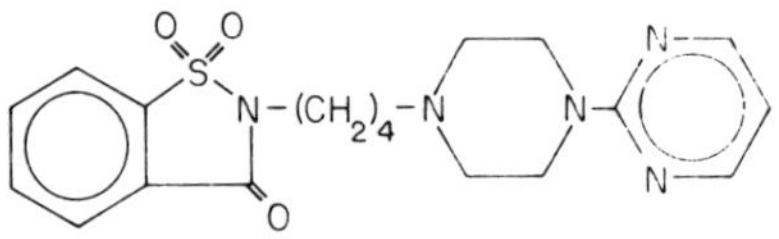

Ipsapirone

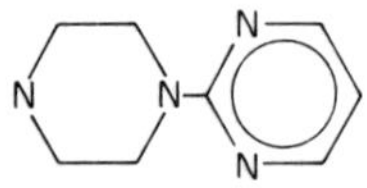

1-Pyrimidylpiperazine
(1-PP) metabolite of buspirone, gepirone
and ipsapirone

Figure 8.4. Chemical structure of some azaspirodecanedione anxiolytics.

which also has a high affinity for alpha$_2$ adrenoceptors. Thus the pharmacological activity of buspirone and related compounds may be the result of a complex interaction between the parent compound and the pharmacologically active metabolite. It seems possible that the antagonist effect of the 1-PP metabolite on alpha$_2$ adrenoceptors might account for the presumed antidepressant action of such drugs, as it is known that some atypical antidepressants such as mianserin and idazoxan also show an antagonistic activity on such receptors. Another interesting aspect of the action of buspirone lies in its specificity of action of 5-HT$_{1A}$ receptors in the brain. Thus experimental studies have shown that it has a more marked effect in reducing the turnover 5-HT in the hippocampus, and to a lesser extent the cortex, than it does in the striatum. From such studies of the effects of buspirone-like drugs on central neurotransmission, it may be concluded that their anxiolytic action is due to a reduction in 5-HT turnover in the limbic region of the brain, while the possible antidepressant effect could be attributed to a selective enhancement of noradrenaline turnover in this region. Such an explanation must be treated with caution, however, as it is well established that alpha$_2$ adrenoceptor antagonists such as yohimbine induce anxiety states in both man and animals. Whether buspirone-like drugs selectively enhance noradrenaline turnover only in the limbic region, and do not cause a hyperarousal state which could induce anxiety, is a matter of conjecture. The pharmacological consequences of the interaction of buspirone with D$_2$ receptor sites is uncertain; there is little evidence that buspirone has neuroleptic properties at those doses which are known to be anxiolytic. The slight abdominal discomfort occasionally associated with the initial administration of buspirone could be due to the stimulation of 5-HT receptors in the gastrointestinal tract.

Clinical trials of buspirone have shown the drug to be slower in onset of action compared with diazepam, but it produces significantly less sedation and fewer detrimental effects on psychomotor function than the benzodiazepines. The main advantage of buspirone would therefore appear to be in its lack of dependence, amnestic and sedative effects. However, its slower onset of action and its lower efficacy in alleviating the somatic symptoms of anxiety make it unlikely that it will replace the therapeutically effective and proven benzodiazepines, despite the greater frequency of their side effects. Whether ipsapirone and gepirone, which are still in clinical development, will be therapeutically superior to buspirone can only be assessed after they become more widely available for clinical use.

Clinical studies show that buspirone is an effective anxiolytic with an advantage over the benzodiazepines of lacking a sedative effect, not interacting with alcohol and not exhibiting any dependence effects following prolonged use. Its main clinical disadvantage lies in the delay in onset of its therapeutic effect (up to 2 weeks in some cases) and its limited efficacy in attenuating anxiety in those patients who had previously responded to benzodiazepines. Furthermore, unlike the benzodiazepines, it does not appear to have beneficial effects in patients with panic disorder.

The failure of buspirone to exhibit cross-tolerance with the benzodiazepines in both animal and man suggests that the drug alleviates anxiety by a different mechanism. Experimental studies have shown that buspirone, gepirone and ipsapirone act as full or partial agonists on 5-HT$_{1A}$ receptor subtypes. Experimental studies show that potent 5-HT$_{1A}$ agonists such as 8-hydroxy-2-(dipropylamino)tetralin (8OH-DPAT) are anxiolytic in some animal models of anxiety. This suggests that this novel class of anxiolytics modulate central serotonergic transmission, which probably accounts for the relative lack of those side effects that the benzodiazepines exhibit due to their facilitating action on GABA receptors (sedation, dependence, etc.).

Modulation of $5\text{-}HT_{1A}$ receptor function may also account for the antidepressant properties which this series of drugs are claimed to show.

In CONCLUSION, evidence has been presented to show that the benzodiazepines produce their variety of pharmacological effects by activating specific receptors that form part of the main inhibitory neurotransmitter receptor system, the GABA receptor, in the mammalian brain. Different classes of benzodiazepine receptor ligands have been developed which can alleviate anxiety or produce anxiety according to the fine structural changes that occur when the drugs interact with the benzodiazepine receptor.

There is some evidence that natural substances occur in the human brain that can cause either an increase or a reduction in the anxiety state by acting on the benzodiazepine receptor. The unique nature of the benzodiazepine receptor, and the disparate properties of the drugs that act on this receptor, should allow plenty of scope for the development of novel compounds with selective anxiolytic and other properties in the future. Despite the evidence from animal studies that benzodiazepine receptor function changes in response to chronic drug treatment, there is little evidence from human brain studies that such changes are relevant to the phenomena of tolerance, dependence and withdrawal effects that have been the recent cause for public concern. Novel anxiolytics such as buspirone that are structurally unrelated to the benzodiazepines and which do not modulate GABAergic function have the advantage of lacking the sedative and dependence-producing effects of the benzodiazepines. Nevertheless, the relative lack of efficacy of such drugs, and the delay in their onset of therapeutic effect, make it unlikely that they will replace the benzodiazepines as the drugs of choice in the treatment of anxiety disorders.

9 Drug Treatment of Insomnia

Introduction

Apart from the benzodiazepines, the sedative hypnotics are a group of drugs that depress the brain in a relatively non-selective manner. This results in a progressive change from drowsiness (sedation), sleep (hypnosis) to loss of consciousness, surgical anaesthesia, coma and finally cardiovascular and respiratory collapse and death. The central nervous system (CNS) depressant drugs include general anaesthetics, barbiturates and alcohols, including ethanol. Before the advent of the benzodiazepines, barbiturates in low doses were widely used as anxiolytics. A *sedative* drug is one that decreases CNS activity, moderates excitement and generally calms the individual, whereas a *hypnotic* produces drowsiness and facilitates the onset and maintenance of sleep from which the individual may be easily aroused.

Historically the first sedative hypnotics to be introduced were the bromides in the mid 19th century, shortly followed by chloral hydrate, paraldehyde and urethane. It was not until the early years of this century that the first barbiturate, sodium barbitone, was developed and this was shortly followed by over 50 analogues, all with essentially similar pharmacological properties. The major breakthrough in the development of selective, relatively non-toxic sedative hypnotics followed the introduction of chlordiazepoxide in 1961. Most of the benzodiazepines in current use have been selected for their high anxiolytic potency relative to their central depressant effects. Because of their considerable safety, the benzodiazepines have now largely replaced the barbiturates and the alcohols, such as chloral hydrate and trichloroethanol, as the drugs of choice in the treatment of insomnia.

The hypnotics are some of the most widely used drugs, over 15 million prescriptions being given for this group of drugs in Britain in 1985; the number of prescriptions for hypnotics has remained fairly constant over the last decade despite the reduction in anxiolytic prescriptions by about 50% over this same period. This situation is hard to reconcile with the fact that all benzodiazepines in current use have hypnotic properties if given in slightly higher therapeutic doses. This implies that what determines their use as anxiolytics, for day-time administration, or hypnotics, for night-time use, is largely a question of dose and marketing. As discussed in considerable detail elsewhere (see p. 157), there is a metabolic inter-relationship between the commonly used 1,4-benzodiazepines and their mode of action is similar. It is of interest that the hypnotic benzodiazepines have received little media attention, in contrast to the anxiolytics of the same class, regarding their possible dependence-forming effects.

Physiology of sleep

Although there is no evidence for a specific sleep "centre" in the brain, it is generally accepted that the level of consciousness is located in the diffuse network of nerve cells that comprise the reticular formation. This region consists of tegmental parts of the medulla, pons and midbrain. Lesions of the reticular formation result in somnolence or coma, sensory stimuli failing to arouse the animal. Such observations led to the conclusion that the brain stem reticular activity system maintains alertness and wakefulness, while lack of sensory stimulation results in sleep. Arousal from sleep by sensory stimuli is attributed to collateral pathways that link the main sensory pathways to the reticular formation. Undoubtedly this is a gross simplification of the anatomical substrate for sleep and wakefulness. There is evidence, for example, that animals may recover consciousness following lesions of the reticular formation and that the forebrain is not completely dependent on inputs from the reticular formation to maintain consciousness. Nevertheless, it is generally accepted that the reticular formation plays an important, if not a key role, in sleep and wakefulness.

A number of *neurotransmitter systems* appear to be involved in the regulation of sleep and wakefulness. The noradrenergic projections from the rostral part of the locus coeruleus are involved in the maintenance of tonic cortical arousal, as are the ascending cholinergic pathways. The inhibitory action of gamma-aminobutyric acid (GABA) on the cholinergic pathways may be important in the regulation of paradoxical (rapid eye movement) sleep. It is also apparent from lesion studies in animals that 5-hydroxytryptamine (5-HT) plays a crucial role in the sleep pattern. Thus destruction of the rostral portion of the raphé nucleus leads to insomnia, while destruction of the dorsal noradrenergic bundle causes hypersomnia. This has led to the suggestion that orthodox (non-rapid eye movement) sleep is initiated by the release of 5-HT originating from the rostral raphé nuclei, while paradoxical sleep involves the release of this transmitter from the caudal raphé; wakefulness and cortical arousal depend on the noradrenergic neurons of the anterior locus coeruleus. The hypnotic effects of the benzodiazepines may be attributed to the modulatory effects of the GABAergic system on the raphé projections and the locus coeruleus, although the precise mechanism whereby these drugs induce sleep is not entirely certain. There is evidence that diazepam binding inhibitor is present in higher concentrations in the brains of animals during the awake state but is absent while the animal is asleep. Whether such factors as the delta sleep-inducing peptide induces sleep by modifying the classical neurotransmitter pathways is unknown.

In animals, two main types of sleep pattern may be identified termed *non-rapid eye movement sleep* (non-REM or slow-wave sleep) and *rapid eye movement sleep* (REM sleep). Normal sleep is composed of several REM and non-REM cycles. *Non-REM sleep* is divided into light sleep (stages 1 and 2) and slow-wave or delta sleep (stages 3 and 4). *Stage 1* sleep is characterized by alpha rhythm on the electroencephalogram (EEG) and forms the transition between wakefulness and sleep; it occupies approximately 5% of the time. Muscle tone is relatively weak and while a certain amount of mental activity persists, concentration and imagination fluctuate. As the sleep deepens, hypnagogic hallucinations may occur. *Stage 2* sleep represents over 50% of the total sleeping time and is marked by characteristic sleep spindles and K complexes in the EEG; delta waves are also present occasionally. Muscle tone is weak and there are no eye movements. *Stages 3 and 4*, slow-wave sleep, occupy approximately 20% of the sleep time. The EEG is characterized by more than 50% of the sleep pattern being in the form of delta waves. This stage of sleep is the recuperative phase which is associated with growth hormone secretion and tissue repair; the secretion of prolactin is not associated with any specific phase of sleep. Dreaming may occur but tends to be of brief duration and of a rational nature. Nocturnal terrors and sleep walking are associated with stage 4 sleep.

REM sleep occupies approximately 20% of the sleep time in the normal adult, up to 30% in the young child and less than 20% in the aged or mentally handicapped. The cortical EEG activity resembles that of wakefulness, but is accompanied by muscular weakness; 4 Hz "sawtooth" waves herald the onset of REM sleep. The precise physiological function of REM sleep is unknown but it is associated with dreaming sleep, the dreams being long, emotional and animated. The physiological changes accompanying REM sleep include hypertension, tachycardia alternating with bradycardia, pelvic congestion in the female and penile tumescence in the male. Cortisol secretion appears to peak during the latter part of the sleep cycle when REM sleep is most pronounced. This type of sleep is also characterized by bursts of eye movement and small sporadic muscular twitches of the face and extremities.

The typical sleep pattern of the young adult is composed of four to six cycles of non-REM sleep alternating with REM sleep at approximately 90 minute intervals. The subject first goes into non-REM sleep and then gradually descends from stage 1 through to stage 4 sleep, the frequency of

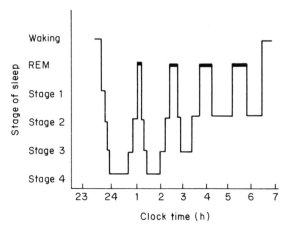

Figure 9.1. Typical hypnogram of a normal young adult.

the waves becoming slower and their amplitude greater. The depth of sleep then briefly (for a few minutes) returns to stage 2, after which the first episode of REM sleep appears. Bodily movements often occur at this stage. This may be illustrated by means of a hypnogram, as shown in Figure 9.1.

It should be noted that stages 3 and 4 are more pronounced during the early part of the sleep period, whereas REM sleep tends to increase during the sleep cycle. The actual period of sleep is to some extent genetically determined, some individuals requiring at least 8 hours while others need only 4 hours to function normally. The sleep pattern becomes more fragile with advancing age, so that in the elderly the number of nocturnal awakenings increases and REM sleep becomes more evenly distributed throughout the night.

The sleep architecture may be modified by disease and by certain drugs. In the healthy individual, the duration of the first phase of REM sleep is usually 3 minutes. In patients with depression or narcoplexy, the time of onset of the first REM phase is shorter than usual, while those with anxiety disorders have a delayed time of onset of the first REM phase. The duration of the first REM phase is also increased in depressed patients.

All hypnotics in current clinical use alter the sleep architecture by reducing the quantity and quality of the REM sleep phase in particular. Thus a single dose of a hypnotic *benzodiazepine* suppresses REM during the period in which it is present, but for up to the two following nights the amount of REM sleep is generally increased (so-called REM rebound). When the hypnotic is given for a prolonged period, the REM sleep gradually returns to normal, but abrupt withdrawal can lead to prolonged rebound in REM sleep, which is often associated with intense and unpleasant dreams and anxiety

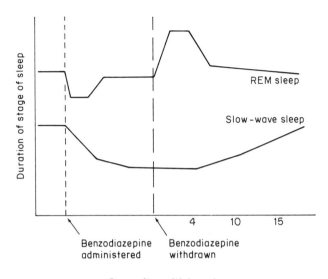

Figure 9.2. Illustration of the rebound effect following 15 days' continuous treatment with a benzodiazepine.

on wakening. Most hypnotics also affect the quality of the non-REM sleep, particularly the slow-wave sleep pattern. Thus stage 3 and stage 4 sleep are suppressed and remain so during the period of drug administration. Following drug withdrawal, the slow-wave sleep gradually returns to normal, but this may take up to 15 days. However, no rebound effect appears to occur in slow-wave sleep. All hypnotics in current use also decrease stage 1 of non-REM sleep and prolong stage 2 sleep; this may be the reason why the nocturnal awakenings decrease, so that the individual feels that the quality of sleep under the influence of the hypnotic has improved! The effect of a hypnotic on the quality of the REM and slow-wave sleep is shown diagrammatically in Figure 9.2.

Disturbance in the sleep pattern commonly occurs in the alcoholic. The sleep pattern in this type of patient is characterized by frequent awakenings and decreased REM and slow-wave sleep. Concomitantly, stages 1 and 2 are increased but shallower than usual. After withdrawal from alcohol, the patient experiences insomnia and REM rebound occurs. The sleep profile of the alcoholic often remains abnormal for 1–2 years following withdrawal.

Most *antidepressants* decrease the quantity of REM sleep in the depressed patient, although it is difficult to say whether this is a reflection of the action of the drugs or due to the underlying pathology. Abrupt withdrawal of antidepressants, particularly the monoamine oxidase inhibitors, is often associated with REM rebound.

Use of hypnotics

Despite the fact that man spends approximately one-third of his life asleep, the purpose of sleep still remains a mystery. The clinical importance of sleep is reflected in the frequency and severity of complaints about insomnia, a condition that signifies unsatisfactory or insufficient sleep. Problems may involve difficulty in getting to sleep, disturbing dreams, early wakening, and day-time drowsiness due to poor sleep at night. In most cases, these symptoms are fairly transient and may be associated with a specific or identifiable event such as a family or work situation, a temporary financial problem, etc. Should the sleep disturbance persist for longer than 3 weeks, specific treatment may be indicated. The Association of Sleep Disorders Centres has classified sleep disorders into two broad classes–*disorders of initiating and maintaining sleep* (DIMS) and *disorders of excessive somnolence* (DOES); these definitions have now been appended to the DSM–IV.

The hypnogram of a patient with an underlying psychiatric illness may be characterized by a delay in sleep onset, the presence of residual muscular activity causing frequent awakenings, fragmented sleep, reduced REM and slow-wave sleep, and day-time drowsiness. Such disorders are generally not associated with a recent or transient event and the cause cannot usually be identified. Often such changes in the sleep architecture are associated with major psychiatric disorders such as depression, mania, psychosis or severe anxiety states.

For the purpose of considering the prescribing of hypnotics, insomnia may be classified into three major types:

1. *Transient insomnia.* This occurs in normal sleepers who experience an acute stress or stressful situation lasting for a few days, for example, air travel to a different time zone or to hospitalization.
2. *Short-term insomnia.* This is usually associated with situational stress caused, for example, by bereavement or which may be related to conflict at work or in the family.
3. *Long-term insomnia.* Studies suggest that insomnia in up to 50% of patients in this category is related to an underlying psychiatric illness. Of the remainder of the patients in this category, chronic alcohol or drug abuse may be the cause of the sleep disruption.

Whenever the use of hypnotics is considered appropriate, it is universally agreed that patients should be given the smallest effective dose for the shortest period of time necessary. This recommendation applies particularly to elderly patients. For transient and short-term insomnia there is no clear consensus, although in practice the use of a medium or short half-life hypnotic for a few days is sometimes recommended when sleep disturbance

Table 9.1. Plasma elimination half-lives of hypnotic benzodiazepines and their active metabolites

Drug	Elimination half-life of parent compound (hours)	Active metabolite	Elimination half-life of metabolite (hours)
Short half-life			
Brotizolam	5.0 (3–5)	1-Methylhydroxy derivative	Short
Triazolam	2.3 (1.4–3.3)	1-Methylhydroxy derivative	Short
Midazolam	2.5 (1–3)	1-Methylhydroxy derivative	Short
Intermediate half-life			
Loprazolam	6.3 (4–8)	None	–
Lormetazepam	9.9 (7–12)	None	–
Temazepam	12.0 (8–21)	None	–
Long half-life			
Flunitrazepam	15.0 (9–25)	7-Amino derivative	23
Flurazepam	Very short	N-Desalkyl-flurazepam	87
Nitrazepam	18 (20–34)	None	–

is associated with shift work or "jet-lag". For chronic insomnia, careful investigation of the underlying cause of the condition is essential before hypnotics are routinely prescribed. Should the insomnia be associated with a psychiatric condition or drug abuse, specific treatment of the core illness will often obviate the need for hypnotics.

For all practical purposes, the benzodiazepines are the group of drugs most widely used to treat insomnia. These may be divided into three classes based on their pharmacokinetic characteristics:

1. *Short half-life drugs*, such as triazolam, midazolam and brotizolam, with elimination half-lives of about 6 hours.
2. *Intermediate half-life drugs*, such as temazepam, lormetazepam and loprazolam, with half-lives of 6–12 hours.
3. *Long half-life drugs*, such as nitrazepam, flurazepam and flunitrazepam, with half-lives over 12 hours.

The elimination half-lives of a number of commonly used hypnotics are shown in Table 9.1. It should be noted that many of the drugs in current use have active metabolites which considerably prolong the duration of their pharmacological effect. This is particularly true for the elderly patient in whom the half-life of the hypnotic is prolonged due to decreased metabolism and renal clearance; such individuals are also more sensitive to the sedative effects of any psychotropic medication.

In general, the efficacy of hypnotics for short-term use is well established and there is a close relationship between their pharmacokinetic and pharmacodynamic profiles. The most widely used hypnotic in the UK, for example, is temazepam, which is relatively slowly absorbed and therefore has only a marginal effect on the sleep latency but facilitates sleep duration. The short elimination half-lives of drugs such as brotizolam ensure that residual sedative effects do not occur during the day. In contrast, fast elimination hypnotics such as midazolam and triazolam, which are effective in treating sleep onset insomnia, often give rise to rebound insomnia on withdrawal. It should be emphasized that the abrupt withdrawal of hypnotics, particularly when they have been given for several weeks or longer, is generally accompanied by REM rebound which results in an increased frequency of dreams and nightmares and can precipitate disturbed sleep and anxiety. Slow reduction in the night-time dose of the hypnotic over several days may reduce the risk of such a rebound.

Regarding the efficacy of hypnotics when used long-term, there is evidence that sleep latency shows more tolerance than sleep time. Furthermore, it is generally accepted that each hypnotic has a minimal effective dose and that increasing this does little to improve the duration of sleep but is more likely to increase the side effects.

Non-benzodiazepine hypnotics

These drugs comprise the barbiturates, alcohols and a new class of cyclopyrrolone hypnotics. Because of the severity of their side effects and their dependence potential, the barbiturates should not be used to treat insomnia.

The alcohol type of hypnotics include the chloral derivatives, of which *chloral hydrate* and *chlormethiazole* are still occasionally used in the elderly, and *ethchlorvynol*. Chloral hydrate is metabolized to another active sedative hypnotic *trichlorethanol*. These drugs all have a similar effect on the sleep profile. They are short half-life drugs (about 4–6 hours) that decrease the sleep latency and number of awakenings; slow-wave sleep is slightly depressed while the overall REM sleep time is largely unaffected, although the distribution of REM sleep may be disturbed. Chloral hydrate and its active metabolite have an unpleasant taste and cause epigastric distress and nausea. Undesirable effects of these drugs include lightheadedness, ataxia and nightmares, particularly in the elderly. Allergic skin reactions to chloral hydrate have been reported. Chronic use of these drugs can lead to tolerance and occasionally physical dependence. Like the barbiturates, overdosage can lead to respiratory and cardiovascular depression. Therapeutic use of these drugs has largely been superseded by the benzodiazepines.

Any new hypnotic should induce and maintain natural sleep without producing residual sedative effects during the day; it should not cause dependence or interact adversely with other sedatives, including alcohol. The *ideal hypnotic* should not cause respiratory depression or precipitate cardiovascular collapse when taken in overdose. *So far no drug fulfils all these criteria.*

Several new anxiolytic and sedative drugs act at the benzodiazepine receptor site, or one of the subsets that comprise this receptor site even though the chemical structure of these molecules differs substantially from the benzodiazepines. One of the first of these compounds to be developed was the cyclopyrrolone *zopiclone*. A structurally somewhat similar molecule *zolpidem*, an imidazopyridine, has also been marketed recently as has the beta-carboline *abercarnil*. Of the newer benzodiazepines, the tetracyclic 2, 4 benzodiazepine *bretazenil* has also been introduced as a short-acting sedative–hypnotic. The chemical structure of these molecules is illustrated in Figure 9.3.

Action of the newer sedative–hypnotic drugs on the benzodiazepine receptor

It is now well established that the GABA-A receptor, upon which both the typical and atypical sedative–hypnotics act to cause hyperpolarization of the central neurons, consists of at least four major subunits. Of these, the alpha, beta and gamma subunits each contain three to six variants. Two major classes of GABA-A receptors have been identified termed type I and II or omega I and II. The omega I site has been associated with the alpha 1 subunit whereas the omega II site appears to be heterogenous and located on GABA receptors with alpha 2, 3 and 5 subunits. Omega I sites predominate in the cerebellum and cortex whereas omega II sites predominate in the spinal cord. However, both omega I and II sites are widely distributed throughout the brain.

Pharmacological studies indicate that the 1, 4-benzodiazepines such as diazepam bind to both the omega I and II receptors with the triazolobenzodiazepines such as alprazolam and triazolam showing a particularly high affinity for these sites. The sedative hypnotic zopiclone, despite its non-benzodiazepine structure, has an affinity for the omega I and II sites that is similar to the typical 1, 4-benzodiazepines whereas zolpidem and abecarnil have a greater affinity for the omega I site.

Because of the adverse effects of the typical 1, 4-benzodiazepines (long-term sedation, dependence), attempts have been made to develop sedative–hypnotic drugs that have a lower propensity to cause these effects. This has led to the development of site-specific sedatives such as zolpidem while other approaches have led to drugs such as bretazenil, which is a partial

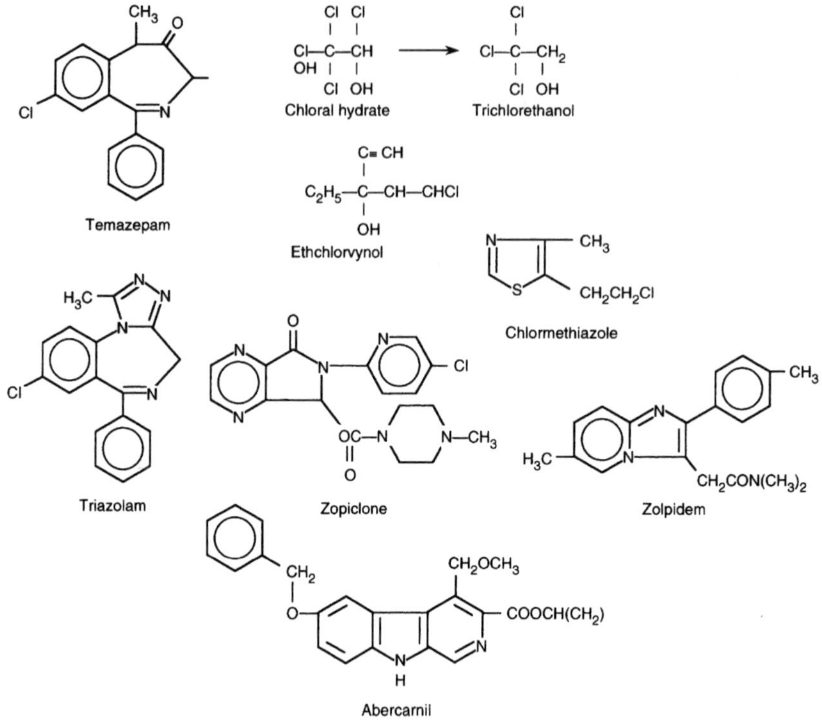

Figure 9.3. Chemical structure of some hypnotics.

agonist of both omega I and II receptors, and abercarnil which are full agonists for the omega I receptor. It is hoped that such novel drugs will lead to a reduction in dependence-producing side effects while maintaining the therapeutic efficacy exhibited by the typical 1, 4-benzodiazepines.

The therapeutic profile and adverse effects of the non-benzodiazepine sedative–hypnotics

Zopiclone was the first of the new sedative–hypnotics to be launched in the late 1970s and has been shown to be equi-effective with the standard sedative–hypnotic benzodiazepines such as flurazepam and temazepam. There is evidence that zopiclone may cause less "hang-over" effects than the conventional benzodiazepines but some studies have shown that this drug does produce performance decrement when this is tested shortly after treatment. A similar profile has been reported for zolpidem while abercarnil has been reported to cause a performance decrement for the first few days of treatment that then largely disappears. Bretazenil has been shown to cause dose-related disruptions in psychomotor performance, but these effects are not as prominent as occurs following an equivalent dose of diazepam or alprazolam. A somewhat unusual side effect has been described by patients taking zopiclone – a bitter, unpleasant taste and a dry mouth. The cause of these effects is presently unknown.

Regarding abuse liability, to date there have been only few studies in which newer sedative–hypnotics have been investigated. Nevertheless there is some evidence that those with a history of sedative abuse preferred high doses of triazolam and zopiclone to placebo. There is some evidence that bretazenil has a lower abuse potential than the benzodiazepines. Abuse liability of these novel sedative hypnotics has also been evaluated in primates. Abercarnil causes a lower incidence of withdrawal effects than conventional benzodiazepines. This may be due to the differences in the intrinsic efficacy rather than the bioavailability of these drugs for the brain. However, zopiclone and bretazenil did lower the seizure threshold to electroshock-induced seizures in mice whereas the seizure threshold was unaffected by zolpidem, tracozalate and C1 218, 872. In baboons zolpidem may cause physiological dependence; similar studies in monkeys show that mild withdrawal effects occur after the abrupt withdrawal of zopiclone, whereas withdrawal from diazepam caused severe symptoms. It may be concluded that sedative–hypnotic drugs with a limited efficacy such as bretazenil and zolpidem are also limited in their ability to cause physiological dependence.

In human studies, there is some evidence that withdrawal signs such as nervousness, anxiety and vertigo, occur following sub-chronic administration of zopiclone but the frequency and intensity of the withdrawal effects are greater after conventional 1, 4-benzodiazepines. No rebound affects have been seen in patients with insomnia who received zolpidem daily for 7–180 days. By contrast, after 3 weeks of abercarnil treatment of patients with generalized anxiety disorder possible signs of withdrawal resulted, the incidence of these withdrawal effects being related to doses of abercarnil administered.

From the published clinical studies, it would appear that the partial agonists bretazenil and abercarnil are less likely to cause physiological dependence, have lower reinforcing effects and a lower incidence of subjective effects associated with abuse liability than the conventional 1, 4-benzodiazepine sedative hypnotics. It is presently unclear whether the full agonists for the GABA-A receptor, zolpidem and zopiclone, offer a real advance in the treatment of insomnia although their adverse effect profiles and abuse liability may be lower than that of the conventional benzodiazepines.

The structure of some of the benzodiazepine and non-benzodiazepine hypnotics is shown in Figure 9.3.

In CONCLUSION, hypnotics are a widely used group of drugs accounting for about 15% of all prescriptions over the last four decades. The condition for which these drugs are prescribed, insomnia, is ill-defined. Various types of insomnia exist, and there are many possible causes. Most short-term insomnia is associated with stress and can be alleviated by the short-term administration of a hypnotic. Most long-term insomnia is associated with psychiatric illness or drug or alcohol abuse and therefore careful investigation and evaluation of the patient is necessary before hypnotics should be considered. As with all psychotropic drugs, the elderly patient is most likely to experience unwanted side effects such as sedation and day-time drowsiness. Of the different classes of hypnotics available, the benzodiazepines, particularly those with medium or short elimination half-lives, are the most widely used. The rule which should always be applied in the prescribing of hypnotics is that the smallest effective dose should be prescribed for the shortest time necessary to treat the sleep disturbance.

10 Drug Treatment of Schizophrenia and the Psychoses

Introduction

Schizophrenia is a group of illnesses of unknown origin that occur in approximately 1% of the adult population in most countries in which surveys have been conducted. The economic and social cost is considerable, as approximately 40% of all hospitalized psychiatric patients in most industrialized countries suffer from schizophrenia and related disorders. At least 25 major family studies have been published in the last three decades that have consistently shown that the risk for the disease in the relatives of schizophrenics is substantially greater than that expected in the general population. While most of these studies have been criticized on methodological grounds, it is generally accepted that schizophrenia does have a genetic basis.

Schizophrenia usually begins during adolescence or young adulthood and is characterized by a spectrum of symptoms that typically include disordered thought, social withdrawal, hallucinations (both aural and visual), delusions of persecution (paranoia) and bizarre behaviour. These symptoms are sometimes categorized as "positive" (e.g. hallucinations) and "negative" (e.g. social withdrawal and apathy). So far, there is no known cure and the disease is chronic and generally progressive. Nevertheless the introduction of the phenothiazine neuroleptic chlorpromazine by Delay and Denecker in France in 1952 initiated the era of pharmacotherapy in psychiatric medicine and has led to the marketing of many dozens of chemically diverse antipsychotic drugs that have played a major role in limiting the disintegration of the personality of the schizophrenic patient. Drugs used to treat psychotic disorders such as schizophrenia are called *neuroleptics, antipsychotics* or *major tranquillizers*.

Although the discovery that chlorpromazine and related phenothiazine neuroleptics were effective in the treatment of schizophrenia was serendipitous, investigators soon attempted to define the mechanism of action of this group of drugs that had begun to revolutionize psychiatric treatment. It was hoped that the elucidation of the mechanism of action of

185

such neuroleptics would not only enable more selective and potent drugs to be discovered, but also give some insight into the pathology of schizophrenia.

A major advance came with the discovery that chlorpromazine, haloperidol and other related neuroleptics not only antagonized the stimulant action of L-dopa (levodopa) in animals but also enhanced the accumulation of the main metabolites of dopamine and noradrenaline in rat brain. These findings led to the suggestion that the neuroleptics must be blocking the postsynaptic receptors for dopamine, and to some extent noradrenaline, thereby leading to a stimulation of the presynaptic nerve terminal through a feedback mechanism. The seminal paper by Carlsson and Lindqvist in 1963 helped to lay the basis for the dopamine hypothesis for schizophrenia and the mode of action of neuroleptic drugs. Later studies in Canada and the United States of America showed that there is a good correlation between the average clinical dose of neuroleptic administered and the affinity of the drug for postsynaptic dopamine receptors. The dopamine hypothesis of schizophrenia has reasonably good support from pharmacological studies, but the supporting evidence from post-mortem material, and from studies on schizophrenic patients using techniques such as positron emission tomography (PET), are more controversial. Whatever the final outcome, however, the dopamine hypothesis has had a major impact on drug development and, even though dopamine may not be the only neurotransmitter involved in the illness, it is leading to an investigation of the interconnection between dopamine and other transmitters which may be more directly involved in the pathology of the illness.

Neuropathological aspects

Variable patchy gliosis and neuronal loss have been reported to occur in the schizophrenic brain, but such changes would not appear to be specific to the disease. It has been suggested that these changes are a manifestation of an inflammatory reaction, possibly due to a virus infection; cytomegalovirus has been specifically implicated. However, there would now appear to be little support for the virus hypothesis of schizophrenia. More recently, detailed analysis of the neuronal architecture of the hippocampal and cortical regions of the schizophrenic brain suggests that a region of the parahippocampal gyrus is abnormal, possibly due to a disturbance of neuronal migration in a late phase of cortical development. Varying degrees of pyramidal cell disorientation in the hippocampus and reduced parahippocampal width suggest structural abnormalities in the basal cortical regions of the temporal lobe.

Computed axial tomography (CAT) scan studies of the brains of schizophrenics have led to a renewed interest in the possibility that neuronal loss is causally connected with the disease. Most studies have implied that the ventricular size is increased, particularly in older patients, such structural changes being associated with neuropsychological impairment and negative symptoms of the disease, but not all investigators have found such correlations. Other CAT studies have shown that in right-handed patients there may be a lesion of the left hemisphere which correlates with the degree of psychological defect and with the occurrence of delusions. PET studies also suggest that the rate of glucose utilization by the left cortical lobe is slightly diminished in the schizophrenic patient. It is of interest that neurochemical studies of transmitters and their synthesizing enzymes also show asymmetry, with a higher concentration of dopamine and a higher activity of choline acetyltransferase in the left basal ganglia of the normal brain. The concentration of dopamine would appear to be greater in the left amygdala of the schizophrenic brain.

Neurotransmitters and the pathogenesis of schizophrenia

In its original form, the dopamine hypothesis of schizophrenia postulated that the positive symptoms of the illness arose as a consequence of the hyperactivity of the dopaminergic system, particularly in the mesocortico-limbic region of the brain that originated in the ventral tegmental area. It is now realized that this is a gross over-simplification and recently attempts have been made to develop the dopamine hypothesis to take into account the neurochemical changes that may underline both the positive and negative symptoms of the condition.

It is well known that atypical neuroleptics, all of which have a high affinity for dopamine receptors (particularly D_2 receptors), do not effectively treat all schizophrenic patients and have only limited beneficial effects on the negative symptoms of the illness. Furthermore, neither typical nor atypical neuroleptics have an immediate effect on the positive symptoms even though it can be shown by both experimental studies in animals and by imaging methods in schizophrenic patients that neuroleptics rapidly bind to dopamine receptors. Thus factors other than an overactive dopaminergic system are probably operative in this disorder. The question is which of the numerous neurotransmitters and modulatory neuropeptides are responsible for both the negative symptoms and the delay in onset of the therapeutic effects of neuroleptics on the positive symptoms?

The deficit syndrome of schizophrenia, characterized by prominent negative symptoms, is presumed to be due to diminished prefrontal cortical activity. In experimental studies in patients, these symptoms often show response to dopaminergic agonists. As there are no dopamine autoreceptors on dopamine terminals in the cortex of the brain, it must be assumed that such agonists are acting on postsynaptic dopamine receptors to alleviate the negative symptoms. A diminished frontal cortical activity, as shown by PET studies for example, appears to be a characteristic feature of the untreated schizophrenic patient which would support the view that, at least in some patients, cortical dopaminergic activity is lower than normal and is not globally increased as was postulated by the original dopamine hypothesis.

Recently, attempts have been made to reconcile the deficiencies in the dopamine hypothesis by focusing on other neurotransmitters that may interact with dopamine in discrete cortical and subcortical neural circuits. In particular, the involvement of the glutamatergic system has received considerable attention. This possibility has arisen from the finding that dissociation anaesthetics such as ketamine and phencyclidine (PCP) can cause a schizophreniform psychosis in normal individuals. Such effects bear a much closer resemblance to the positive and negative symptoms of schizophreniform psychosis than the changes elicited by amphetamine which produced changes that more closely resemble the positive symptoms of the condition. In schizophrenic patients, PCP has also been shown to exacerbate a psychotic episode.

As will be discussed in detail later (see Chapter 14) PCP is a non-competitive inhibitor of the N-methyl-D-aspartate (NMDA) subtype of the glutamate receptor. This has led to the suggestion that schizophrenia may be associated with a decreased glutamatergic activity particularly in cortical regions of the brain.

Glutamate is the most important excitatory neurotransmitter in the brain, probably influencing more than 50% of all synapses. The major glutamatergic system involves a projection from the cortex to the striatum. Thus the hypofunctioning of the cortex may be a reflection of the diminished glutamatergic and dopaminergic activity in that area of the brain. It has been suggested that dopamine hetero receptors may regulate the release of glutamate in the striatum which could help to verify the hypothesis implicating both glutamate and dopamine in the aetiology of schizophrenia. This forms the basis of the hypothesis proposed by Arvid Carlsson that schizophrenia arises due to an abnormality in the dopamine–glutamate systems in the corticostriatal pallido-thalamic circuit.

In addition to an abnormality in the corticostriatal system, it is also possible that a disorder in the dopamine–glutamate system occurs in other subcortical regions which could account for some of the symptoms seen in schizophrenia. The hippocampus and the associated entorhinal cortex are important areas of the brain concerned in memory formation, information processing and the generation of specimen-specific behaviours. Neuropsy-chological tests in schizophrenic patients have occasionally been shown to be abnormal and the cytoarchitecture and other morphological changes in the hippocampus and entorhinal cortex suggest that the positive symptoms of the illness may originate within the hippocampus. These regions of the brain are innervated by the dopaminergic system while glutamate is the predominant intrinsic excitatory transmitter in the hippocampus. Thus a dysfunction of the hippocampal dopamine–glutamate system in these areas could also account for the positive symptoms of the illness.

In Chapter 14, the complexity of the glutamatergic system is briefly outlined. Four distinct families of glutamate receptors were described of which the alpha-amino-3-hydroxy-5-methyl-4-isoxazole proprionic acid (AMPA) and the NMDA glutamate receptors have been most extensively studied. Recently the cloning of both NMDA and non-NMDA (for example, AMPA) receptor genes has enabled receptor expression at the transcriptional level to be made. Such techniques are much more sensitive than those used previously that relied on the binding of a radioactive ligand to a glutamatic receptor. Using this technique of *in situ* hybridization it has been shown that, after 2 weeks of treatment of rats with either haloperidol or clozapine (representing a typical and an atypical neuroleptic respectively) substantial alteration occurs in non-NMDA receptors in the hippocampus. It has been postulated that one of the functions of neuroleptics is to "up-regulate" some types of non-NMDA glutamate receptors in the cortex and hippocampus, thereby leading to an amelioration of the symptoms of schizophrenia. It is of interest that there were some subtle differences in the changes in the glutamate receptor subtypes between haloperidol and clozapine which may account for the greater efficacy of clozapine in the treatment of the negative features of schizophrenia. It now remains to be shown that similar changes occur in the schizophrenic patient following therapeutically effective doses of typical and atypical neuroleptics. Nevertheless such studies do help to extend the dopamine hypothesis to explain the neurochemical basis of the positive and negative symptoms, the selectivity of the atypical neuroleptics in ameliorating the negative symptoms and, partly, the reason why it is necessary to administer neuroleptics for several weeks before optimal therapeutic benefit is obtained by the patient.

Effects of neuroleptics on dopaminergic and other neurotransmitter systems

Because of the discovery that all neuroleptics in clinical use are dopamine receptor agonists, and that an abnormality in the dopaminergic system might underlie the pathology of the condition, the action of neuroleptics on the dopaminergic system has been extensively studied over the past two decades. Four major anatomical divisions of the dopaminergic system have been described:

1. *The nigrostriatal system*, in which fibres originate from the A9 region of the pars compacta and project rostrally to become widely distributed in the caudate nucleus and the putamen.
2. *The mesolimbic system*, where the dopaminergic projections originate in the ventral tegmental area, the A10 region, and then spread to the amygdala, pyriform cortex, lateral septal nuclei and the nucleus accumbens.
3. *The mesocortical system*, in which the dopaminergic fibres also arise from the A10 region (the ventral tegmental area) and project to the frontal cortex and septo-hippocampal regions.
4. *The tuberoinfundibular system*, which originates in the arcuate nucleus of the hypothalamus and projects to the median eminence.

Following its release, dopamine produces its physiological effects by activating postsynaptic receptors which have been classified into the D_1 and D_2 families. The D_1 *receptors* are linked to adenylate cyclase which, when activated, produces cyclic AMP as a secondary messenger. The D_2 *receptors* are not positively linked to adenylate cyclase and may owe their physiological effects to their ability to inhibit this enzyme. The D_2 receptors are probably the most important postsynaptic receptors mediating behavioural and extrapyramidal activity. Most therapeutically effective neuroleptics block the D_2 receptors, while drugs like bromocriptine, which is a dopamine receptor agonist used in the treatment of parkinsonism, activate them. The correlation between the antagonist effect of a series of neuroleptics on brain D_2 receptors and their appropriate therapeutic potency is shown in Figure 10.1. It should be emphasized that recent studies on the effects of atypical neuroleptics on the D_2 *receptors* in mammalian and D_4 brain show an even better correlation between receptor antagonism and the therapeutic dose.

Agonist stimulation of D_1 receptors results in cyclic adenosine monophosphate (cyclic AMP) synthesis followed by phosphorylation of intracellular proteins, including dopamine- and AMP-regulated phosphoprotein (DARPP-32). The receptor binding affinity of a dopamine agonist is dependent on the degree of association of the receptor and the guanine nucleotide binding regulatory protein, which is regulated by guanosine triphosphate (GTP) and calcium or magnesium ions. Thus the D_1 receptor may exist in a high or low agonist affinity state depending on the balance between CTP (which favours low affinity) and the divalent cations (which favour high affinity). The high affinity D_1 receptor is classified as a D_5 receptor.

The D_3 and D_4 receptors appear to be largely restricted to the limbic areas of the rat and human brain. These receptors are of particular interest as they have a high affinity for such atypical neuroleptics as clozapine. Such findings suggest that the D_3 and D_4 receptors in the human brain may mediate the

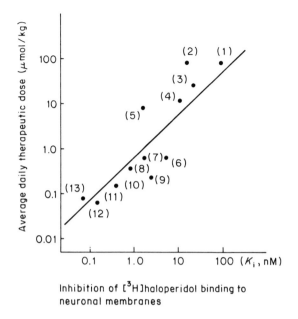

Inhibition of [³H]haloperidol binding to
neuronal membranes

Figure 10.1. Correlation between the average daily dose of various neuroleptics and their affinity for D_2 receptors. (1)= promazine; (2)=chlorpromazine; (3)=thioridazine; (4)=clozapine; (5)=triflupromazine; (6)=penfluridol; (7)=trifluoperazine; (8)=fluphenazine; (9)=haloperidol; (10)=pimozide; (11)=fluspirilene; (12)=benperidol; (13)=spiroperidol (spiperone).

antipsychotic actions of many typical and atypical neuroleptics. The restriction of these receptors to the limbic regions may also lead to the development of neuroleptics which are specifically targeted to these areas. This may assist in the development of drugs that combine antipsychotic potency with reduced extrapyramidal side effects.

In the mammalian brain, the D_1 receptors are located postsynaptically in the striatum, nucleus accumbens, olfactory tubercle, substantia nigra, etc., but their precise physiological function in the brain is currently unclear. The partial D_1 receptor agonist SKF 38393 stimulates grooming and stereotypic motor behaviour in rodents, effects that are blocked by the D_1 antagonist SCH 23390. This antagonist also blocks the behaviour initiated by the selective D_2 receptor agonist quinpirole (LY 171555), which suggests that there is a functional interaction between the D_1 and the D_2 receptors.

Unlike the D_1 receptor, the function of the D_2 receptor in the brain is at least partially understood. The anterior lobe mammotrophs of the pituitary control lactation via prolactin release, and dopamine acting on the D_2 receptor in this area acts as the *prolactin release inhibitory factor*. In the intermediate lobe of the rat, dopamine inhibits alpha melanocyte-stimulating hormone release. In the striatum, D_2 receptors inhibit acetylcholine release, while on the dopaminergic nerve terminals the D_2 receptors function as autoreceptors and inhibit the release of dopamine. D_2 receptors occur on the dopaminergic neurons in the substantia nigra where they inhibit the firing of the neurons. In man, these receptors stimulate growth hormone release. Lastly, in the *chemoreceptor trigger zone*, stimulation of the D_2 receptors elicits emesis. The selective agonist for D_2 receptors is quinpirole (LY 171555), while the selective antagonist is spiroperidol (spiperone).

Increased motor activity and stereotypic behaviour arises as a result of the activation of central D_2 receptors in rodents, while in man psychosis, stereotypic behaviour and thought disorders occur. Conversely, neuroleptic drugs with selective D_2 antagonist properties (e.g. the benzamides such as sulpiride) are antipsychotic and can lead to parkinsonism in man or catalepsy in rodents, although the propensity of the benzamide neuroleptics to cause these effects is much less than the phenothiazine neuroleptics that have mixed D_1 and D_2 receptor antagonist properties. The butyrophenone neuroleptics such as haloperidol are approximately 100 times more potent in acting as D_2 receptor antagonists than as D_1 antagonists.

The results of such studies suggest that the major classes of neuroleptics in therapeutic use owe their activity to their ability to block D_2 and/or D_1 receptors, particularly in the mesocortical and mesolimbic regions of the brain. Side effects, such as parkinsonism and increased prolactin release, would seem to be associated with the antagonistic effects of these drugs on D_2 and/or D_1 receptors in the nigrostriatal and tuberoinfundibular systems.

While the precise importance of D_1 and D_2 receptors in the clinical effects of neuroleptics is still uncertain, there is experimental evidence from studies in primates that oral dyskinesia (which may be equivalent to tardive dyskinesia in man) is related to an imbalance in D_1 and D_2 receptor function, the dyskinesia arising from a relative overactivity of the D_1 receptors. Thus the elucidation of the precise function of these receptor subtypes may be important not only in determining the mode of action of neuroleptics but also in understanding their side effects.

The relationship between pre- and postsynaptic receptors and a summary of the suspected sites of action of the different classes of drugs that modulate the functioning of the dopaminergic system in the striatum are shown in Figure 10.2.

While there is extensive experimental evidence showing that all clinically effective neuroleptic drugs block dopamine receptors, and a general agreement that blockade of the D_2 receptors in the mesocortical regions is particularly important for antipsychotic activity, only with the advent of PET has it been possible to determine the relative importance of these receptor subtypes in schizophrenia patients on neuroleptic therapy. Using PET the

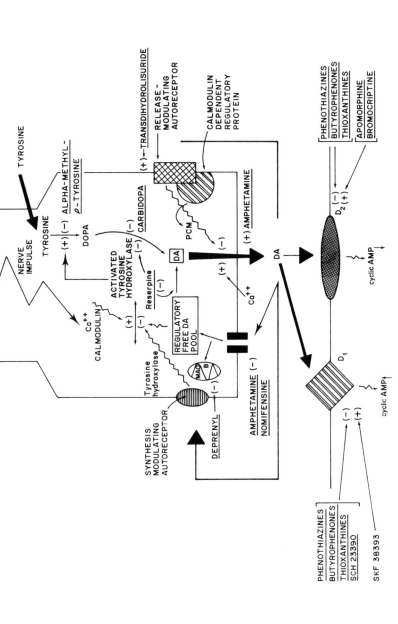

Figure 10.2. Schematic diagram of the possible sites of action of drugs that modify dopaminergic function in striatal and other non-mesocortical regions of the mammalian brain. PCM=protein;O-methyltransferase, which catalyses the transfer of methyl groups from S-adenosylmethionine to the calmodulin-dependent regulatory protein and may regulate calcium–calmodulin dependent transmitter synthesis and release. (−)=inhibition; (+)=stimulation; DA=dopamine. Sites of action of drugs are underlined.

Table 10.1. Classification of dopamine receptors

D_1-like receptors	
DIA	This is the "classical" D_1 receptor. "Classical" neuroleptics such as the phenothiazines and butyrophenones act as antagonists of these receptors.
DIB/$_{D5}$	These receptors are present in a low density in most brain regions. The highest density of these receptors is in the corticolimbic area of the brain. So far, their function is obscure and no selective antagonists are known.
D_2-like receptors	
D_2 "long" and "short" forms (D_{2A}, D_{2B})	These are the "classical" D_2 receptors. All effective neuroleptics act as antagonists of these receptors. Some atypical neuroleptics such as remoxipride may show selectivity for the D_{2B} receptors which are present in limbic regions of the brain.
D_3	These are largely restricted to the corticolimbic region of the brain. No specific functions have been elucidated nor have selective antagonists so far been developed.
D_4	Novel receptors that are largely restricted to the corticolimbic region. No specific functions have been elucidated. Clozapine, the atypical neuroleptic, blocks these receptors.

occupancy of D_2 receptors in the cortical regions of the brains of schizophrenics treated with phenothiazines (chlorpromazine, trifluoperazine or perphenazine), a thioxanthine (flupenthixol), butyrophenones (haloperidol or melperone), a diphenylbutylpiperazine (pimozide) or the atypical neuroleptics sulpiride, raclopride or clozapine has been calculated. The results of this study with this structurally disparate group of drugs showed that 65–89% of the D_2 receptors were occupied. Other investigators have also shown that over 70% of D_2 receptors are occupied in the brains of schizophrenics following effective treatment with melperone. In contrast, no D_1 receptors were occupied by sulpiride or perphenazine, while 42% of these receptors were occupied by clozapine. From such a study it may be speculated that a D_2 receptor antagonist action may be essential for the therapeutic effect of neuroleptics.

A summary of the new families of dopamine receptors and their distribution and properties is shown in Table 10.1.

Mechanism of action of neuroleptics

Laborit in the early 1950s is credited with the observation that chlorpromazine had a "calming" effect in disturbed schizophrenic patients and since that time psychopharmacologists have sought to explain the mechanism of action of neuroleptic drugs. Carlsson and Linquist in 1963 demonstrated a link between the therapeutic effects of the phenothiazine neuroleptics and an inhibition of dopamine receptor function. This led to the dopamine hypothesis of schizophrenia which postulated that psychosis was associated with an increase in dopaminergic function in the brain and that neuroleptics alleviate the symptoms of the illness by blocking the receptors that are specifically activated by dopamine. Later, during the 1970s, it was shown that the antipsychotic action of neuroleptics was correlated with their affinity to block dopamine receptors *in vitro*. It was discovered, by Kebabian and Calne in 1979, that dopamine receptors could be classified into two specific types, D_1 and D_2, and that there was a good correlation between the therapeutic potency of the phenothiazine neuroleptics and haloperidol and their affinity for the D_2 receptors. With the introduction of molecular cloning techniques it has now been possible to define at least five distinct subtypes of the dopamine receptor in the human brain as well as two variants (termed isoforms) of the original D_2 receptor. These different subtypes of the dopamine receptor may be broadly classified into those resembling the original D_1 receptor (D_1 and D_5) and those resembling the D_2 receptor (D_2, D_3 and D_4).

The neuroleptics that are widely available may be divided into two general categories, those with low potency (such as chlorpromazine and thioridazine) and those with a high potency (exemplified by haloperidol, trifluoperazine and pimozide). The former groups have a lower propensity to cause extrapyramidal side effects but are more sedative and likely to cause postural hypotension and have anticholinergic side effects. *In vitro* studies have shown that chlorpromazine has an affinity for all five types of dopamine receptor and has some preference for D_2 and D_3 receptors. By contrast, haloperidol is more potent than chlorpromazine for the D_2, D_3 and D_4 receptors with a low affinity for the D_1 and D_5 receptors (see Table 10.2).

In addition to their affinity for dopamine receptors, which appears to be essential for their therapeutic activity, all neuroleptics in current clinical use have affinities for other types of neurotransmitter receptor. Mention has already been made of the side effects of the weaker neuroleptics such as chlorpromazine, for histamine-1, muscarinic and alpha-1 adrenoceptors. However, it is now apparent that many of the newer, atypical, neuroleptics have an affinity for subtypes of 5-hydroxytryptamine (5-HT) receptors which may be beneficial in reducing the frequency of extrapyramidal side effects. Thus neuroleptics may now be broadly classified into those which are selective antagonists of D_2 receptors, those that are D_2 and D_3 receptor antagonists, those blocking both D_1 and D_2 receptors and, a most important group of novel neuroleptics, those that are antagonists of $5-HT_2$ and D_2 receptors.

Table 10.2. Receptor affinities for some atypical neuroleptics

Receptor type	Clozapine	Olanza-pine	Remoxi-pride	Risperi-done	Haloperidol
Dopamine					
D_1	85	31	n.a.	75	10
D_{2L}	60	11	125	1.5	0.5
D_{2S}	35	11	54	1.5	0.5
D_3	300	–	n.a.	6.7	2.0
D_4	9	27	n.a.	–	2.0
D_5	35	–	–	–	27
5-Hydroxytryptamine					
5-HT_{1A}	875	n.a.	n.a.	16	n.a.
5-HT_{2A}	8	5	n.a.	0.6	74.
5-HT_{2C}	12	23	n.a.	16	n.a.
5-HT_3	170	140	n.a.	n.a.	n.a.
5-HT_6	4	2.5	n.a.	425	n.a.
5-HT_7	6.3	104	n.a.	1.4	263
Cholinergic					
M_1	1.8	1.9	n.a.	n.a.	n.a.
M_2	21	18	n.a.	n.a.	n.a.
M_3	13	25	n.a.	n.a.	n.a.
M_4	12	13	n.a.	n.a.	n.a.
M_5	3.7	–	n.a.	n.a.	n.a.
Adrenergic					
$Alpha_1$	7	19	n.a.	2	46
$Alpha_2$	8	280	n.a.	3	360
$Beta_1$	n.a.	n.a.	n.a.	n.a.	n.a.
Others					
$Histamine_1$	6	7	n.a.	155	n.a.
Sigma	n.a.	–	60	–	5

Values expressed as the inhibition constant (m nM) which reflects the affinity of the drug for the receptor, i.e. the lower the value the greater the affinity.
n.a.=no affinity at concentrations lower than 2000 nM.
–=no data available.

Atypical neuroleptics

An important breakthrough in the development of novel neuroleptics arose over 25 years ago with the discovery of the dibenzazepine neuroleptic clozapine. This neuroleptic was novel because it attenuated both the positive and negative symptoms of schizophrenia without causing extrapyramidal side effects on elevating serum prolactin concentrations, effects which characterize most typical neuroleptics such as chlorpromazine and haloperidol.

Despite its novel therapeutic profile, it was soon evident that clozapine occasionally caused agranulocytosis, a potentially fatal immune condition, in approximately 3% of patients. The use of clozapine was therefore restricted largely to patients who suffered severe side effects with the typical neuroleptics, who were resistant to conventional neuroleptics or who had a high proportion of negative symptoms. Thus, clozapine has served as a useful prototype for the development of new neuroleptics and these will be briefly described.

   Clozapine binds with a high affinity (in the nanomolar range) to D_4 and D_2 receptors and with lower affinity for the D_1, D_3 and D_5 receptors. The finding that clozapine had a high affinity for the D_4 receptors was particularly exciting when it was discovered that an elevated expression of D_4 receptors occurred in the brains of schizophrenic patients. However, more recent studies have shown that clozapine also binds with a high affinity to the short form of the D_2 receptor. Further evidence for the relative lack of specificity of clozapine, not only for different types of dopamine receptors but also for 5-HT, muscarinic, adrenergic and histaminergic receptors, suggests that it is a neuroleptic with a very broad basis of action. However, the beneficial effects of clozapine (and other atypical neuroleptics such as risperidone, seroquel and sertindole), may be due to its selective effects on mesolimbic and mesocortical dopaminergic neurons. Clinical and experimental studies suggest that such atypical neuroleptics decrease the negative symptoms of schizophrenia by enhancing prefrontal dopaminergic activity while decreasing the activity of this transmitter in the mesolimbic system, thereby attenuating the psychotic symptoms of schizophrenia. Experimental studies also show that clozapine, and other novel atypical neuroleptics, have little effect on the activity of the nigrostriatal dopaminergic system which probably accounts for the low incidence of extrapyramidal side effects seen with these drugs. Clozapine and several other atypical neuroleptics are also potent inhibitors of 5-HT$_2$ type receptors, particularly the 5-HT$_{2A}$ and 5-HT$_{2C}$ subtypes (see Table 10.2) and it has been postulated that their antipsychotic action combined with a low propensity to cause extrapyramidal side effects may be attributable to the antagonism of 5-HT$_{2A}$ receptors combined with an inhibition of mesocortical D_2 receptors. The experimental evidence to support this view arises from findings that stimulation of 5-HT$_{2A}$ receptors enhances the synthesis and release of dopamine in the rat brain. Conversely 5-HT$_{2A}$ receptor antagonists reduce the stimulant effects of amphetamine, a drug that in high doses can produce symptoms of paranoid schizophrenia, possibly due to its ability to release dopamine in the mesocortical and mesolimbic regions of the brain.

   Partly as a result of the extensive experimental and clinical studies which have been carried out on clozapine in recent years there have been two major approaches to the development of atypical neuroleptics. The first approach has been to develop drugs which broadly simulate the pharmacological profile of clozapine but which lack the adverse haematological effects. Olanzapine is an example of a drug in the advanced stage of development which is based on this principle. The second approach has involved targeting specific dopamine receptors located in the forebrain. Remoxipride is an example of a drug which appears to have a selectivity for the D_2 receptor subtype (D_{2S}) located in the limbic forebrain. Clearly the aim of such developments is to produce neuroleptics that attenuate both the positive and negative symptoms of schizophrenia without causing extrapyramidal side effects.

Pharmacological profiles of some novel atypical neuroleptics

Olanzapine, like clozapine, has a broad spectrum of action on dopamine, 5-HT, adrenergic, histamine$_1$ and muscarinic receptors (see Table 10.2). While the precise significance is presently unclear, it is of interest that whereas clozapine binds with a high affinity to 5-HT$_6$ and 5-HT$_7$ receptors, olanzapine only shows a high affinity for 5-HT$_6$ receptors.

Clinical studies have demonstrated that olanzapine has a similar profile to clozapine without causing agranulocytosis; preliminary studies also show that it does not cause extrapyramidal side effects or increase prolactin release.

Risperidone has been developed as a combined D_2/5-HT$_{2A}$ receptor antagonist. In addition, it has a high affinity for 5-HT$_{1A}$ and 5-HT$_7$ receptors. Whether such an effect has any relevance to its beneficial effects on the negative symptoms of schizophrenia, and lack of extrapyramidal side effects at moderate therapeutic doses, is unknown. An important advantage of risperidone over clozapine lies in its lack of antagonism of muscarinic receptors.

Remoxipride is a selective D_2 antagonist with higher affinity for the D_{2S} subtype of receptors. It has no affinity for 5-HT, adrenergic, muscarinic or histamine receptors but, unlike the other atypical neuroleptics, does bind to sigma receptors (see p. 345 for possible importance of sigma receptors).

In clinical studies, remoxipride has been shown to improve both positive and negative symptoms of schizophrenia and may have a place in the treatment of resistant schizophrenic patients. In addition such side effects as the neuroleptic-induced deficit syndrome, sedation and extrapyramidal side effects are apparently absent in patients treated with the drug. Unfortunately, a few cases of aplastic anaemia have been reported which may be drug related. This has led to the untimely withdrawal of the drug from the European market.

These three examples of atypical neuroleptics with different pharmacological profiles to clozapine merely serve as an illustration of the structural and pharmacological diversity of atypical neuroleptics. In addition to olanzapine, risperidone and remoxipride other novel neuroleptics in various stages of clinical development include *seroquel, sertindole, ziprasidone, amperozide* and *fluperlapine* all of which have antagonistic effects on 5-HT$_{2A}$/D_2 receptors.

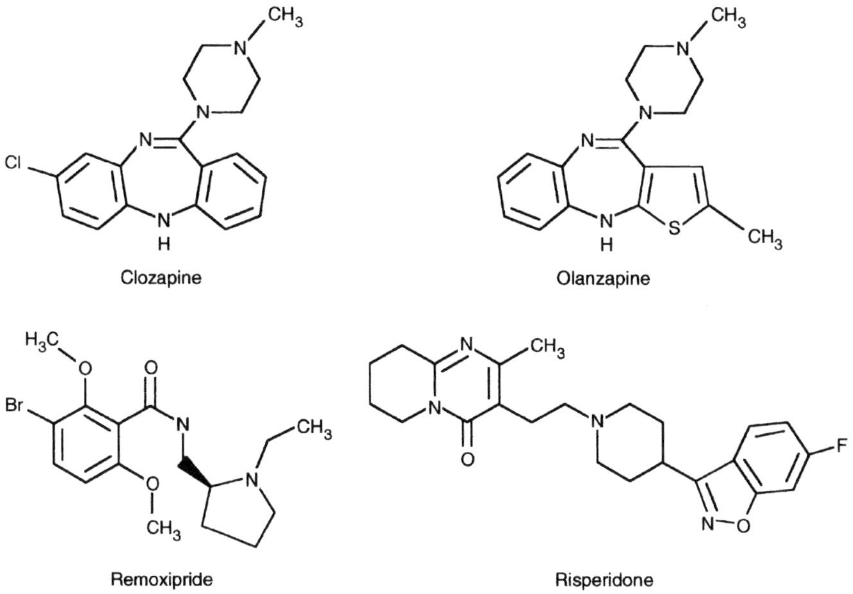

Figure 10.3. Chemical structure of selected atypical antipsychotics.

The chemical structures of these atypical neuroleptics is shown in Figure 10.3.

Tardive dyskinesia

This syndrome was first described by Schonecker within 5 years of the introduction of the neuroleptics. It comprises involuntary movements of the tongue, lips and face (such as protrusion or twisting of the tongue, lip smacking, puffing of the cheeks, sucking of the lips and chewing) often combined with abnormal involuntary movements of the trunk and limbs, termed choreiform or choreoathetoid movements. Despite the association of tardive dyskinesia with the introduction of neuroleptics, it is evident that 5–15% of elderly people who have never received neuroleptics also show an orofacial dyskinesia, the prevalence rate of the condition in schizophrenic patients on neuroleptics being variously reported to be between 0.5 and 56% (mean of 20%).

Factors predisposing a patient to tardive dyskinesia include age, sex (female patients show a greater prevalence), presence of brain damage, early susceptibility to drug-induced extrapyramidal side effects and the presence of a primary affective disorder. In patients with such predisposing factors, the presence of neuroleptics may precipitate the onset of the syndrome. In addition, the schizophrenic illness itself may be a risk factor as there is evidence from clinical reports published long before the advent of neuroleptics that abnormal movements similar to tardive dyskinesia occurred. Recent evidence further suggests that schizophrenic patients with pronounced negative symptoms (e.g. blunting of affect and social withdrawal) are more likely to develop the syndrome than those with primarily positive symptoms (hallucinations, delusions, etc.). Clearly the somewhat simplistic view advanced some years ago that tardive dyskinesia was due to dopamine receptor supersensitivity resulting from prolonged dopamine receptor blockade by a neuroleptic is now redundant.

Despite the diversity of drugs which have been tried for the *treatment of tardive dyskinesia*, no satisfactory drug therapy exists to date. In some cases the short-acting reserpine analogue tetrabenazine has been used with limited success. More recently, some success has been claimed for the calcium channel blockers verapamil and diltiazem, and for the antioxidant alpha-tocopherol (vitamin E), but double-blind controlled studies are still needed to validate the efficacy of such treatments. Clearly, since neuroleptics may precipitate this syndrome, it is essential that such drugs be prescribed only when clearly indicated, at a minimum effective dose and for only as long as their beneficial effects are clearly needed. Concurrent anticholinergic drug administration leads to a worsening of the symptoms of tardive dyskinesia, and the possibility of the syndrome arising is much greater in patients over the age of 50.

Recently it has been found that haloperidol and several putative atypical neuroleptics such as rimcazole, BMY 14802 and HR 375 have a high affinity for sigma receptors in the mammalian brain. It is now established that the sigma receptors (see p. 347) are different from the phencyclidine receptors which are located in the ion channel of the NMDA receptor complex. Drugs like N-allylnormetazocine (NANM) and (+) pentazocine for example, bind specifically to sigma sites but not to the phencyclidine sites thereby enabling the two receptor sites to be distinguished. However, it must be emphasized that not all neuroleptics have an affinity for the sigma receptors and furthermore drugs such as rimcazole and BMY 14802 have questionable antipsychotic activity. Nevertheless it is possible that some atypical neuroleptics may owe some of their therapeutic activity to their action on sigma receptors. The possible significance of sigma receptors to the action of different classes of psychotropic drugs is discussed in Chapter 18.

It may be concluded that despite the importance of the dopamine hypothesis of schizophrenia in serving to unify the mechanism of action of both typical and atypical neuroleptics, it is apparent that some serotonin receptor subtypes, and glutamate receptors of the NMDA subtype, may also play a crucial role.

Action of neuroleptics on different types of neurotransmitter receptor: relevance to side effects

In recent years traditional neuroleptics, as exemplified by chlorpromazine, have been structurally modified to produce drugs with greater affinity for dopamine receptors while retaining some of their activity on other receptor systems (e.g. on alpha$_1$ adrenoceptors, 5-HT$_2$ receptors and histamine$_1$ receptors). In the non-phenothiazine series, a high degree of specificity for the D$_2$ receptors has been achieved with sulpiride and pimozide, with haloperidol showing antagonistic effects on the 5-HT$_2$ and alpha$_1$ adrenoceptors in addition to its selectivity for D$_2$ receptors. The cis-(Z) isomers of the thioxanthines are potent neuroleptics that, in addition to their selectivity for D$_2$ receptors, also show antagonistic effects on D$_1$, 5-HT$_2$ and alpha$_1$ adrenergic receptors; cis-(Z)-flupenthixol has a greater effect on D$_1$ receptors than cis-(Z)-clopenthixol.

In the phenothiazine series of neuroleptics, thioridazine has less antimuscarinic potency than chlorpromazine, but appears to be equally active as an antagonist of 5-HT$_2$ and D$_2$ receptors; like chlorpromazine, however, it is a potent alpha$_1$ adrenoceptor antagonist. In contrast, the potent phenothiazine neuroleptic perphenazine is only slightly less selective in blocking D$_2$ receptors than haloperidol but, unlike the latter, has a greater antagonistic effect on histamine receptors.

The *atypical neuroleptics*, exemplified by clozapine and fluperlapine, have relatively low affinity for either D$_1$ or D$_2$ receptors but a major antagonistic action on 5-HT$_2$ receptors. It should be noted, however, that clozapine has some preferential, although unselective, action *in vivo* as a D$_1$ receptor antagonist. Clozapine also shows a high affinity for the D$_4$ receptors. Both these drugs are fairly potent antihistamines and alpha$_1$ adrenoceptor antagonists; fluperlapine also has antimuscarinic properties. Extreme selectivity for neurotransmitter receptors is shown by SCH 23390, which is highly selective as a D$_1$ receptor antagonist with only a slight antagonistic effect on 5-HT$_2$ receptors.

As the clinical effects of the specific D$_1$ antagonist SCH 23390 are presently unknown, it is difficult to draw any firm conclusion regarding the relative importance of the D$_1$/D$_2$ receptor interaction and the antipsychotic effect of these drugs. It is clear that all neuroleptics in current use are D$_2$ receptor antagonists and, while the selective D$_2$ antagonist sulpiride appears to have low antipsychotic potency, other benzamides (e.g. remoxipride and raclopride) are at least 100 times more potent than sulpiride in animal behavioural tests, which might indicate their greater antipsychotic potency. With the *typical neuroleptics* in wide clinical use (e.g. chlorpromazine, thioridazine, haloperidol, pimozide, flupenthixol and clopenthixol), there would appear to be a correlation between their D$_2$ antagonistic potency and their clinical potency; presumably the ability of these drugs to block 5-HT$_2$

receptors to varying extents is also evidence that the serotonergic system is involved in their clinical activity in some way.

The actions of neuroleptics on histamine, muscarinic and alpha$_1$ adrenergic receptors explain the side effects of these drugs, i.e. sedation, anticholinergic effects and hypotensive effects, respectively, which are generally considered to be undesirable and can lead to poor patient compliance.

Clinical pharmacology of the typical ("classical") neuroleptics

Despite the wide differences in the potency of the neuroleptics in current use, and the differences in specificity regarding their effects on various neurotransmitter systems in the mammalian brain, there is little evidence to suggest that their overall efficacy in treating the symptoms of schizophrenia, mania and other psychoses markedly differs. Thus the "classical" neuroleptics appear to be effective in attenuating the positive symptoms of schizophrenia (e.g. hallucinations and delusions) without affecting appreciably the negative symptoms of the illness (lethargy and social withdrawal), although a critical analysis of the actions of neuroleptics on the positive and negative symptoms suggests that both types of symptoms, which may coexist in the patient simultaneously or occur at different times during the course of the illness, may be favourably influenced by those drugs. Whether these effects on the positive and negative symptoms can be explained in terms of changes in the functional activity of different subtypes of dopamine and other neurotransmitter receptors is presently uncertain.

Dopamine receptor adaptation occurs in response to chronic neuroleptic treatment, and this may be important in understanding both the efficacy and side effects of the drugs. Thus while the blockade of dopamine receptor functions is quite rapid, the clinical response does not occur for several days. Further, the extrapyramidal side effects which occur as a consequence of dopamine receptor blockade in the basal ganglia cause a sequence of changes beginning with *dyskinesia* and followed by *akathisia* and *parkinsonism-like* movements after several weeks or months of treatment. *Tardive dyskinesia*, should it occur, may take months or even years to be manifest. While attempts have been made to explain the complexity of these adverse neurological effects in terms of changes in dopamine receptor sensitivity arising as a consequence of prolonged dopamine receptor blockade in the basal ganglia, knowledge that the commonly used neuroleptics also interact with many other neurotransmitter systems in that region of the brain make such an explanation implausible. Furthermore, orofacial dyskinesias occur to a significant extent in untreated schizophrenic patients and it is now well established that neuroleptics combined with the ageing process increase the prevalence of such disorders. Nevertheless, there is clear evidence from clinical studies on schizophrenic patients being treated with neuroleptics that changes in central dopaminergic function are related to the clinical response to treatment. Thus it has been shown that the free plasma concentration of homovanillic acid (HVA), the main metabolite of dopamine, correlates significantly with the antipsychotic effect of the phenothiazines. Undoubtedly the increased use of PET techniques to study neurotransmitter receptors in schizophrenic patients during neuroleptic treatment will provide invaluable information regarding the precise sites of action of these drugs in the patient's brain.

The *serum concentrations* of "classical" neuroleptics and their metabolites vary considerably in patients, even when the dose of drug administered has been standardized. Such interindividual variation may account for the differences in the therapeutic and side effects. High interindividual variations in the steady-state plasma levels have been reported for pimozide, fluphenazine, flupenthixol and haloperidol, some of these differences being attributed to differences in absorption and metabolism between patients.

Various factors may account for the *variability in response* to neuroleptics. These include differences in the diagnostic criteria, concurrent administration of drugs which may affect the absorption and metabolism of the neuroleptics (e.g. tricyclic antidepressants), different times of blood sampling, and variations due to the different type of assay method used. In some cases, the failure to obtain consistent relationships between the plasma neuroleptic concentration and the clinical response may be explained by the contribution of active metabolites to the therapeutic effects. Thus chlorpromazine, thioridazine, levomepromazine (methotrimeprazine) and loxapine have active metabolites which reach peak plasma concentrations within the same range as those of the parent compounds. As these metabolites often have pharmacodynamic and pharmacokinetic activities which differ from those of the parent compound, it is essential to determine the plasma concentrations of both the parent compound and its metabolites in order to establish whether or not a relationship exists between the plasma concentration and the therapeutic outcome.

Even in the case of drugs like haloperidol which do not have active metabolites, an unequivocal relationship cannot be found between the clinical effects and the plasma concentrations.

Fluphenazine enanthate, fluphenazine decanoate and haloperidol decanoate were developed as *depot* preparations to overcome many of the problems of oral neuroleptic administration, particularly lack of compliance, which has been estimated to be as high as 60% in outpatients. Depot neuroleptics produce a fairly predictable and constant plasma level and have the advantage of not being metabolized in the gastrointestinal tract or liver before reaching the brain. Despite the clear advantages of depot over oral preparations, the relapse rate among schizophrenic patients on such preparations over a 2-year period approaches 30%. The incidence of extrapyramidal side effects would also appear to be similar, but the longer half-life of the depot neuroleptic means that there is a longer delay before such symptoms may be controlled.

The relationship between plasma levels, drug doses and clinical response gives no clear guidelines for clinical practice. There is no convincing evidence that a "therapeutic window" exists for neuroleptics. Furthermore, there is little evidence to show that very high doses of neuroleptics improve the overall level of response or speed of resolution of an acute psychosis. High doses of neuroleptics may benefit those patients who fail to achieve optimal plasma concentrations on standard doses. Regarding the depot preparations, in a study in which patients treated with a low dose of fluphenazine decanoate (range 1.25–5.0 mg every 2 weeks) were compared with a group on a standard dose (range 12.5–50.0 mg every 2 weeks) over a 12-month period, the relapse rates were significantly higher in the low dose group (56% versus 7%). Furthermore, there was no clear advantage in the lower dose regarding the frequency of side effects or improved social functioning. The only advantage of the low dose of depot neuroleptic was a lower incidence of tardive dyskinesia. It would seem that depot neuroleptics may be the appropriate method of drug administration for short-term treatment, just as orally administered neuroleptics have a place in long-term maintenance treatment.

Classification of the neuroleptics

In addition to their well-established antipsychotic properties, the neuroleptics have a number of clinically important properties that include their antiemetic and antinauseant actions, their antihistaminic effects and their ability to potentiate the actions of analgesics and general anaesthetics.

Reserpine is unique among the neuroleptics in that it is a naturally occurring alkaloid obtained from the snake plant *Rauwolfia serpentina*. The use of aqueous extracts of the root of this plant for the treatment of "hysteria" was known to the native practitioners in the Indian subcontinent for centuries before the main active principal, reserpine, was isolated in the early 1950s. The marked antihypertensive effect of the drug, combined with its tranquillizing activity, led to its use in the treatment of schizophrenia. However, as has already been discussed in an earlier chapter, reserpine depletes all transmitters that are contained in storage vesicles in nerve terminals by selectively blocking their uptake by the magnesium-dependent adenosine triphosphatase (ATPase) linked transport site on the vesicle membrane. This renders the transmitter susceptible to intraneuronal catabolism. However, the side effects of long-term reserpine administration in schizophrenic patients were so numerous that its use has been discontinued. These side effects, which can be predicted from the action of reserpine on the storage vesicles for noradrenaline, 5-HT, dopamine and acetylcholine, include sedation, parkinsonism, predisposition to seizures, hypotension and a general impairment of peripheral sympathetic activity associated with parasympathetic hyperactivity (e.g. nausea, diarrhoea, gastric hypersecretion with susceptibility to gastric ulceration, bradycardia and hypersalivation).

Of the *phenothiazines*, chlorpromazine was the first drug to be introduced for the treatment of schizophrenia and is still the most widely used worldwide. All phenothiazines have antihistaminic, anticholinergic, anti-dopaminergic and adrenolytic properties, the potencies of the drugs for these different types of receptors depending upon the structure of the side chain which is attached to the tricyclic ring system. In general terms, it appears that the substitution of a halogen atom in the tricyclic ring (position "R" in Figure 10.4) is essential for neuroleptic activity. Thus *promazine*, which lacks a halogen substituent, has weak neuroleptic properties but it is a potent antihistaminic and anticholinergic agent. The side chain (position "B" in Figure 10.4) is important for the neuroleptic potency and also the anticholinergic, antihistaminic and adrenolytic side effects. Of the three main chemical classes of phenothiazines in clinical use, the *aliphatic* type are the least potent neuroleptics but are the most sedative, with pronounced anticholinergic, antihistaminic and adrenolytic properties. These effects are related to the structure of aliphatic side chain. The *piperidine* type are slightly more potent as neuroleptics and also have anticholinergic and adrenolytic side effects. The most potent, and least sedative, phenothiazines are in the *piperazine* group. This type of neuroleptic largely lacks anticholinergic, antihistaminic and adrenolytic activity.

The aliphatic phenothiazine chlorpromazine is the prototype neuroleptic with a wide range of pharmacological effects. Its antipsychotic and antiemetic properties are attributed to its antagonist action at central dopamine receptors in the mesocortical and vomiting centres, respectively, while the hypotensive action of chlorpromazine and related phenothiazines is associated with their alpha$_1$ adrenoceptor antagonist properties combined with their ability to reduce hypothalamic and central vasomotor function. The depression of hypothalamic activity also accounts for the hypothermia which may occur at therapeutic doses, particularly in the elderly patient. The antimuscarinic and antihistaminic activity, which can be predicted from the structure of the aliphatic side chain, accounts for the sedative and peripheral anticholinergic effects of this group of drugs. The aliphatic phenothiazine

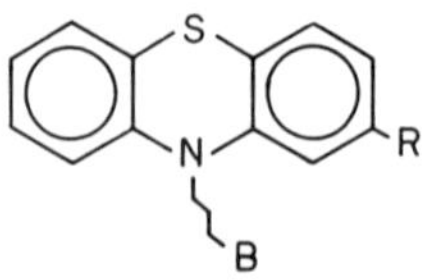

R	B	
H	$N(CH_3)_2$	Promazine
Cl	$N(CH_3)_2$	Chlorpromazine
Cl	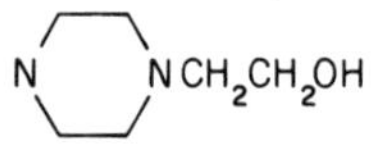 N⎯⎯N CH_2CH_2OH	Perphenazine
CF_3	$N(CH_3)_2$	Triflupromazine
CF_3	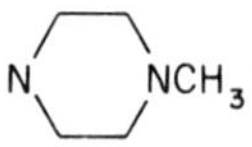 N⎯⎯NCH_3	Trifluperazine
CF_3	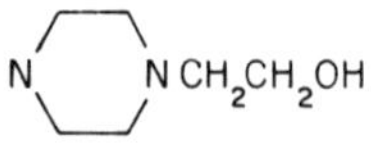 N⎯⎯N CH_2CH_2OH	Fluphenazine
SCH_3	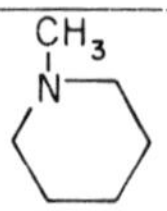 CH_3 N⎯⎯	Thioridazine

Figure 10.4. Chemical structure of the phenothiazine series of neuroleptics.

triflupromazine is a more potent neuroleptic than chlorpromazine due to substitution of $-CF_3$ for the $-Cl$ group in the ring.

The piperidine phenothiazines, as exemplified by the most widely used member of this series *thioridazine*, are approximately equivalent to the aliphatic phenothiazines but tend to be more sedative. Members of this series are therefore widely used for the more agitated, anxious psychotic patient. As their ability to cause parkinsonism appears to be less than with the other

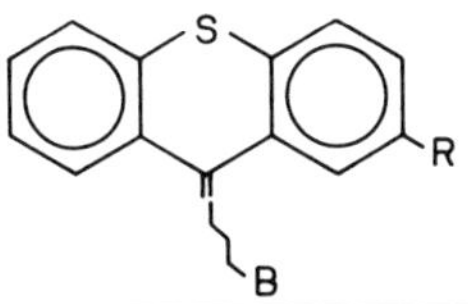

R	B	
Cl	N(CH$_3$)$_2$	Chlorprothixene
Cl	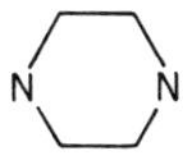 N◯N CH$_2$CH$_2$OH	Clopenthixol
CF$_3$	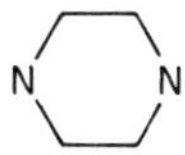 N◯N CH$_2$CH$_2$OH	Flupenthixol
CF$_3$	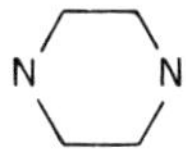 N◯N CH$_3$	Thiothixene

Figure 10.5. Chemical structure of the thioxanthine series of neuroleptics.

phenothiazines, possibly because of their potent central anticholinergic effects and slightly greater selectivity for mesocortical dopamine receptors, they are widely used to treat elderly psychotic patients.

The *piperazine* phenothiazines, as exemplified by *fluphenazine,* are the most potent members of the phenothiazine group, being at least 50 times more potent than chlorpromazine. Because of the structure of their side chain, members of this series lack anticholinergic, antihistaminic, adrenolytic and sedative effects. However, they are more likely to cause extrapyramidal side effects.

The *thioxanthines* are structurally closely related to the phenothiazines (see Figure 10.5) and may be divided into three separate series of compounds with aliphatic (e.g. *chlorprothixene*), piperazine (e.g. *clopenthixol, flupenthixol*) or piperidine side chains. Their potency and side effects are essentially similar to the corresponding phenothiazine neuroleptics.

The *butyrophenones* and *diphenylbutylpiperidines* differ from the phenothiazines and thioxanthines in that they are not tricyclic structures. The first butyrophenone to be developed was *haloperidol*, and this is the most widely used, potent neuroleptic. Unlike many of the phenothiazines, these neuroleptics largely lack antihistaminic, anticholinergic and adrenolytic activity; they are also non-sedative in therapeutic doses. Their potent antidopaminergic activity renders them likely to cause extrapyramidal side effects. Of the various butyrophenones shown in Figure 10.6, *benperidol* has been selectively used to suppress asocial sexual behaviour.

The diphenylbutylpiperidines are structurally related to the butyrophenones and have essentially similar properties. *Pimozide* is the most well-established member of this series and is a potent neuroleptic that, like other potent neuroleptics, is likely to cause extrapyramidal side effects.

Sulpiride is a member of a series of neuroleptics, the benzamides, of which the antiemetic drug metoclopramide is another example. The benzamides have a lower propensity to cause extrapyramidal side effects, probably because they show a high degree of selectivity for the D_2 dopamine receptors.

The chemical structure of clozapine and sulpiride is shown in Figure 10.7.

Atypical neuroleptics and their effects on serotonin and dopamine receptors: relevance to clinical action

Imaging techniques such as CAT have shown that enlargement of the lateral ventricles is a frequent feature of schizophrenia. Such structural changes do not appear to be associated with the nature or duration of neuroleptic therapy and are found in affective disorders. The changes found in the schizophrenic brain may be triggered by environmental factors such as birth complications. In addition, selective reduction in the size of the temporal lobe commonly occurs in schizophrenics and such changes appear to be lateralized in the left hemisphere. Regional blood flow studies, and the measurement of regional glucose metabolism, has provided evidence of reduced frontal lobe function (hypofunctionality).

Atypical neuroleptics such as clozapine, remoxipride, risperidone and sulpiride have been developed because it was found that up to 20% of schizophrenic patients did not respond to "classical" neuroleptics of the phenothiazine or butyrophenone type, while those patients who do initially respond to such medication frequently relapse during the first 2 years of treatment. Another reason for developing novel neuroleptics has been motivated by the finding that the "classical" neuroleptics have little beneficial effect either on the chronic course of the illness or on the negative symptoms. The negative symptoms of schizophrenia are frequently problematic to the patient and tend to be persistent, disabling and difficult to treat. In addition, the side effects of the "classical" neuroleptics which are

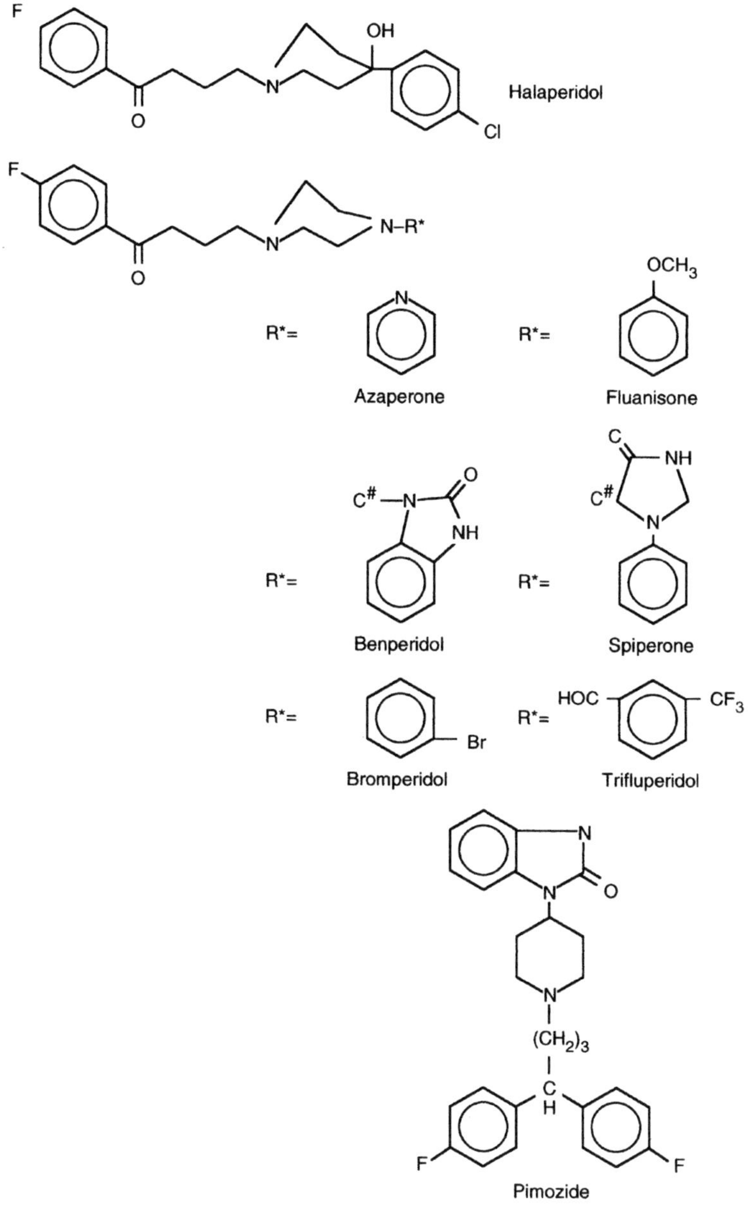

Figure 10.6. Chemical structure of the butyrophenone and diphenylbutylpiperidine series of neuroleptics indicates that N has been replaced by C.

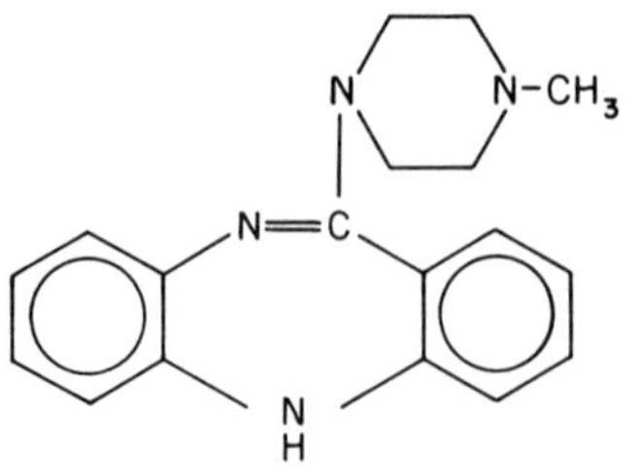

Clozapine

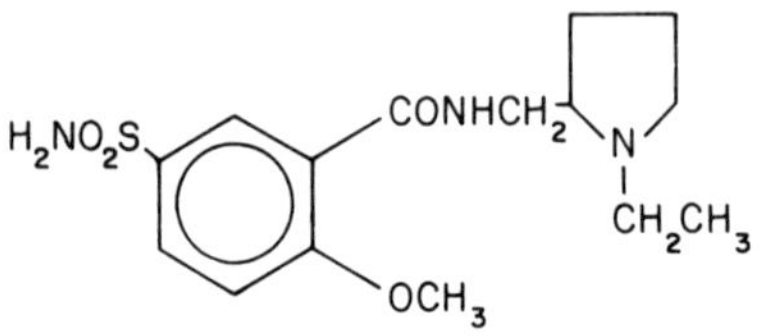

Sulpiride

Figure 10.7.   Chemical structure of the atypical neuroleptics clozapine and sulpiride.

associated with the sedative, anticholinergic and extrapyramidal effects of these drugs, often result in poor compliance.

The potential advantage of the atypical neuroleptics arises from their ability to act on both positive and negative symptoms, to have a reduced tendency to cause extrapyramidal side effects, to be less sedative and to have little antimuscarinic activity. In terms of their actions on central neurotransmitters, the atypical neuroleptics can be divided into broad classes, namely those drugs such as remoxipride which are highly selective as D_2 receptor antagonists and those that have a relatively weak D_2 antagonistic action but which are potent inhibitors of $5\text{-}HT_{2A}$ receptors. This latter group includes clozapine, risperidone, zotepine, sertindole, olanzapine and amperozide.

It has been postulated that the $5\text{-}HT_2$ antagonistic action of the atypical neuroleptics plays an important role in their efficacy in reducing the negative symptoms. There is evidence from PET studies in man that atypical neuroleptics such as clozapine occupy 80–90% of $5\text{-}HT_2$ receptors whereas the "classical" neuroleptics, such as haloperidol, occupy hardly any $5\text{-}HT_2$ receptors even at high therapeutic doses. The precise mechanism whereby such a high affinity of the atypical neuroleptics leads to a reduction in the negative symptoms and schizophrenia is uncertain. It is hypothesized that hypofrontality is associated with the negative symptoms and that the blockade of $5\text{-}HT_2$ receptors in the corticolimbic region of the brain reduces such symptoms. Experimental studies in rats have shown that serotonin modifies the pattern of dopamine release. When treated with the psychotomimetic drug phencyclidine, which can induce both positive and negative symptoms of schizophrenia in man under experimental conditions, the activity of the dopaminergic terminals in the frontal cortex is reduced. This hypofunctioning dopaminergic system can be normalized by treatment with 5-HT$_2$ antagonists. It therefore appears that 5-HT$_2$ antagonists cause an indirect activation of midbrain dopaminergic cell activity, together with an increase in dopamine release in the frontal cortex.

The consequence of the combination of D$_2$ and 5-HT$_2$ receptor antagonism is therefore the selective enhancement of dopaminergic activity in the prefrontal cortex and, as a consequence, a correction of the regional imbalance between the cortical and midbrain dopaminergic systems.

Regarding the extrapyramidal side effects commonly found after treatment with the "classical" neuroleptics, PET studies of schizophrenia patients have shown that such drugs occupy 70–80% of D$_2$ receptors in the basal ganglia at therapeutic doses. It has been calculated that a D$_2$ receptor occupancy in the basal ganglia of approximately 80% carries a high risk that the patient will develop extrapyramidal side effects. Furthermore, Canadian studies have shown that the occurrence of extrapyramidal side effects was a major predictor for the subsequent development of tardive dyskinesia.

Thus the atypical neuroleptics with their lower affinity for D$_2$ receptors in the basal ganglia, and their high affinity for 5-HT$_2$ receptors in the frontal cortex, appear to combine therapeutic efficacy with a reduced tendency to cause neurological side effects.

The main pharmacological properties of some atypical neuroleptics are summarized in Table 10.3. A comparison of the affinities of some atypical neuroleptics with that of the typical neuroleptic haloperidol is given in Table 10.2.

Efficacy of high doses of "classical" neuroleptics in the treatment-resistant patient

There is no published evidence for the efficacy of high dose medication as an effective strategy either to accelerate therapeutic response or to increase the number of patients who respond to medication. Neither is there any objective evidence to show that escalating the dose of a "classical" neuroleptic is likely to produce a beneficial response in chronically resistant patients. Furthermore, there are anecdotal reports that high dose neuroleptics can cause sudden death (due to cardiotoxicity), severe parkinsonism and/or akathisia with the possibility of paradoxical and violent behaviour (possibly associated with akathisia). The possibility of the neuroleptic malignant syndrome occurring following high dose neuroleptics

Table 10.3. Efficacy, tolerability and mechanism of action of some atypical neuroleptics

Drug	Antipsychotic efficacy	Adverse effects	Mechanism of action
Clozapine	Useful in therapy-resistant schizophrenia; ameliorates negative symptoms	Neutropenia, seizures, salivation, weight gain, sedation, *but* few EPS	Antagonist. Affinity for D_4 receptors and $5-HT_2$ receptors. Also blocks $5-HT_{2C}$, histamine$_1$ and ACh muscarinic receptors
Remoxipride	Equipotent with "classical" phenothiazine neuroleptics. Ameliorates negative symptoms	Agranulocytosis reported: Named patient basis only. Little sedation. Few EPS	Selective D_2 receptor antagonist in cortex; less antagonism of D_2 receptors in basal ganglia
Risperidone	As for remoxipride	Side effects less frequent and severe than "classical" phenothiazines. Few EPS	High affinity for D_2 and $5-HT_2$ receptors as an antagonist
Zotepine	As for remoxipride	As for risperidone	High affinity for D_2, D_1 and $5-HT_2$ receptors
Sertindole	Preliminary clinical data suggests that sertindole is equiactive with "classical" phenothiazine but more likely to attenuate negative symptoms	Preliminary data suggests that it has similar adverse effects to risperidone with lower EPS profile	Potent $5-HT_2$ receptor antagonist but weak D_2 antagonist
Amperozide	Preliminary clinical data suggests similarity to remoxipride	As for sertindole	Potent $5-HT_2$ receptor antagonist and selectivity for mesolimbic D_2 receptors
Olanzapine	Preliminary clinical data suggests that it has similar efficacy to clozapine	Low EPS profile in preliminary studies	Potent $5-HT_2$ and D_2 antagonist

is more closely related to the rate of dose escalation than to the quantity of neuroleptic administered.

However, despite the absence of firm evidence for efficacy because of the real dangers that may arise, it is occasionally justified to consider administering a high therapeutic dose of a "classical" neuroleptic to a patient who is responding poorly to a normal dose of the drug. It is well established that the blood concentration of a neuroleptic varies considerably between patients given the same oral dose. Such variation probably arises from differences in compliance, in first-pass metabolism and in the rate of elimination. Where possible, the plasma concentrations should be determined before proceeding with the dose escalation of a standard neuroleptic. Assuming that pharmacologically active concentrations of the drug have been achieved, it is possible that poor therapeutic response is due to an insufficient population of the D_2 receptors in the mesocortical areas of the brain being blocked by the neuroleptics. However, it must be emphasized that the use of high doses of neuroleptics should be the last resort for carefully selected and supervised patients. It may be argued that as the new atypical neuroleptics are equi-effective with the "classical" antipsychotics, and certainly superior in their tolerability and side-effect profile, such drugs (despite their high unit cost) should be considered before escalating the dose of a non-response patient on a "classical" neuroleptic.

Hormonal changes resulting from neuroleptic treatment

Acute dopamine receptor blockade by neuroleptics has long been known to induce a dose-dependent increase in *prolactin* as a consequence of the decreased activity of the inhibitory D_2 receptors that govern the release of this hormone from the anterior pituitary. However, dose–response studies show that the dose of a neuroleptic required to raise the plasma prolactin concentration is lower than that necessary to have an optimal therapeutic effect. Furthermore, the time of onset of the rise in prolactin is short (hours), whereas the antipsychotic effect of a neuroleptic takes many days or even weeks. There is also evidence that raised serum prolactin levels persist throughout drug treatment, which suggests that tolerance of the tubero-infundibular dopaminergic system to the action of neuroleptics does not occur; it should be noted that not all investigators agree with such a view. There is little evidence to suggest that a relationship exists between the symptoms of schizophrenia, or the response to drug therapy, and changes in plasma prolactin concentrations.

The secretion of *growth hormone* is under the control of the dopaminergic, noradrenergic, serotonergic and possibly other neurotransmitter systems. The acute apomorphine growth hormone challenge test has been used to assess D_2 receptor function in untreated schizophrenics and in patients during neuroleptic treatment. Apomorphine-stimulated growth hormone secretion is reported to be higher in untreated schizophrenics and to be blunted following both acute and chronic neuroleptic treatment, returning to control values within a few weeks of drug withdrawal.

Sexual dysfunction in schizophrenic patients on long-term neuroleptic therapy is well established and may result from hyperprolactinaemia. Menstrual cycle disruption is a common feature of neuroleptic treatment which may be complicated in hyperprolactinaemia. However, it seems unlikely that the changes in gonadotrophin secretion are a unique feature of schizophrenia, as patients with depression and anorexia nervosa also show such abnormalities. Furthermore, detailed studies of the luteinizing hormone and follicle-stimulating hormone levels in a group of male and female patients on very long-term neuroleptic therapy could not confirm an abnormality in sex hormone dysfunction due to drug treatment. Thus it must be concluded that unequivocal evidence showing that prolonged neuroleptic treatment results in sexual dysfunction due to a defect in gonadotrophin release is not yet available.

Changes in cognitive function during neuroleptic treatment

The effects of long-term neuroleptic administration on cognitive and psychomotor function have been the subject of many studies. Some of the early studies undertaken during the 1960s reported that acute doses of phenothiazine neuroleptics caused cognitive impairment in schizophrenic patients, whereas chronic treatment led to improvement. More recent studies, however, have reported improvement in attention and in cognitive function following short-term administration. Detailed studies revealed that memory and fine motor coordination were impaired by many neuroleptics, the amnesic effects probably being related to the central anticholinergic effects of the drugs while the effects on motor control may be ascribed to the blockade of dopamine receptors. In general, it would appear that the hyperarousal state that occurs in schizophrenia is reduced by neuroleptics, thereby leading to an improvement in attention. However, the consensus would now appear to be that a general decrease in brain stem arousal does not account for the beneficial effect of neuroleptics, and it seems more probable that these drugs correct a frontal lobe dysfunction. It should be noted that tardive dyskinesia is almost invariably associated with a deterioration of intellectual function.

Thus it would appear that neuroleptics have little effect on higher cognitive functioning in schizophrenic patients and that the improvement in attention is facilitated by a non-mesocortical–mesolimbic mechanism. There is also evidence that neuroleptics improve asymmetry in hippocampal function which may be deranged in the illness. It is generally agreed that studies of the effects of neuroleptics on normal subjects, which frequently show impaired cognitive and psychomotor function, are of only limited relevance to our understanding of the beneficial effects which these drugs produce in schizophrenic patients.

In CONCLUSION, the use of the "classical" neuroleptics, as exemplified by the phenothiazines, thioxanthines, butyrophenones and diphenylbutylpiper- idines, has been a landmark in the pharmacotherapy of schizophrenia and psychotic disorders. The efficacy of such drugs in the alleviation of the symptoms of schizophrenia is universally accepted. However, it is also evident that they have a spectrum of adverse effects that frequently renders their long-term use problematic. Side effects such as akathisia, parkinsonism, tardive dyskinesia and the all too frequent changes in peripheral autonomic activity are largely predictable from the structure of the molecules and the basic animal pharmacology data. Such adverse effects, and the difficulties encountered when attempting to reduce their frequency and severity by concurrent medication, has stimulated the development of "atypical" neuroleptics such as clozapine and risperidone which, hopefully, will combine efficacy with a reduction in side effects.

11 Drug Treatment of the Epilepsies

Introduction

Hughlings Jackson, reputed to be the "father" of the modern concept of epilepsy, defined epilepsy about 100 years ago as "an episodic disorder of the nervous system arising from the excessively synchronous and sustained discharge of a group of neurons". Such a definition implies that, in addition to the seizure, there are disturbances in both motor and cognitive function. Hughlings Jackson also noted that a single seizure is not indicative of epilepsy, but he did not exclude seizures that are secondary to systemic metabolic disorders – such seizures would not be included in the classification of epilepsy today. The main importance of this definition is that it emphasized for the first time that epilepsy has a neuropathological basis and suggested that excitatory and inhibitory neurotransmitter processes are probably involved in the causation of the symptoms.

The term "epilepsy" applies to a group of disorders that are characterized by sudden and transient episodes (seizures) of motor (convulsions), sensory, autonomous or psychic origin. The seizures are usually correlated with abnormal and excessive discharges in the brain and can be visualized on the electroencephalogram (EEG).

The epilepsies are estimated to affect 20–40 million individuals worldwide and are more common in children than in adults. They are classified into two broad groups: *primary* or *idiopathic* epilepsy is the term applied to those types for which no specific cause can be identified, and *secondary* or *symptomatic* epilepsy arises when the symptoms are associated with trauma, neoplasm, infection, cerebrovascular disease or some other physically induced lesion of the brain. Seizures that accompany severe metabolic disturbances are not classified as epilepsy.

For the purpose of drug treatment, the epilepsies are classified according to the seizure type. The classification generally used is based on that proposed by the Commission on Classification and Terminology of the International League against Epilepsy. The main groups are:

1. *Partial (focal) seizures*, or seizures initiated locally in the brain. These include:
   (a) Simple partial seizures, which encompass focal motor attacks and seizures with somatosensory signs or psychic symptoms.

217

(b) Complex partial seizures, including temporal lobe or psychomotor seizures where consciousness is impaired; these may begin as simple partial seizures.

(c) Secondary generalized seizures, which commence as (a) or (b) but later develop into generalized tonic–clonic, clonic or tonic seizures.

2. *Generalized seizures*, including bilateral symmetrical seizures or seizures without local onset. This group includes:

(a) Clonic, tonic and tonic–clonic seizures

(b) Myoclonic seizures.

(c) Absence and atypical absence seizures.

(d) Atonic seizures.

This classification does not take into account the frequency, duration or causes of precipitation of the seizure. Any type of attack that is maintained for more than 1 hour is termed *status epilepticus*, which may be qualified as focal or generalized.

Pathological basis of the epilepsies

The pathophysiology of epilepsy is poorly understood and so far there is no clear association between the abnormal function of a specific group of neurons and the genesis of seizures. It is generally agreed that epileptogenesis involves the complex interaction of multiple factors. In some cases lesions such as those arising from traumatic haemorrhage can cause secondary seizures, whereas other forms of brain damage, for example that caused by ischaemic stroke, are less likely to cause seizures. Microscopic changes involving glial proliferation and loss of neurons have been identified in epileptic patients, and a loss of those neurons containing inhibitory neurotransmitters has been particularly implicated in the aetiology of the disease. Whether such changes are the cause or the consequence of the seizures is uncertain.

There is considerable controversy regarding the possible *genetic* basis of the epilepsies. It has been calculated that there are at least 100 different trait markers that may predispose some individuals to the disease, and it has been shown that identical seizure disorders may be present in patients who either have, or do not have, a particular genetic marker. Clearly this is an important area of research for the future.

Animal models

Animal models have been developed not only in an attempt to screen potential antiepileptic drugs but also to define more precisely the possible aetiology of the condition. In mice, there are at least 12 single locus mutations that produce neurological syndromes with spontaneous seizures. One particular species, the "tottering mouse", shows spontaneous seizures which resemble absence attacks both in terms of the behavioural and the EEG changes. The only specific cellular pathology which has been found in this model is a selective outgrowth of axons from the locus ceruleus which results in an increase in the noradrenaline content of the neocortex, hippocampus, cerebellum and thalamus. The seizures are attenuated in this species by the local injection of the neurotoxin 6-hydroxydopamine, which destroys the noradrenergic terminals. However, it should be noted that this neurotoxin usually results in the lowering of the seizure threshold in most species of animal, so the precise relevance of these findings in the "tottering mouse" to the human condition is unclear.

Strong sensory stimuli (e.g. 90 dB sound) can precipitate tonic–clonic seizures in some strains of mice, the DBA/2 strain being particularly susceptible, while posturally induced seizures in "epileptic-like" mice have been extensively studied and have been shown to be associated with abnormalities in both the adenosine triphosphatases (ATPases) and various biogenic amine neurotransmitters.

Beagle dogs show a high incidence of epileptic seizures, including those of the secondary type; complex partial and generalized tonic–clonic seizures frequently occur in this species. However, the nearest model to human epilepsy is undoubtedly photically induced seizures in the Senegalese baboon.

Chronic focal epilepsy can be induced in rats, cats and monkeys by the topical application of metals such as aluminium, cobalt and iron. Alumina paste applied to the motor cortex of the monkey initiates spontaneous convulsive seizures that eventually generalize to the rest of the brain. It has been shown that neurons in the vicinity of the seizure focus have a reduced glutamate decarboxylase activity, which suggests that gamma-aminobutyric acid (GABA) synthesis in this area is impaired. Not all animal models of epilepsy show such changes in GABA content, however. Some strains of Mongolian gerbil exhibit myoclonic and clonic–tonic seizures in early adulthood, but in such species the GABA content of the hippocampus has been shown to increase, which suggests that a process of disinhibition of inhibitory transmitter pathways may occur in this model.

Recently there has been much interest in the *kindling* of epileptic seizures in rodents. This occurs following focal electrical stimulation of cortical regions, usually the temporal region, by a current that is sufficient to cause an after-discharge but insufficient to cause a direct seizure. When such stimuli are repeated at regular intervals for several days, a stage is reached whereby a subthreshold stimulus results in a full seizure. This suggests that kindling is associated with the lowering of the seizure threshold consequent upon the induction of enhanced neurotransmitter receptor sensitivity. There is no evidence that brain damage is responsible for such changes but it has been suggested that the alterations in receptor sensitivity are similar to those occurring in long-term potentiation, a phenomenon produced by high frequency stimulation of afferent inputs to the hippocampus that leads to enhancement of excitatory synaptic potentials and increased memory formation.

Whereas the genetic and kindling models have been widely used to investigate possible neurotransmitter defects that cause different types of epilepsy, rodent models in which seizures are induced by electroshock, or by convulsant drugs such as pentylenetetrazol (also called pentetrazol, leptazol), picrotoxin or bicuculline, are mainly used in screening procedures to identify potential anticonvulsants.

Biochemical changes in human epilepsy

Membrane-bound enzymes, particularly the ATPases involved in the ionic pumps for calcium, sodium and potassium, have been found to function abnormally in the brains of epileptic patients and animals. A reduction in Na^+K^+-ATPase activity has been reported in human focal epileptogenic tissue, but it is uncertain whether such changes are due to the disease itself or a reflection of drug treatment. Similar changes have, however, been reported in experimental animals following the localized application of alumina cream and in DBA/2 mice that exhibit sound-induced seizures; a reduction in calcium-dependent ATPase has also been found in the brain of DBA/2 mice. Such findings are consistent with the hypothesis that a defect in ion channels may occur in epilepsy.

Another possibility is that endogenous epileptogenic compounds may be produced in the brain of the epileptic patient. Both tetrahydroisoquinolines and beta-carbolines have been detected in the human brain, as has the tryptophan analogue quinolinic acid, which all have convulsant and excitotoxic properties. The enzymes that synthesize quinolinic acid have also been identified in human brain tissue.

Of the various amino acid neurotransmitters which have been implicated in epilepsy, the inhibitory transmitter glycine has been shown to be present in normal concentrations, or even slightly elevated, in the vicinity of the epileptic focus. Conversely, the concentration of GABA has been found to be reduced in the cerebrospinal fluid (CSF) of chronic epileptics and in patients with febrile seizures. The central role of GABA in epilepsy is further suggested by the observation that drugs that reduce the GABA concentration are epileptogenic, while those that raise the GABA concentration are generally anticonvulsants. The observation that the concentration of glutamate may be reduced in the epileptic focus lends further support to the view that there may be a defect in GABA synthesis which predisposes the individual to the disease.

Despite early studies suggesting that the acetylcholine concentration was raised in epileptogenic foci, which would be consistent with the finding that anticholinesterases cause seizures in both animals and man, it now appears that overactivity of the central cholinergic system is unlikely to be the cause of seizures in the human epileptic. Other candidates that have been implicated in the aetiology of epilepsy include adenosine and the enkephalins, but conclusive evidence for their involvement is presently lacking.

Action of anticonvulsants on central neurotransmitters

The anticonvulsants in clinical use may be divided into eight major groups. These are:

1. The *barbiturates*, such as phenobarbitone and primidone.
2. The *hydantoins*, such as diphenylhydantoin (phenytoin) and ethytoin.
3. The *dibenzazepines*, such as carbamazepine.
4. The *oxazolidinediones*, such as trimethadione (troxidone).
5. The *succinimides*, such as ethosuximide.
6. The *benzodiazepines*, such as diazepam, clobazam and clonazepam.
7. The *sulphonamides*, such as acetazolamide and sulthiame.
8. The *short chain fatty acids*, such as sodium valproate.

The chemical structure of representative drugs from each of these groups is shown in Figure 11.1.

Of the various animal models of epilepsy that have been developed to screen compounds for their potential therapeutic activity, antagonism of maximal electroshock seizures is generally indicative of the drug being useful in the control of partial seizures; drugs such as diphenylhydantoin and carbamazepine are active in such tests. Conversely, antagonism of pentylenetetrazol seizures is usually associated with the effective control of absence (petit mal) seizures, the succinimides and oxazolidinediones being particularly effective in antagonizing such seizures. Drugs such as sodium valproate and the benzodiazepines have a broad spectrum of action and are effective against primary generalized seizures (including petit mal) as well as partial seizures (including temporal lobe epilepsy).

The actions of anticonvulsants at the cellular level are complex and include facilitation of inhibitory feedback mechanisms, membrane stabilization and changes in synaptic transmission to reduce excitatory transmission. Of these various possibilities, it is widely accepted that anticonvulsants enhance GABA-mediated inhibitory processes. Such a mechanism has been clearly demonstrated for the benzodiazepines, barbiturates, diphenylhydantoin and sodium valproate.

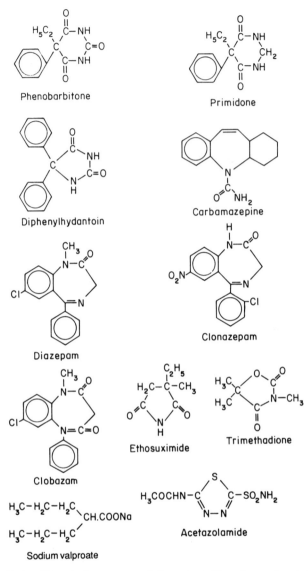

Figure 11.1. Chemical structure of the principal anticonvulsant drugs.

Enhanced GABAergic transmission

Electrophysiological studies show that benzodiazepines, barbiturates and sodium valproate facilitate GABAergic transmission in the animal brain. Further evidence comes from studies on the GABA-benzodiazepine receptor complex, the order of potency of a series of benzodiazepines to displace [^{3}H] diazepam from its receptor site being clearly correlated with the antagonism of pentylenetetrazol seizures, but not with electroconvulsive seizures. However, most classes of anticonvulsants appear to facilitate GABAergic transmission via the picrotoxin-binding site on the GABA-benzodiazepine receptor complex (see p. 57).

The precise mechanism of action of valproate in facilitating GABA transmission is still uncertain. There is evidence that the drug can facilitate GABA synthesis, probably by inhibiting GABA transaminase activity, but the dose of drug necessary to achieve this effect is very high and not relevant to the clinical situation. One possibility is that valproate desensitizes GABA autoreceptors and thereby facilitates the release of the transmitter.

A reduction in the activity of excitatory neurotransmitters as a possible mechanism of action is largely confined to experimental studies on the barbiturates and benzodiazepines. *In vitro* studies have shown that drugs such as phenobarbitone can reduce the release of glutamate and acetylcholine, probably by impairing the entry of calcium ions into presynaptic terminals.

Membrane and ionic effects

The hydantoins have been most widely studied for their effects on ion movements across neuronal membranes. In the brain, these drugs have been shown to decrease the rise in intracellular sodium that normally occurs following the passage of an action potential; a reduction in calcium flux across excitable membranes also occurs.

In cell culture preparations, diphenylhydantoin, carbamazepine and valproate have been shown to reduce membrane excitability at therapeuti-cally relevant concentrations. This membrane-stabilizing effect is probably due to a block in the sodium channels. High concentrations of diazepam also have similar effects, and the membrane-stabilizing action correlates with the action of these anticonvulsants in inhibiting maximal electroshock seizures. Intracellular studies have shown that, in synaptosomes, most anti-convulsants inhibit calcium-dependent calmodulin protein kinase, an effect which would contribute to a reduction in neurotransmitter release. This action of anticonvulsants would appear to correlate with the potency of the drugs in inhibiting electroshock seizures. The result of all these disparate actions of anticonvulsants would be to diminish synaptic efficacy and thereby reduce seizure spread from an epileptic focus.

Pharmacokinetic aspects

Unlike most classes of psychotropic drugs where there is no direct correlation between the blood concentration and the therapeutic effect, for most of the commonly used anticonvulsants there is a high degree of correlation between the blood and brain concentrations and the therapeutic effect. A knowledge of the pharmacokinetic properties of the anticonvulsant drugs is therefore essential if their therapeutic efficacy is to be maximized and side effects minimized.

The anticonvulsants are metabolized in the liver by the microsomal oxidative pathway, although some drugs, such as phenobarbitone and ethosuximide, are partially eliminated unchanged. Most anticonvulsants act as inducers of the liver microsomal enzyme system and thereby enhance their own rate of destruction. In patients on a combination of anticonvulsants, this can result in shorter elimination half-lives for some of the drugs and a corresponding wide fluctuation in the plasma drug concentrations. Sodium valproate is an exception in that it does not act as a microsomal enzyme inducer.

Some anticonvulsants are metabolized in the liver to pharmacologically active metabolites which, if they have long half-lives, may accumulate and have neurotoxic effects. The following commonly used anticonvulsants are known to produce active metabolites:

Primidone   – Phenobarbitone and phenylethylmalonamide
Carbamazepine – Carbamazepine 10, 11-epoxide
Trimethadione   – Dimethadione (long half-life)
Methsuximide   – N-Desmethylmethsuximide (long half-life)

Most anticonvulsants have relatively long half-lives, which is clearly a major therapeutic advantage in achieving steady blood levels. Sodium valproate is exceptional in that it has a relatively short half-life, while phenobarbitone has the longest half-life of those drugs in general use. As with most psychotropic drugs, the half-life varies with the age of the patient; the older the patient, the longer the half-life. Slow absorption of a drug generally favours stable blood levels and to achieve this several anticonvulsants have been formulated into slowly absorbed formulations. Clearly it is important that the patient is treated with the same formulation of the drug. For patients being treated with diphenylhydantoin for example, changing formulations can lead to a sudden change in the steady-state drug concentration due to differences in the bioavailability of the preparations. This can lead to large fluctuations in the tissue drug concentrations with an increasing possibility of neurotoxicity and lack of seizure control despite similar peak blood concentrations being reached.

Most anticonvulsants have linear elimination kinetics, which means that an increase in the dose of drug administered leads to a proportional increase in the blood concentration and pharmacological activity. However, diphenylhydantoin and valproate are exceptions; the former does not follow linear kinetics so that the blood concentration is not directly related to the dose administered, while valproate is highly bound to serum proteins so that the total blood concentration may not directly reflect the quantity of drug available to the brain.

Drugs used in the treatment of epilepsy

The clinical applications of some of the most widely available anti-convulsants may be summarized as follows:

Febrile seizures	Phenobarbitone, benzodiazepines
Idiopathic Lennox–Gastaut syndrome	Valproate, benzodiazepines, adreno-corticotrophic hormone
Absence seizures (petit mal)	Ethosuximide, valproate, benzodiazepines, acetazolamide
Generalized tonic–clonic seizures (grand mal)	Valproate, phenobarbitone, carbamazepine, diphenylhydantoin
Juvenile myoclonic epilepsy	Valproate, ethosuximide, primidone
Reflex epilepsy	Benzodiazepines, valproate, phenobarbitone, methsuximide
Status epilepticus	Benzodiazepines, diphenylhydantoin

Benzodiazepines

Benzodiazepines used to treat epilepsy include diazepam, clonazepam, clobazam and lorazepam. Of these, diazepam and lorazepam have been most widely used to control status epilepticus, while use of clonazepam is usually restricted to the chronic treatment of severe mixed types of seizures (e.g. Lennox–Gastaut syndrome and infantile spasm). The major problem with most of the benzodiazepines, with the possible exception of clobazam, is sedation.

Lorazepam is less lipophilic than diazepam and there is evidence that it has a longer duration of anticonvulsant action than diazepam after intravenous administration. This could be due to the fact that diazepam is more rapidly removed from the brain compartment than lorazepam, which limits its duration of antiepileptic activity. In practice, when diazepam is used to control status epilepticus it is often necessary to continue treatment with diphenylhydantoin, which has a longer duration of action in the brain. The principal hazards of benzodiazepines when given intravenously include respiratory depression and hypotension. Diazepam may be administered rectally, its ease of absorption leading to peak plasma levels within about 10 minutes.

Clonazepam is the most potent of the benzodiazepine anticonvulsants and is particularly indicated in the treatment of the more difficult cases of epilepsy, especially those of the multiple seizure type. More recently, *clobazam*, which at therapeutic doses has the advantage of causing little sedation, has been advocated as an "add-on" anticonvulsant in those cases where the seizures cannot be readily controlled by more conventional drug treatment.

Carbamazepine

Carbamazepine is a unique anticonvulsant in that it has a tricyclic structure, which may account for its usefulness in the treatment of some affective disorders such as mania and atypical pain syndromes as well as epilepsy. Its primary use is in the treatment of partial elementary, partial complex and tonic–clonic seizures.

Like many anticonvulsants, carbamazepine is a hepatic microsomal enzyme inducer, an effect which can lead to a doubling of its elimination half-life. Coadministration with phenobarbitone, diphenylhydantoin and valproate causes a significant elevation in the plasma levels of carbamazepine, and its active metabolite carbamazepine epoxide. Drugs inhibiting hepatic microsomal enzymes, such as the macrolide antibiotics (e.g. erythromycin) also increase the plasma levels of this drug. Other drug interactions may occur as carbamazepine is partially plasma protein bound.

Sedation occurs in up to 30% of all patients on prolonged therapy, but tolerance to this effect develops, particularly if the dose of the drug is escalated slowly. Other side effects of carbamazepine include allergic rashes, movement disorders, hyponatraemia and blood dyscrasias (neutropenia and rarely agranulocytosis).

Succinimides

Of the succinimide anticonvulsants, *ethosuximide* is particularly effective in the control of absence seizures. The main side effects of this drug are singultus (hiccups) and sedation at high doses. Hallucinations have also been reputed to occur. Ethosuximide has no beneficial effect in generalized tonic–clonic seizures. A close analogue of ethosuximide, *methsuximide*, has largely been reserved as a "second-line" drug and as a useful adjunct to the treatment of refractory partial complex seizures. It is, however, more sedative than ethosuximide.

Diphenylhydantoin

Diphenylhydantoin is the most widely used drug in the treatment of all types of partial seizures, generalized tonic–clonic seizures and status epilepticus. It is relatively non-sedative. There is a good correlation between the increase in the blood levels of the drug and the occurrence of neurotoxicity, concentrations about $25 \mu g/ml$ usually being associated with such symptoms.

The well-known dose-related side effects include gingival hyperplasia (due to altered collagen metabolism), cerebellar-vestibular effects (nystagmus, vertigo, ataxia), behavioural changes (confusion, drowsiness, hallucinations), increased seizure frequency, gastrointestinal disturbances (nausea, anorexia), osteomalacia (due to reduced calcium absorption and increased vitamin D metabolism) and megaloblastic anaemia (due to reduced folate absorption).

The main problem arising from the routine use of diphenylhydantoin relates to its non-linear elimination kinetics. This means that as the blood concentration is increased the apparent half-life is progressively prolonged. Thus at the therapeutic range of $10–20 \mu g/ml$ blood, the half-life is in the range of 6 to 24 hours, but it increases to 20–60 hours when the blood concentration exceeds $20–25 \mu g/ml$. Furthermore, significant differences in the bioavailability of the oral preparations of the drug have been found, leading to a variation in the time of peak drug concentration from 3 to 12 hours. Because of the non-linearity of the drug elimination kinetics, formulations of the drug with different absorption rates are not bioequivalent, so that it is important that the patient should always be maintained on the same form of the drug. About 90% of the drug is bound to serum proteins (mainly serum albumin) which is an important consideration if the patient is given other drugs concurrently that may compete for the protein binding sites. The main metabolite of diphenylhydantoin is inactive.

Phenobarbitone and primidone

Phenobarbitone is the oldest anticonvulsant in common use but suffers from a high incidence of behavioural and cognitive effects, particularly in children. While tolerance may develop to the sedative effects of the drug, high blood levels are associated with a measurable deterioration in motor performance, and learning difficulties are likely to occur in children as a consequence of the central depressant properties of the drug. Phenobarbitone has the longest half-life of all the anticonvulsants in common use (30–150 hours).

Primidone has a relatively short half-life (4–15 hours), but it is metabolized to phenobarbitone and phenylethylmalonamide, which prolongs the duration of the anticonvulsant effect.

Sodium valproate

Sodium valproate is useful in the control of most seizure types and has the shortest half-life of the commonly used anticonvulsants (4–15 hours); a slowly absorbed form of the drug, divalproex sodium, is sometimes preferred. Valproate is relatively free from cognitive and behavioural side effects, but alopecia and weight gain frequently occur. The most severe side effect is idiosyncratic hepatotoxicity and pancreatitis, particularly in younger patients. However, these side effects are more frequent in patients taking valproate as a co-medication with other anticonvulsants.

Some novel anticonvulsant drugs

Gabapentin is a newly introduced anticonvulsant drug that has been approved for the treatment of partial seizures, with or without secondary seizures, in adults. It is recommended to be used as an addition to standard anticonvulsant therapy. The chemical structure of gabapentin is unique in that it consists of a molecule of GABA covalently bound to a lipophilic cyclohexane ring (Figure 11.2). Thus gabapentin was designed as a centrally active GABA agonist, the high lipophilicity of the molecule facilitating its transport across the blood–brain barrier. However, when gabapentin is applied microiotophoretically to GABA receptors *in vitro* it does not mimic the action of the inhibitory transmitter but appears to act by an as yet unknown mechanism to enhance the release of GABA. Recent evidence suggests that gabapentin acts on a specific binding site in the brain to bring about this effect. There is no evidence that gabapentin reduces the active firing of action potentials nor does it significantly affect any of the calcium channels. Thus it would appear to have a pharmacological profile that differs substantially from any of the more conventional antiepileptic drugs.

Double-blind placebo-controlled trials of patients with refractory partial seizures demonstrate that the addition of gabapentin to standard anti-convulsants was superior to placebo. To date there is little published information on the use of gabapentin as a monotherapy.

The pharmacokinetic properties of gabapentin also differ from most of the standard anticonvulsants. Thus the drug is not metabolized in man; it has a half-life of 5 to 9 hours and does not affect the plasma concentrations of phenytoin, carbamazepine, phenobarbitone or valproate. Overall, clinical studies show that gabapentin is well tolerated, the most common adverse effects being sedation, dizziness, ataxia and fatigue that tend to resolve within the first 2 weeks of the start of therapy.

Lamotrigine is a novel phenyltriazine derivative which has also recently been introduced as an addition to other standard anticonvulsant drugs for

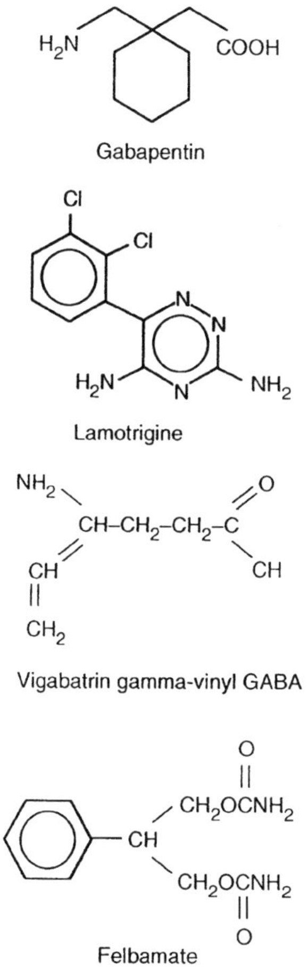

Gabapentin

Lamotrigine

Vigabatrin gamma-vinyl GABA

Felbamate

Figure 11.2. Chemical structure of some novel anticonvulsants.

the treatment of partial seizures in adults. The chemical structure is shown in Figure 11.2.

Lamotrigine is unique in its mode of action in that it acts as an antagonist of the excitatory amino acid glutamate by blocking the N-methyl-D-aspartate (NMDA) receptors. Its action has also been attributed to a block of voltage-sensitive sodium channels, an effect which is also seen with phenytoin and carbamazepine.

Double-blind placebo-controlled trials in patients with refractory partial seizures have demonstrated that the addition of lamotrigine to other standard anticonvulsants was superior to placebo. There is also preliminary clinical evidence to show that lamotrigine is effective as a monotherapy for patients newly diagnosed with partial or generalized seizures, the drug being equieffective with carbamazepine. Lamotrigine may also be effective in the treatment of absence seizures.

Lamotrigine is completely absorbed from the gastrointestinal tract and has a half-life of elimination of about 24 hours. It is metabolized in the liver and its elimination rate is substantially increased by such standard anti-convulsants as phenytoin, carbamazepine, primidone and phenobarbitone. Conversely, lamotrigine will reduce the plasma concentration of valproate by approximately 25% when the drugs are given concurrently. The most common adverse effects are dizziness, blurred vision, nausea, vomiting and rashes when lamotrigine is added to a standard anticonvulsant therapy. A few cases of Stevens–Johnson syndrome and disseminated intravascular coagulation have also been reported.

Gamma-vinyl GABA (GVG) is the first anticonvulsant drug which was developed on the basis of an understanding of the possible pathology of epilepsy. Thus GVG is an irreversible inhibitor of GABA transaminase, the main degradative enzyme of GABA. Experimental studies show that GVG increases brain GABA concentrations at doses that inhibit maximal electroshock seizures and kindled seizures. The chemical structure is shown in Figure 11.2.

Double-blind studies have indicated that GVG is efficacious in the treatment of both partial and secondary generalized seizures. It is marketed in most European countries under the approved name of *vigabatrin*. The principal adverse effects are depression and psychosis in a small percentage of patients. In animals, high doses of GVG have been associated with microvacuolation of myelin; there is currently no convincing evidence that this occurs in therapeutic use.

Although *felbamate* was withdrawn from the market in the USA because of a few cases of aplastic anaemia that were associated with its use, it was found to be particularly effective in the treatment of children with Lennox–Gastaut syndrome. This is a severe disorder characterized by multiple types of seizure which are largely refractory to conventional antiepileptic treatment. In addition the children are generally mentally retarded. Double-blind placebo-controlled trials also showed that felbamate was effective in patients with poorly controlled partial and secondary generalized seizures.

In experimental studies felbamate was shown to be effective in the control of both the maximal electroshock and leptazol induced seizure models. At the cellular level, felbamate was found to be unique in its action as it inhibited the action of glutamate on NMDA receptors and, at the same concentration that was relevant to its clinical effect, potentiated GABA-evoked responses. It is believed that this dual action of felbamate on both excitatory and inhibitory transmission may account for its wide spectrum of therapeutic action. The dicarbamate structure of felbamate is shown in Figure 11.2.

Which type of anticonvulsant should be used for which type of seizure?

This is often a question of clinical choice but the following summary may be of practical use. In the case of a child with infantile spasms the use of adrenocorticotrophic hormone (ACTH) or glucocorticoids would appear to be essential. Similarly ethosuximide has a high degree of specificity for the treatment of generalized absence seizures. However, in the majority of seizure types there is a considerable overlap between the various antiepileptic drugs. Apart from carbamazepine which may be superior to the other drugs for the treatment of complex partial seizures, the choice of drug will largely depend on the tolerance of the patient to the adverse side effects. For example, phenytoin is often unsuitable because of its frequent, and often intolerable, side effects. Teratogenic effects are common with most anticonvulsant drugs although there is some evidence that carbamazepine is less teratogenic than most of these drugs. It should also be emphasized that in pregnancy the metabolism of most anticonvulsants is increased so that the plasma drug concentrations should be monitored should the therapeutic efficacy of the drug be in doubt.

In CONCLUSION, epilepsy is a term used to describe a variety of recurrent symptoms which result from the synchronous or sustained discharge of a group of neurons. It is not clear which specific abnormality in synaptic function is associated with epilepsy, but there is some evidence that an impairment of inhibitory transmission in the neocortex and hippocampus may be primarily involved. The possible causative role of GABA is supported by the fact that many clinically useful anticonvulsants facilitate GABA transmission. Other anticonvulsants may owe their efficacy to their ability to stabilize cation movements across neuronal membranes and/or to affect the phosphorylation of membrane proteins.

With regard to the antiepileptic drugs that are currently available, no attempt has been made to be entirely comprehensive. There are a number of exciting developments in the search for novel anticonvulsants, of which selective GABA transaminase inhibitor *gamma-vinyl GABA* (vigabatrin) is particularly interesting. However, we must await the outcome of the extensive clinical trials before a proper assessment may be made of its efficacy and lack of toxicity. Another novel approach to the treatment of epilepsy has been to reduce the functional activity of the glutaminergic pathway in the cortical and limbic regions of the brain. *Lamotrigine* has recently been introduced for the treatment of partial seizures and generalized tonic–clonic seizures that are not satisfactorily controlled by standard medication. *Lamotrigine* acts by reducing the excitatory effects of glutamate by acting as a NMDA receptor antagonist. Perhaps the most unique antiepileptic drug to be developed so far is *gabapentin,* the mechanism of action of which still remains elusive.

12 Drug Treatment of Parkinson's Disease

Introduction

Idiopathic Parkinson's disease was first described by James Parkinson in 1817 as paralysis agitans, or the "shaking palsy". It is a relatively common neurodegenerative disease afflicting approximately 1% of all adults over the age of 65. The primary neurological features of the disease include difficulty in walking, a mask-like facial expression, and impairment of speech and of skilled acts such as writing. Without effective treatment, these symptoms progress to a rigid akinetic state in which the patients are incapable of caring for themselves and which inevitably ends in death due to complications of immobility such as pneumonia. There have been major advances in the drug therapy of parkinsonism in recent years which have markedly reduced the morbidity from this disease.

Parkinsonism is a clinical syndrome that comprises four main features: *bradykinesia* (a slowness and poverty of movement), *muscular rigidity* (increased resistance of muscles to passive movement), *resting tremor*, which usually disappears during voluntary movement, and *abnormalities in posture and gait*.

It is now widely accepted that the term *Parkinson's syndrome* refers to a collection of neurodegenerative diseases, all of which are characterized by movement disorders. It also applies to drug-induced disorders of the parkinsonian type. A schematic representation of this syndrome is shown in Figure 12.1.

Most of these disorders are related to degenerative processes that are confined to the neuromelanin-pigmented nuclei of the basal ganglia (the substantia nigra), the locus ceruleus and parts of the dorsal vagal nucleus and reticular formation. While the cause of idiopathic parkinsonism is unknown, neuroleptics, viral infections and metals such as manganese are known to precipitate non-degenerative forms of the disorder. In addition to defects of movement, parkinsonian patients often show symptoms such as depression and lack of concentration, an inability to associate ideas, a tendency to perseveration and a general slowness of thought which may progress to a true dementia. Abnormal endocrine function, involving for example prolactin and growth hormone secretion, has also been reported to occur in this disorder.

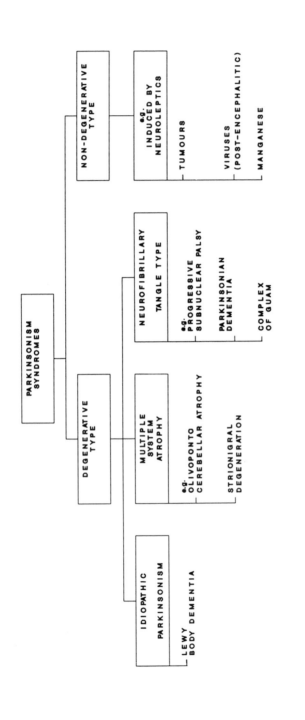

Figure 12.1. Neurobiological diseases in which parkinsonian symptoms occur.

Idiopathic parkinsonism is distinguished from the other syndromes by the presence of Lewy bodies in the substantia nigra and locus ceruleus, and to a lesser extent in the substantia innominata, hypothalamus, dorsal medulla and sympathetic ganglia.

While the aetiology of idiopathic parkinsonism is unknown, the underlying pathology is established. In 1960, Hornykiewicz demonstrated that patients with the disease showed a deficit in the concentration of dopamine in the zona compacta and substantia nigra, the reduction in the concentration of this transmitter correlating with the severity of the symptoms. Genetic factors do not appear to play an important role, although familial forms of the disease have been described. The lack of genetic factors that predispose patients to the disease has prompted research into possible environmental causes. So far no specific environmental toxins have been identified, but there has been considerable interest in the discovery that N-methyl-4-phenyl-1,2,4,6-tetrahydropyridine (MPTP), a toxic metabolite formed during the synthesis of pethidine, can cause a syndrome in man and primates which is indistinguishable from true parkinsonism (see p. 304 for further discussion). This experimentally induced form of the disease responds to anti-parkinsonian therapy and has been of considerable importance in the development of a useful animal model of the disease. It has been speculated that substances that are structurally related to MPTP may occur in the environment (e.g. some herbicides can produce such compounds), and the possibility arises that repeated exposure to small quantities of such toxins, combined with the effects of ageing, may be sufficient to cause the disease.

While there is little evidence to suggest that endogenous excitotoxic mechanisms play a role in the neuronal degeneration found in parkinsonism, there is experimental evidence that the excitotoxic action of methamphetamine against dopaminergic nigrostriatal neurons is blocked by the N-methyl-D-aspartate (NMDA) receptor antagonist MK-801. As these neurons degenerate selectively in parkinsonism it may be postulated that an endogenous excitotoxin is instrumental in causing the disease. Thus it may be speculated that nigrostriatal neurons are sensitive to a sequence of events in which either physical trauma or some toxic agent induces oxidative stress resulting in the release of excitatory amino acids that damage the nigrostriatal dopaminergic cells.

The striatal dopaminergic system and parkinsonism

The classical studies of Hornykiewicz and colleagues in the early 1960s clearly established that the symptoms of parkinsonism were correlated with a defect in the dopamine content of the striatum. The pigmented neurons of the substantia nigra contain dopamine as the major neurotransmitter, accounting for 80% of the total dopamine content of the brain, and the principal motor abnormalities of the disease occur when the transmitter has been depleted by about 80%. While it is now established that acetylcholine, gamma-aminobutyric acid (GABA), glutamate and a number of neuropeptides (e.g. somatostatin, the enkephalins and substance P) also occur in the basal ganglia, so far only dopamine and acetylcholine appear to be of significance with regard to the drug treatment of this disorder. A simple, but useful, model of basal ganglia function suggests that the neostriatum, containing the caudate nucleus and the putamen, normally contains a balance between the inhibitory dopaminergic and the excitatory cholinergic components. As the cholinergic neurons in the basal ganglia do not appear to be damaged in parkinsonism, it is postulated that the symptoms of the disease arise as a consequence of the lack of inhibitory control of the excitatory cholinergic neurons. This provides a rational basis for the use of L-dopa (levodopa), the precursor amino acid of dopamine, and of anticholinergic drugs for the symptomatic relief of this disorder. The interrelationship between the numerous transmitters that play a role in the function of the basal ganglia is shown diagrammatically in Figure 12.2.

Patients with Parkinson's disease show changes in the pre- and postsynaptic dopaminergic neurons which try to compensate for the progressive disappearance of the transmitter. Thus the surviving presynaptic terminals become hyperactive, while the postsynaptic D_2 receptors become hypersensitive in an attempt to compensate for the reduced dopaminergic function. These compensatory changes probably account for the relative lack of symptoms of the disease until the dopamine content has been depleted by more than 80%.

In addition to changes in the basal ganglia, a disruption of the mesocortical limbic dopaminergic system also occurs. Thus in parkinsonism the ventral tegmental area, a dopamine-rich region of the mesocortical system, has been shown to have a reduced dopamine content, as have the terminals that project to the cortex from this region. However, there is no evidence to show that the D_2 receptors in the limbic region become hypersensitive as a consequence of dopamine cell loss. The impaired dopaminergic transmission in the limbic and cortical regions may play a crucial role in the psychiatric symptoms (e.g. perseveration, slowness of thought) that occur in the advanced stage of the illness. Similarly, the hallucinations which occasionally occur in patients on long-term L-dopa therapy may be a consequence of overstimulation of D_2 receptors in these regions of the brain.

Selective degeneration of dopamine neurons in the hypothalamus also occurs, which probably accounts for the rise in the release of prolactin, growth hormone and melanocyte-stimulating hormone; dopamine is known to inhibit the release of these hormones under normal physiological conditions.

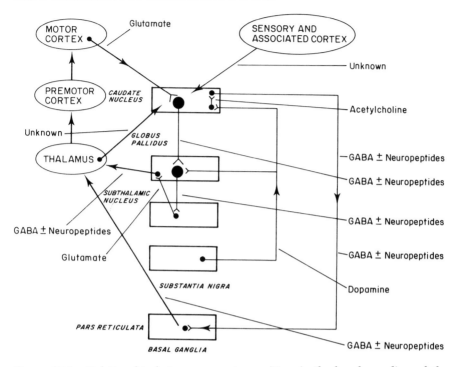

Figure 12.2.   Relationship between neurotransmitters in the basal ganglia and the cortex.

In addition, to the well-established degenerative changes in the dopaminergic system which are the main neuropathological features of Parkinson's disease, it is now known that aminergic and cholinergic ascending subcortical neurons, and peptidergic pathways, are also affected in this disease. Thus lesions of the locus ceruleus occur, with a loss of noradrenaline and its main synthesizing enzyme, dopamine beta-oxidase, in both cortical and subcortical regions of the brain. It would appear that the dorsal bundle from the locus ceruleus is most severely damaged, while the ascending pathways are largely unaffected. In patients at an advanced stage of the disease, cortical alpha$_1$ and beta adrenoceptors show an increase which may be correlated with the onset of some of the symptoms of dementia in these patients. Similarly, a defect in serotonergic transmission has been reported in parkinsonism, a change that may contribute to the depressive symptoms that often occur in the advanced stage of the disease.

Regarding the cholinergic system, there is evidence that the pathway from the substantia innominata to the cortex degenerates in parkinsonism, and that the septohippocampal pathway is also functioning suboptimally. As more than 30% of parkinsonian patients exhibit intellectual deterioration with deficits in cognitive function and memory, it is possible that these cholinergic deficits may account for at least some of the symptoms of parkinsonian dementia.

The enkephalins, somatostatin and substance P all appear to be depleted in idiopathic parkinsonism, which may be a consequence of neuronal degeneration rather than a cause of any of the symptoms of the disease. Thus these changes do not correlate with the severity of the motor symptoms, although there is some indication that the loss of somatostatin may be associated with intellectual impairment.

In SUMMARY, the parkinsonian syndromes all show a marked degeneration of the nigrostriatal dopaminergic system which Hornykiewicz has designated the "striatal dopaminergic deficiency syndromes". Nevertheless, other neurotransmitter systems, such as those involving the cortical noradrenergic, serotonergic, cholinergic and somatostatin-containing neurons have also been shown to be defective. Such systems may be responsible for the intellectual deterioration which frequently occurs in the advanced stage of the disease.

Drugs used in Parkinson's disease

L-dopa

The discovery that dopamine was depleted in the basal ganglia of patients who suffered from parkinsonism at the time of death led to the rational development of the therapeutic treatment, namely the use of L-dopa. Since dopamine does not cross the blood–brain barrier, and is rapidly catabolized in the wall of the intestinal tract by monoamine oxidase (MAO) the amine itself cannot be administered. However, L-dopa is rapidly decarboxylated in the brain to dopamine and it was found that high doses of the precursor could reverse many of the symptoms of the disease. Such high doses (up to 10 g were sometimes necessary) caused serious peripheral side effects because up to 95% of the drug was decarboxylated in the peripheral tissues and therefore never reached the brain. To prevent the peripheral catabolism of L-dopa, and to also reduce the dose of the drug that had to be given to produce a beneficial effect, a peripherally acting dopa decarboxylase inhibitor is now routinely combined with the drug. Decarboxylase inhibitors such as carbidopa or benserazide are structural analogues of L-dopa and thereby act as false substrates for dopa decarboxylase. Being charged molecules at physiological pH they cannot cross the blood–brain barrier and thereby permit parenterally administered dopa to reach the brain unchanged. The use of such inhibitors enables the dose of L-dopa to be reduced to a few grams or less, and thereby reduces the frequency and severity of the peripheral side effects which were so apparent in the early stages of its application. It should be noted, however, that an interaction occurs between dopa and pyridoxine due to the fact that pyridoxine is an essential cofactor for the enzyme metabolizing this drug. This can occasionally be a problem in patients who are concurrently taking a multi-vitamin preparation that contains pyridoxine. Despite the progress which has been made in recent years regarding the reduction in the effective dose of L-dopa that is administered, approximately 80% of patients have gastrointestinal disturbances on the drug. These take the form of nausea and occasionally vomiting. Orthostatic hypotension is also apparent in some patients. The structure of L-dopa and the peripheral dopa decarboxylase inhibitors is shown in Figure 12.3.

Approximately 75% of patients with idiopathic parkinsonism respond satisfactorily to L-dopa therapy with a reduction in their symptoms of at least 50%. In addition to a beneficial change in their motor symptoms, the mood changes associated with the disease also improve. In some patients, L-dopa has an alerting effect and occasionally more disturbing mental symptoms arise. These take the form of hallucinations, paranoia, mania, insomnia, anxiety and nightmares. Older patients being treated with L-dopa appear to be more prone to these effects. In addition, enhanced libido may occur in male patients, which may be socially unacceptable! Approximately 15% of patients may show such symptoms, which are often controlled by lowering the dose of the drug. The more severe psychotic episodes appear to be more frequent in those patients who are dementing.

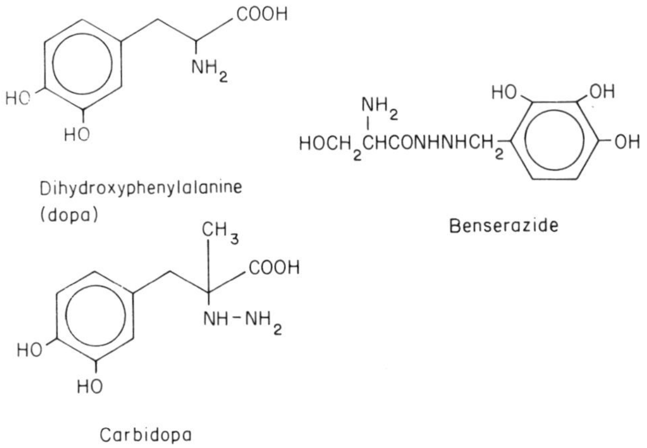

Figure 12.3. Chemical structure of dopa and two peripheral dopa decarboxylase inhibitors.

Abnormal involuntary movements appear in approximately 50% of patients within the first few months of the commencement of L-dopa therapy, these effects being correlated with the dose of the drug and the degree of clinical improvement. The frequency of the abnormal involuntary movements increases with the duration of administration and can reach 80% of patients after 1 year of therapy. Such abnormal movements are presumed to be due to postsynaptic dopamine receptor hyperactivity and include buccolingual movements, grimacing, head-bobbing, and various choreiform and dystonic movements of the extremities. Tolerance does not appear to develop to these effects and there is no known treatment apart from reducing the dose of L-dopa, a situation which inevitably leads to the likelihood of a return of the parkinsonian symptoms.

Other side effects involve changes in gastrointestinal function, which may be reduced by increasing the dose of the decarboxylase inhibitor and/or giving the peripheral antiemetic drug domperidone. Postural hypotension arises as a consequence of the increase in the dopamine content of the sympathetic ganglia; in these ganglia dopamine acts as an inhibitory transmitter, so that the decreased ganglionic transmission inevitably leads to reduced peripheral sympathetic tone and a drop in blood pressure.

Figure 12.4 illustrates the relationship between the efficacy of L-dopa therapy and time.

Drug-induced parkinsonism may arise following the long-term administration of neuroleptics that block central dopamine receptors or reserpine-like drugs that deplete dopamine stores. Because of their mode of action, neuroleptics should never be coadministered to patients being treated with L-dopa or vice versa.

Non-specific MAO inhibitors such as phenelzine, isocarboxazid or tranylcypromine are contraindicated in patients on L-dopa therapy as they are likely to precipitate hyperpyrexia and hypertension. However, recently the selective MAO-B inhibitor *deprenyl* (also called selegiline) has been shown to be a useful adjunct to L-dopa therapy. Deprenyl, by preventing the catabolism of dopamine in the basal ganglia, enables a lower dose of dopa to be administered and also appears to delay the onset of the more serious side effects of dopa. There is also experimental evidence to show that deprenyl can prevent the occurrence of the symptoms of parkinsonism induced by the neurotoxin MPTP (see Chapter 14). There is evidence that MPTP is converted to its active metabolite the 1-methyl-4-phenylpyridinium ion (MPP^+) by MAO-B. By inhibiting MAO-B, deprenyl therefore protects the basal ganglia from the degenerative effects of MPP^+. The low incidence of the "cheese effect" and the synergistic interaction between deprenyl and L-dopa suggest that MAO-B type inhibitors will play an increasingly important role in the management of parkinsonism in the future.

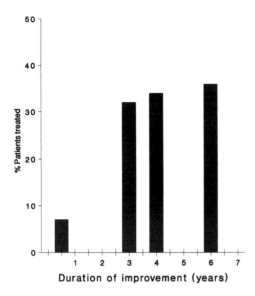

Figure 12.4. Relationship between the efficacy of L-dopa treatment and time. It should be noted that patients who fail to show any improvement ($<50\%$) after short-term (<1 year) treatment with L-dopa are probably not suffering from idiopathic parkinsonism.

Dopamine receptor agonists

Because of the side effects commonly associated with L-dopa treatment, a number of directly acting dopamine receptor agonists have been tried in the hope that they may combine therapeutic efficacy with reduced adverse effects. *Apomorphine* was one of the first drugs to be tried and while it was shown to have some effect on the symptoms of parkinsonism, its short duration of action and the frequency and severity of its side effects precluded its further use. Of the more recently developed dopamine agonists, the *ergolines* have received particular attention. These drugs include *bromocriptine, pergolide* and *lisuride*. Like apomorphine, these drugs are not specific agonists for the D_2 type receptors and all have side effects which are related to their ergot type of structure. Nausea and vomiting are particularly prominent side effects, even at low doses, while psychiatric reactions and postural hypotension of the type associated with L-dopa are also features of the ergolines.

Of the ergolines that have been developed, *bromocriptine* has received most attention. Since the first report in 1974 of its use as an adjunct to L-dopa therapy, more than a decade of clinical experience with bromocriptine has failed to establish a distinct role for the drug in the treatment of parkinsonism. Experience with the use of bromocriptine alone in newly diagnosed cases is even more limited. Unacceptable adverse reactions are frequent and even in those patients who can tolerate the gastrointestinal side effects the beneficial effects decline rapidly. It seems unlikely that the rapid onset of tolerance to the therapeutic effects is only due to changes in dopamine receptor sensitivity, as L-dopa is generally effective in patients who cease to respond to bromocriptine. It is also of interest that the abnormal involuntary movements which frequently occur following dopa therapy are seldom found after treatment with the ergolines. The reason for this is unknown but may be associated with differences in the action of these drugs on dopamine receptor subtypes. Bromocriptine, for example, acts as a partial agonist at D_1 receptors and as a full agonist at D_2 receptors. Whether the development of a specific D_2 agonist will combine therapeutic efficacy with a reduced frequency of side effects remains to be seen. The structure of some of the ergolines that have been used in the treatment of parkinsonism is shown in Figure 12.5.

Amantadine

This is an antiviral agent which was accidentally discovered to be of some value in the initial treatment of Parkinson's disease. While the precise mechanism of action of this drug is uncertain, there is experimental evidence to show that it increases the release and synthesis of dopamine and inhibits its reuptake, thereby facilitating the action of the neurotransmitter in those dopaminergic terminals that are still able to function. It has been found that patients soon develop a tolerance to the beneficial effects of the drug, which has largely precluded its long-term use.

Anticholinergic drugs

These drugs, initially as the crude extract of *Atropa belladonna* and more recently as specific anticholinergic drugs such as *benztropine* or *biperiden*, have been used for over a century to reduce the tremor seen in patients with parkinsonism. The mechanism of action of these drugs lies in their ability to reduce the functional activity of the excitatory cholinergic system in the basal ganglia; centrally acting anticholinesterases such as physostigmine are known to exacerbate the tremor associated with the disease.

In the past 40 years a wide variety of synthetic and semi-synthetic anticholinergic agents have been developed for their selectivity in blocking muscarinic receptors in the brain (see Figure 12.6 for the structure of some of those in current clinical use), but all are associated to some degree with the typical peripheral anticholinergic effects of blurred vision, dry mouth, urinary retention and constipation. The popularity of *benzhexol* lies in its additional ability to inhibit striatal dopamine reuptake.

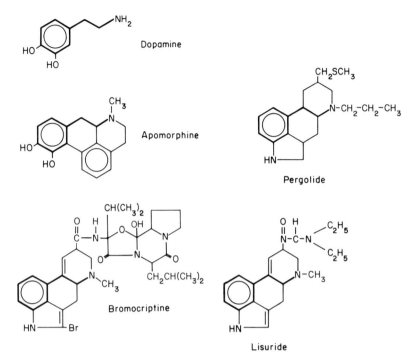

Figure 12.5. Chemical structure of some ergolines that have been or are currently used in the treatment of parkinsonism. The outline structure of dopamine is also given to show why these drugs act as dopamine receptor agonists. The extended side chains in lisuride may also account for the action of the drug on 5-HT (particularly 5-HT$_2$) receptors. The hallucinogenic effects of lisuride may be attributed to its action on central 5-HT$_2$ receptors.

The anticholinergic agents attenuate the tremor associated with parkinsonism and relieve the muscular rigidity, but have no effect on the akinesia. This suggests that the features of increased tremor and rigidity are the result of disinhibited cholinergic efferent activity, whereas the negative symptoms of reduced motor function correlate with the dopamine deficiency. There is evidence of tolerance development after several years of treatment with these drugs, so that their use is largely restricted to the more acute phase of the disease.

It must be stressed that elderly patients are particularly sensitive to the anticholinergic effects of drugs, whether they be tricyclic antidepressants, phenothiazine neuroleptics or central anticholinergics. Such drugs can cause toxic confusional states and impaired memory and intellectual function; these effects are particularly apparent following long-term therapy. For this

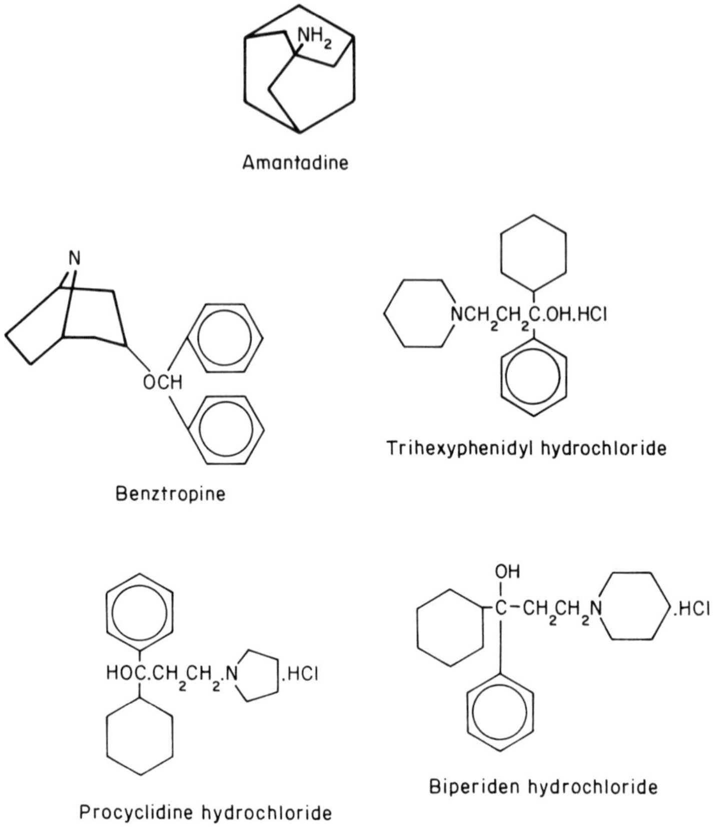
NH2
Amantadine
N
OCH
Benztropine
NCH2CH2C.OH.HCl
Trihexyphenidyl hydrochloride
HOC.CH2CH2.N
.HCl
Procyclidine hydrochloride
OH
C–CH2CH2N
.HCl
Biperiden hydrochloride

Figure 12.6. Chemical structure of amantadine and of centrally acting anticholinergic agents used in the treatment of parkinsonism. The antiviral compound amantadine is a dopamine-releasing agent with some anticholinergic activity.

reason, such drugs should only be used sparingly in the elderly and then only when other therapeutically effective agents cannot be used.

Table 12.1 summarizes the drugs which have been used to treat the symptoms of Parkinson's disease.

Limitations in the use of L-dopa in the treatment of parkinsonism: the "on-off" phenomenon

The combination of L-dopa with a peripheral dopa decarboxylase inhibitor is generally considered to be the most effective therapy for idiopathic parkinsonism. A major controversy concerns the timing of the initiation of drug treatment. Some investigators favour delaying treatment for as long as possible since there is evidence that drug-induced dyskinesias and

Table 12.1. Drugs used in the treatment of Parkinson's disease

Mechanisms of action	Drugs
L-dopa	Levodopa, levodopa+carbidopa, levodopa+ benserazide, levodopa+carbidopa (controlled release formulation), levodopa infusion
Direct-acting dopamine receptor agonists	Apomorphine, bromocriptine, lisuride, pergolide
Dopamine releasing agent	Amantadine
Monoamine oxidase B inhibitor	Selegiline (deprenyl)
Centrally acting anticholinergic drugs	Benzotropine, trihexyphenidyl, procydidine
Free radical scavengers (of doubtful clinical efficacy)	Ascorbate; tocopheol

In addition, antidepressants are sometimes necessary to reduce the depressive symptoms which frequently occur in these patients.

fluctuations in response to treatment (the "on-off" phenomenon) are related to the early initiation of drug treatment. However, there is increasing clinical evidence that the dyskinesias and fluctuation in treatment response are a reflection of the degenerative changes caused by the disease. It has also been shown that there is a reduction in the mortality and a slower progression in the severity of the disease when treatment is initiated relatively soon after the disease has been diagnosed.

Two main phases of treatment with L-dopa have been distinguished. The initial induction phase lasts several weeks and is followed by the maintenance phase. During the induction phase the daily dose of L-dopa should be increased slowly to minimize the likelihood of side effects. However, following 2–5 years' successful therapeutic control of the symptoms, the dyskinesias and abnormal involuntary movements often occur. Such changes are attributed to striatal dopamine receptor super-sensitivity, possibly occurring as a consequence of denervation of the dopaminergic tracts in the nigrostriatal area. When they occur, the dyskinesias are superimposed on the waxing and waning of the response to treatment, and may be associated with the peak therapeutic effect (called "peak-dose" dyskinesia). Eventually the patient becomes unable to achieve any degree of mobility without experiencing some involuntary movement. Dietary factors and erratic gastric emptying may further complicate the picture so that the response to L-dopa may seem random and unrelated to the time of administration of the drug. At this stage, the patient may suddenly switch from a state of good therapeutic control to severe parkinsonism (the "on-off" effect); such a situation occurs in up to 50% of patients after 5 or more years of treatment and may eventually occur in 90% of patients after more than a decade of treatment.

The fluctuating motor performance can be partly explained by the pharmacokinetics of L-dopa. Most patients have a critical plasma dopa concentration above which the therapeutic effects are apparent. Presumably this reflects the dose necessary to raise the concentration of dopamine in the brain. However, as the degeneration of the nigrostriatal pathway continues, the capacity of dopaminergic neurons to synthesize and store the amine becomes progressively compromised so that the neurons that continue to function are increasingly dependent on the presence of L-dopa for immediate brain dopamine synthesis. Fluctuations in motor performance therefore reflect this dependency on plasma dopa. Thus the beneficial effects of L-dopa decrease with the increasing severity of the motor symptoms, despite the fact that the elimination half-life is relatively uniform throughout the period of treatment. This means that lowering the dose of L-dopa administered in an attempt to reduce the dyskinesia will inevitably lead to a shortened duration of therapeutic effect.

Management of the motor fluctuations has largely been concentrated on attempts to prolong the duration of action of the drug, either by the use of controlled release preparations to obtain "smooth" concentration-time curves or by combining dopa with deprenyl or bromocriptine. Long-term (about 16 years) follow-up studies of patients have shown that the mean "functional" status of the patient approaches pretreatment levels after 5 years, and by 16 years all surviving patients were functionally less well than at the initiation of therapy. From such studies it may be concluded that L-dopa does not cure Parkinson's disease but does produce significant relief for many years and still remains the most effective treatment for the illness.

Use of brain transplants

Despite the compensatory changes which occur amongst surviving cells in the brain of the patient with parkinsonism, once approximately 80% of the nigrostriatal neurons die the clinical deficits of the disease become apparent. The possible mechanisms whereby cell death occurs due to the actions of endogenous neurotoxins has been discussed elsewhere (see pp. 252).

In recent years, experimental evidence has accumulated to suggest that fetal tissue containing aminergic cells may grow on implantation into the mammalian brain. Preliminary studies in patients with parkinsonism have shown that implants of human fetal tissue can grow and innervate the basal ganglia. So far fetal adrenal tissue has been used with beneficial results. While there are many ethical and technical problems regarding the use of adrenal tissue in this way (e.g. several years after receiving such implants some of the patients have developed gliomas), such an approach may point the way to a more successful and permanent method of treating patients with Parkinson's disease in the future.

There is evidence that trophic factors, which are essential for the development of neurons and their maintenance in the adult brain, could play a role in delaying the degenerative changes in the brain of a patient with Parkinson's disease. Such trophic factors include the epidermal growth factor, basic fibroblast growth factor, brain-derived neurotrophic factor and the glia-derived neurotrophic factor. These factors have been shown to enhance the survival and growth of dopaminergic neurons in cell culture. The glia-derived neurotrophic factor appears to be particularly specific in stimulating the growth of dopaminergic neurons. It is now possible to add the appropriate factors to fetal dopaminergic cells prior to their transplantation to ensure their long-term viability and differentiation.

In CONCLUSION, the last 30 years have witnessed many important advances in our understanding of Parkinson's disease. Based on this understanding drugs have been developed that have led to a significant reduction in the mortality of patients with the disease. However, despite these advances there is no evidence that the drugs available prevent the progression of the disease. Perhaps the application of growth factors will provide the clinician with the means whereby this can be achieved.

13 Alzheimer's Disease and Stroke: Possible Biochemical Causes and Treatment Strategies

Introduction

Alzheimer's disease is the most common dementing disease in the industrialized countries affecting approximately one in five persons over the age of 80 years. It is characterized by memory loss, personality changes and signs of cortical malfunction such as apraxia, aphasia and agnosia. Substantial pathological changes have been found in cortical and subcortical areas, including neurofibrillary tangles and amyloid-containing neuritic plaques. The hippocampus appears to be particularly vulnerable to such changes, which probably accounts for the gross disturbance in memory function that occurs early in the onset of the disease.

Alzheimer's disease was first described in 1907 by Alois Alzheimer who identified and described the presence of numerous *neurofibrillary tangles* in the brain of a 51-year-old woman who had suffered from progressive dementia over a number of years. These neurofibrillary tangles were predominantly found in the hippocampus, amygdala, nucleus basalis, hypothalamus and several other subcortical structures. Further studies clearly showed that the density of those tangles correlated with the degree of cognitive impairment shown by the patient prior to death. The other characteristic pathological feature of the brain of the patient with Alzheimer's disease is the presence of *senile* or *neuritic plaques*. Such structures are large, lie within the neurophil, and occur throughout the neocortex and hippocampus. The density of these plaques is also correlated with the degree of cognitive impairment shown by the patient at the time of death. In addition to the tangles and plaques, *Hirano bodies* are also a feature of the post-mortem brain of the Alzheimer patient. These bodies were first described in the brains of patients suffering from a rare dementing disease called amyotrophic lateral sclerosis of Guam.

Gross changes are also apparent in the brain of an Alzheimer's patient, but do not appear to be specific for Alzheimer's disease. Thus the brain weight is reduced compared with age- and sex-matched non-demented individuals, although it must be emphasized that there is considerable overlap between the controls and demented patients. A moderate degree of lateral and third ventricular dilatation is also apparently associated with a thinning of the cortex. Loss of the underlying white matter also occurs in the brains of Alzheimer's patients. In contrast, the deeper subcortical nuclei of the basal ganglia and thalamus appear to retain their normal appearance.

Although it has been postulated that the presence of amyloid protein in the Alzheimer's brain could be specifically involved in the causation of the disease, there is now evidence that amyloid deposits also occur in the brains of patients with other types of neurological disorder and it is therefore doubtful whether amyloid protein is a primary pathogenetic factor for this illness. However, it is also possible that the structure of the amyloid protein in the brain of the Alzheimer patient differs from that in the brain of the aged individual.

Genetic factors

Epidemiological studies have identified two major risk factors in the causation of Alzheimer's disease, namely advanced age and the presence of relatives who are, or have been, afflicted with the disease. Over 50 familial pedigrees of Alzheimer's disease have so far been identified and investigated. Analysis of these pedigrees reveals that in some of these families a predisposition of the disease may be transmitted as an autosomal dominant trait. These families are characterized by an early age of onset of the disease (40–60 years) in those affected. By contrast, in population studies such an early onset of Alzheimer's disease occurs only infrequently, which either suggests that there is a relatively rare, genetically linked form of familial Alzheimer's disease or that more extensive and detailed studies of these families may show that the disease also occurs in the more typical form in the older (70 years or more) members of the family. Recent studies conducted in the United States in which a large number of elderly patients were screened for Alzheimer's disease have suggested that there is evidence of an autosomal dominant genetic transmission of the disease. These studies further suggest that the expression of this dominant gene is late, with the maximum probability of its appearance being in the ninth decade! Thus it seems possible that there are at least two forms of genetic transmission, one form producing the early onset, and the more common form the late onset of the disease. In addition, exogenous factors such as a slow virus, an abnormal immunoglobulin that may target nervous tissue, particularly the amyloid protein associated with plaques, or an increased sensitivity to environmental toxins such as aluminium may also be causally involved.

The similarity between the neuropathological changes seen in Alzheimer's disease and in Down's syndrome suggests that there may be a common genetic factor underlying both diseases. Several research groups have recently identified a beta-amyloid protein-producing gene located on chromosome 21 in both Down's syndrome and some patients with Alzheimer's disease. Preliminary data have also shown that patients with Alzheimer's disease show the presence of a gene for the amyloid protein on chromosome 9 which appears to be absent in patients with Down's syndrome.

One of the most exciting findings, however, concerns the identification of a specific mutation in the gene coding for amyloid precursor proteins on chromosome 21 in a small group of patients with familial Alzheimer's disease. However, it must be emphasized that some patients with this form of the disease do not show such mutations, neither do those patients with the late onset form of familial Alzheimer's disease. This suggests that there may be another gene on chromosome 21 that predisposes to the familial form of Alzheimer's disease. Other forms of inherited neurological disease that may be associated with a mutation in amyloidogenic proteins include familial amyloidotic polyneuropathy, Gerstmann–Straussler syndrome and some forms of Creutzfeldt–Jakob disease. Despite the recent exciting discovery of a gene mutation that may be responsible for some forms of Alzheimer's disease, more data must be obtained before it can be finally established that the amyloid precursor protein gene is the causative factor in this condition.

The last 10 years have witnessed an astonishing increase in knowledge concerning the pathogenic mechanisms in Alzheimer's disease. It is widely acknowledged that the amyloid beta protein plays an important role in the pathogenesis of the disease. It is also apparent that a number of genes have been identified that are clearly linked to Alzheimer's disease, particularly the familial (or early onset) form of the disease. Mutations in the amyloid precursor protein gene on chromosome 21, and point mutations on chromosomes 14 and 3, have now been identified. Such mutations account for approximately 70% of familial Alzheimer's disease among patients with the early onset illness. In addition, a potent susceptibility locus on chromosome 19 associated with apolipoprotein E has been strongly associated with an increased risk of the late onset form of the disease with the presence of the apolipoprotein E_4.

The question arises how an overproduction of a naturally occurring protein, the amyloid beta protein, can be the main causative event in the development of Alzheimer's disease. It is known that in Down's syndrome the triplicated chromosome 21 is associated with increased synthesis of amyloid beta protein and that Alzheimer's disease is an inevitable occurrence in those patients by the time they reach early middle age. It would now appear that these individuals with mutations on chromosome 14 and 1 also have an increased synthesis of amyloid beta protein, particularly in the form of the protein that contains the 1–42 amino acid (termed $A\beta1$–42) sequence.

In recent years the mechanism by which amyloid beta protein causes neurotoxicity has received much attention. Recent studies have suggested that Aβ1–42 induces its neurotoxicity by a process of apoptosis or programmed cell death. Cell death proceeds by two general mechanisms, namely necrosis or apoptosis. Necrosis is a passive response of the cell to a lethal stressful insult whereas apoptosis usually follows a defined series of events which includes the formation of swellings (blebs) on the cell surface, condensation and destruction of the chromatin, division of the nucleus and nuclear extrusion. Proteolysis disrupts the cellular cytoskeleton and activates various nucleases. Several genes are now known to be activated during this process, the immediate response genes termed *C-Jun* and *C-fos* being particularly important. It would now appear that the increase in the synthesis of Aβ1–42 is responsible for neuronal destruction by increasing apoptosis.

The question arises how these changes caused by Aβ1–42 are linked with the appearance of neurofibrillary tangles which are also a characteristic pathological feature of the disease. The answer to this question is so far unclear. It does not appear that neurofibrillary tangle formation is simply the end stage of a neurodegenerative process brought about by Aβ neurotoxicity as other neurodegenerative processes are not associated with tangle formation. Tangle formation is therefore unlikely to be a non-specific event that occurs as a result of the death of brain cells.

The recent discovery of the association between apolipoprotein E₄ (APOE₄) and the increased risk of late onset Alzheimer's disease is of considerable importance as it could act as an easy marker of the disease. The relationship between the four main alleles of APOE and the pathogenesis of Alzheimer's disease has still to be determined. It has been hypothesized that some apolipoproteins are involved in transporting Aβ which could enhance the susceptibility to the disease; APOE₄ may be particularly important in this regard.

A detailed account of the pathological changes involved in Alzheimer's disease are outside the boundary of this text. The advances that have been made in the last decade do, however, serve to illustrate how the powerful techniques of molecular biology have helped to evaluate the pathological mechanism underlying Alzheimer's disease which will, hopefully, lead to the development of drugs that can reduce the excessive synthesis of Aβ which appears to be responsible for the premature destruction of brain cells.

Neurochemical changes associated with Alzheimer's disease

There has been considerable interest in the involvement of the major neurotransmitters in the possible aetiology of Alzheimer's disease. Thus it is

Table 13.1. Changes in the neurotransmitters in the brain of an Alzheimer patient

Neurotransmitter system	Changes occurring in Alzheimer's disease
Cholinergic system	Decreased choline acetyltransferase and acetyl-cholinesterase activity in cortex. Reduced choline uptake and acetylcholine synthesis. Loss of cells in nucleus basalis and occurrence of tangles in remaining cells in the brain area
Noradrenergic system	Decreased dopamine beta-oxidase and reduced noradrenaline synthesis. Loss of cells in the locus ceruleus and occurrence of tangles in remaining cells
Dopaminergic system	Slight reduction in dopamine
Serotonergic system	Some reduction in 5-HT synthesis with a loss of cells in the raphé nuclei and the occurrences of tangles in remaining cells
Peptidergic system	Reduction in somatostatin and corticotrophin releasing factor immunoreactivity in cortex. No convincing evidence of change in the concentration of substance P, enkephalins, cholecystokinin, neuropeptide Y, glutamate, aspartate or GABA

well established that the nucleus basalis of Meynert and related areas of the basal forebrain show a distinct loss of cholinergic cell bodies in patients with Alzheimer's disease. Similarly, serotonergic neurons of the midbrain raphé area and noradrenergic neurons of the locus ceruleus have been shown to be significantly diminished, particularly in early onset Alzheimer's disease. A summary of the pathological changes in the neurotransmitter systems in the brain of the Alzheimer patient is given in Table 13.1.

The finding that a gross deficit occurs in *central cholinergic transmission* in Alzheimer's disease, the degree of dementia being correlated with the relative deficit in central cholinergic transmission, has led to the suggestion that this is the primary cause of the dementia of Alzheimer's disease. However, it is now increasingly accepted that a cholinergic deficit is unlikely to be the only or indeed a major causative factor. Thus not all patients with the disease, and showing the typical neuropathological changes, show a reduction in the activity of choline acetyltransferase, the enzyme concerned in the synthesis of acetylcholine. Additionally, other patients show normal cholinergic cell numbers in the nucleus basalis of Meynert. More recently it has been shown that patients with a rare neurological disorder, olivopontocerebellar atrophy, exhibit a gross loss of cholinergic neurons in the basal forebrain and yet show no signs of dementia.

It might also be argued that if Alzheimer's disease was primarily due to a cholinergic deficit, it should be possible to correct the deficit by suitable centrally acting cholinomimetic drugs. Despite the numerous studies in which different types of cholinomimetic drugs have been administered, there is no overwhelming evidence to suggest that these drugs have any substantial benefit to the patient (see below). Thus it would appear that, despite the widely confirmed findings that various "classical", peptide and amino acid neurotransmitters are defective in Alzheimer's disease, it is debatable whether a defect in one specific neurotransmitter system is responsible for the clinical signs and symptoms of the disease. There is also some debate about whether the site of the lesion is primarily cortical or subcortical.

The involvement of the excitatory amino acid neurotransmitters, particularly *glutamate*, in post-stroke epilepsy and possibly multi-infarct dementia has led to the suggestion that they may also be involved in the aetiology of Alzheimer's disease. Glutamate is the principal excitatory amino acid neurotransmitter in cortical and hippocampal neurons. In the hippocampus, glutamate has been implicated in memory; it is widely believed that its ability to elicit long-term potentiation is of fundamental importance in memory formation. One of the major excitatory amino acid receptors activated by glutamate is the N-methyl-D-aspartate (NMDA) receptor. Antagonists of the NMDA receptor block the action of glutamate and impair spatial discrimination learning in animals and also memory formation. A disruption in the pre- and postsynaptic excitatory amino acid pathways has been found in patients with Alzheimer's disease. It has been suggested that initial hyperactivity of the glutaminergic input to the hippocampus results in excessive hyperexcitability of the hippocampal cells, leading eventually to cell death.

The primary mechanism whereby glutamate can cause excessive cellular hyperactivity, and ultimately cell death, is via a loss of calcium homeostasis. Calcium ions serve as an intracellular signal that mediates the actions of neurotransmitters and growth factors. The increase in intracellular free calcium is normally transient and is rapidly restored to resting levels by membrane extrusion mechanisms and calcium-binding proteins such as calmodulin. Sustained increases in intracellular calcium, as could occur following excessive glutamate release, result in cytoskeletal disruption, neuritic degeneration and cell death.

In addition to glutamate, various growth factors and amyloid have also been shown to destabilize the intracellular calcium concentration and to induce neurofibrillary-like degeneration in cultured brain cells. An attractive feature of the calcium hypothesis of Alzheimer's disease is that it helps to explain the heterogeneity of the disorder. In addition to functional abnormalities in excitatory amino acids, growth factors, amyloid protein, etc., calcium channels and binding proteins may also be involved. It is not without interest that various dietary and environmental factors (such as aluminium) may also contribute to the calcium defect, so leading to the disorder.

In support of this hypothesis, experimental studies have shown that glutamate neurotoxicity can produce biochemical changes similar to those seen in Alzheimer's disease. Furthermore, the widely publicized finding that the anticholinesterase drug *tetrahydroaminoacridine* (THA, tacrine) is beneficial in ameliorating some of the symptoms of Alzheimer's disease, and the fact that most potent anticholinesterases appear to have minimal beneficial activity, has led to the suggestion that THA could modulate the action of glutamate on the NMDA receptors. Preliminary experimental evidence has shown that THA may act in this way.

It should be emphasized, however, that not all investigators agree that the degenerative changes in cortical neurons are due to glutamate excitotoxicity. Thus, three groups of British and Swedish investigators have suggested that the glutaminergic system is hypoactive rather than hyperactive in Alzheimer's disease. Nevertheless, the development of drugs that block NMDA receptors may be of value in the treatment of multi-infarct dementia, in which there is evidence that excessive glutamate release, with the consequent neuron degeneration, follows the cerebral hypoxia.

It may be concluded that it is not possible at present to identify any one neurotransmitter system as being of primary importance in any of the dementias and that the recorded neurochemical changes are possibly secondary to more fundamental disturbances, the nature of which is unclear. Nevertheless, significant correlations have been shown to exist between neurotransmitter disturbances and behavioural symptoms which may be of value in formulating treatment strategies.

Excitotoxins

The concept of excitotoxicity

The amino acids glutamic and aspartic acids are known to be present in high concentrations in the mammalian brain, where they have been shown to act as excitatory neurotransmitters (see p. 52 *et seq.*). Over 20 years ago, it was shown that the systemic administration of glutamic acid to newborn rodents resulted in a destruction of retinal cells and also some cells in the central nervous system. Later studies showed that high oral doses of this amino acid also caused brain damage in primates, such toxic effects being particularly apparent on the postsynaptic dendrosomal membranes where the excitatory amino acid receptors are located. Such findings led to the concept of excitotoxicity and, later, to the view that some neurological diseases such as epilepsy could be a consequence of nerve cell damage due to the excessive release of glutamate within the brain.

At least three types of excitatory amino acid receptors have been identified, termed the NMDA, alpha-amino-3-hydroxy-5-methyl-4-isoxazole proprionic acid (AMPA) and kainate receptors according to their affinity for specific excitatory amino acids (see p. 61). Antagonists of some of these receptor types, such as MK 801 and D-2-amino-5-phosphonopentanoate (AP 5), were then shown to protect neurons *in vivo* against the neurotoxic effects of glutamate or NMDA. Table 13.2 lists some of the compounds that have been developed as antagonists of the most important of the excitatory amino acid receptors, the NMDA receptor.

So far, only the non-competitive antagonists of the NMDA receptors such as phencyclidine and MK 801 can readily penetrate the blood–brain barrier and therefore protect animals against the toxic effects of exogenous excitatory amino acids. The barbiturates (e.g. thiopentone) have an additional action in blocking both NMDA and non-NMDA (e.g. kainic acid) receptors and are therefore of some interest as broad-spectrum excitotoxin antagonists, while the quinoxalinedione derivative cyanonitro-quinoxalinedione (CNQX) was the first compound to be synthesized that showed a greater potency in blocking non-NMDA excitatory amino acid receptors.

The essential features of the NMDA receptor are illustrated diagramma-tically in Figure 13.1. The NMDA receptor controls the opening of the sodium/calcium ion channel, which may be blocked by dissociation anaesthetics such as phencyclidine and ketamine or by magnesium ions. In addition to glutamate, glycine can also facilitate the opening of the ion channel by activating a strychnine-insensitive receptor site. It should be remembered that in the spinal cord glycine acts as an inhibitory transmitter by acting on a different type of glycine receptor; strychnine causes characteristic convulsions by blocking the action of glycine on these spinal cord receptors. Zinc ions can reduce the effects of glutamate and glycine on the NMDA receptor. In view of the complex inter-relationships between the various agonists that act on the NMDA receptor, it may be speculated that a pathological process affecting any of these factors might create an imbalance which leads to a malfunctioning of excitatory amino acid transmission in the brain.

Environmental excitotoxins

It is well established that *monosodium glutamate*, a widely used food additive and major component of soya sauce, can destroy nerve cells when administered orally to young animals. Those neurons lying immediately outside the blood–brain barrier, e.g. in the arcuate nucleus of the hypothalamus, are the most vulnerable. It is therefore possible that ingestion of a diet high in glutamate may contribute to degenerative changes in the brain later in life.

Table 13.2. Potencies of some antagonists of NMDA receptors in chick embryo retina *in vitro*

	Potency
Competitive NMDA antagonists	
D-2-Amino-5-phosphonopentanoate (AP 5)	25 μM
D-2-Amino-5-phosphonoheptanoate (AP 7)	75 μM
Non-competitive NMDA antagonists	
MK 801	0.01 μM
Phencyclidine	0.5 μM
Ketamine	5 μM
(+/−) Cyclazocine	5 μM
(+/−) N-Allylnormetazocine (SKF 10047)	10 μM
Dextromethorphan	50 μM
Mixed excitatory amino acids	
Cyanonitroquinoxalinedione (CNQX)	50 μM
Kynurenic acid	300 μM
Barbiturates	
Amylobarbitone	50 μM
Thiopentone	200 μM

Potencies of compounds expressed as the minimal concentration (μM) required to provide total protection against the excitotoxic effects of NMDA.

Neurolathyrism occurs in some tropical countries as a result of consuming large quantities of the legume *Lathyrus sativus*, which contains a potent excitatory amino acid analogue that can cause paralysis. In certain South Sea Islands, particularly the island of Guam, ingestion of the seeds of the cycad plant leads to the occurrence of a specific neurological disease with the combined features of amyotrophic lateral sclerosis, parkinsonism and dementia. The analogue of alanine that causes this neurological disease has been identified.

Excitotoxins and neurodegenerative diseases

Epilepsy and related disorders may arise as a consequence of a dramatic release of glutamate from central nerve terminals. Sustained seizures of the limbic system in experimental animals result in brain damage that resembles that due to glutamate toxicity. Similar pathological changes are seen at autopsy in patients with intractable epilepsy. In animals, such seizure-related brain damage may be reduced by the administration of non-competitive NMDA antagonists (such as MK 801, phencyclidine or ketamine), but it would appear that not all seizure activity is suppressed by such drugs.

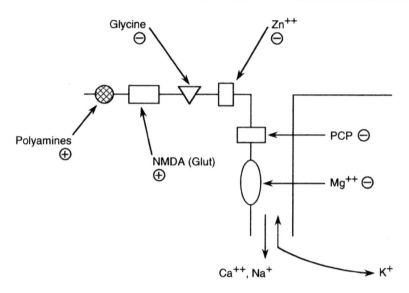

Figure 13.1. Sites of action of endogenous ligands and drugs that modulate the action of excitatory amino acids on the NMDA receptor. Recent evidence shows that glutamate (Glut) and possibly other excitatory amino acids released from presynaptic terminals activate the NMDA receptor site on postsynaptic membranes, resulting in the opening of the Na^+/Ca^{++} channels. Glycine acts on a strychnine-insensitive receptor while polyamines (e.g. spermine and spermidine) also have a modulatory role. Conversely Zn^{++} and Mg^{++} and drugs like phencyclidine (PCP) block the ion channel by acting at various sites on the NMDA receptor complex or the ion channel.

The precise mechanism whereby persistent seizure activity results in neuronal degeneration is incompletely understood. It seems possible that repetitive depolarization and repolarization of the nerve membrane eventually leads to an energy-deprived state within the cell, thereby preventing the restoration of the cell membrane potential. Each depolarization will also lead to an influx of calcium ions, and an efflux of potassium ions, which if prolonged can result in cell death. The reduced efficiency of glial cells to remove potassium ions and the ability of high extracellular concentrations of potassium ions to depolarize neurons and cause neurodegenerative changes also play a critical role in causing the degenerative changes that are a feature of status epilepticus and intractable epilepsy.

Hypoxia and ischaemia may also cause neurodegenerative changes in the mammalian brain. In animals, cerebral ischaemia has been shown to cause a marked elevation in the extracellular concentrations of glutamate and aspartate, particularly in the hippocampus. Such pathological changes can be prevented by the prior administration of NMDA receptor antagonists. The hypoxic state results in energy deficiency within the brain, so that the mechanism responsible for the maintenance of transmembrane potentials may become compromised. The net effect of the elevation in the extracellular concentrations of excitatory amino acids could be a failure of magnesium ions to reduce the functional activity of the NMDA receptor. This could result in persistent membrane depolarization, excessive intracellular accumulation of calcium ions and the extracellular accumulation of potassium ions. The movement of sodium ions, accompanied by water, into the cell further compromises cellular function and results in cell death. Somewhat similar pathological changes have been postulated to occur following *brain and spinal cord injury* and in *dementia pugilistica*, a concussive brain injury associated with boxing.

Other neurological diseases in which a disorder of central excitatory amino acid function has been implicated include *Huntington's disease*, *Alzheimer's disease* and *parkinsonism*. Experimental studies have shown that the injection of excitatory neurotoxins such as kainic and ibotenic acids into the rat brain results in pathological changes that resemble those seen in Huntington's disease. More recently, an endogenous neurotoxin, quinolinic acid, has been found in human brain which, if present in excessive quantities, selectively destroys the striatum but leaves other regions largely unaffected. While it now seems unlikely that quinolinic acid is the endogenous excitotoxin responsible for the pathological changes found in Huntington's disease, it remains a possibility that some other excitotoxin with similar properties and selectivity of action on striatal function may be involved. The possible involvement of excitotoxins in the pathology of Alzheimer's disease and parkinsonism is considered in the appropriate chapters.

Treatment strategies based on correcting neurotransmitter defects

The cholinergic system

Following the dramatic improvement of a small group of patients with Alzheimer's disease after the administration of THA, there has been a renewed interest in the administration of anticholinesterases and directly acting cholinomimetic drugs to try to reverse some of the behavioural deficits associated with the disease. Five major approaches have been used:

1. Use of *acetylcholine precursors*. Administration of high oral doses of choline or phosphatidylcholine (lecithin) have failed to produce any beneficial effects in any of the studies so far published.

2. Use of drugs that *release acetylcholine*. There is preliminary evidence to suggest that 4-aminopyridine and 3,4-diaminopyridine have some beneficial effects in patients; the use of phosphatidylserine, which increases acetylcholine synthesis and release *in vivo*, has so far proved to be of limited benefit in a small number of patients in two double-blind trials.

3. Use of directly acting *cholinomimetic drugs*. These drugs stimulate the postsynaptic muscarinic receptors, which appear to be relatively normal in patients with Alzheimer's disease. The major practical problems that arise when such drugs are used, however, are related to their short half-lives and their poor penetration into the brain even when administered intravenously. Arecoline, for example, has been administered by multiple intravenous infusions and may have slight benefit, but the use of this drug is obviously limited by the difficulty of administration. Similarly the cholinergic agonist bethanechol has been administered directly into the cerebrospinal fluid (CSF) by intraventricular injection, but the results of a multicentre trial are disappointing.

4. Use of *acetylcholinesterase inhibitors*. The administration of drugs such as physostigmine has been tried since the late 1970s. Some 20 of the 31 studies conducted show modest improvement in the memory of the Alzheimer patients following physostigmine. Nevertheless, the improvements have largely been short-lived, even when the anticholinesterase was combined with the acetylcholine precursors choline or lecithin.

5. Use of *THA*. Following the positive results of Summers and coworkers in 1986, several studies have been undertaken in an attempt to replicate those findings. It must be stated that this trial has been severely criticized on methodological grounds (diagnosis, patient selection, etc.). Furthermore, to date none of the trials undertaken in France or Sweden has shown a dramatic improvement in any of the patients treated, 15–34% of the patients showed signs of hepatotoxicity due to the drug. A large multicentre study of the efficacy of THA sponsored by the National Institutes of Health, the Alzheimer Association and the Warner Lambert Company in the United States was temporarily suspended because of the high incidence of raised liver enzymes. Nevertheless, there was some evidence that a minority of patients showed some benefit from the treatment during the initial titration phase of the study. This drug is now marketed in the USA and several European countries.

Biogenic amines

Despite the well-established deficit in central noradrenergic and serotonergic function in patients with Alzheimer's disease, there is little evidence to suggest that any of the drugs known to enhance central noradrenergic or serotonergic transmission are of benefit to Alzheimer's patients. There is clinical evidence, however, that some antidepressants such as the *5-hydroxytryptamine (5-HT) uptake inhibitor* alaproclate improve the emotional state of some elderly demented patients. There is no evidence that neuroleptics such as haloperidol or thioridazine, widely used to reduce the symptoms of hostility, irritability and emotional lability in demented patients, have any specific effects on the core symptoms of the illness.

Noötropic drugs

The term "noötropic" was introduced by Giurgea to describe a group of drugs which have an ability to improve integrative brain mechanisms associated with mental performance. The main features of noötropic agents, as exemplified by the prototype compound *piracetam*, are:

1. An ability to enhance memory and learning.
2. Facilitation of the flow of information between the cerebral hemispheres.
3. Enhancement of the resistance of the brain to physical and chemical assault.
4. Lack of effect on the peripheral system and lack of sedative, analgesic or neuroleptic activity.

The precise mechanism of action of piracetam (and some of the more recently introduced analogues such as *pramiracetam, aniracetam* and *oxiracetam*) appears to involve enhanced release of acetylcholine, particularly in the hippocampus. However, despite the dramatic and reproducible finding that such noötropic agents enhance learning and memory in rats, the clinical studies in patients with dementia have been uniformly disappointing.

Co-dergocrine

Although *co-dergocrine* ("Hydergine"), a mixture of three dihydrogenated ergot alkaloids, is generally classified as a specific cerebral vasodilator agent, there is recent evidence to suggest that, in rats, it can cause a dose-related and selective increase in choline acetyltransferase activity in the forebrain. Nevertheless, while improvement in social functioning has been demonstrated in many studies in which patients with dementia were treated with this agent, there is little evidence to show that an improvement in memory or cognitive function occurs.

A major deficiency in all the studies in which these drugs have been assessed lies in the lack of pharmacokinetic data, the well-recognized pharmacokinetic changes in the elderly seldom being taken into account in the clinical studies of noötropic agents and related drugs. A summary of the pharmacological agents that have been used to treat various types of dementia, and their possible therapeutic benefits, is given in Table 13.3.

Table 13.3. Drugs that have been used in the treatment of Alzheimer's disease and other dementias

Drug category	Agent	Benefit to patient
Cerebral vasodilatory	Papaverine	None
	Cyclandelate	None
	Isoxsuprine	None
	Vincamine	?
Metabolic enhancers	Nafronyl	?
	Meclofenoxate	None
	Pyritinol	?
Noötropics	Piracetam	None
	Pramiracetam	None
	Aniracetam	None
	Oxiracetam	?
	Suloctidil	None
Psychostimulants	Methylphenidate	None
	Amphetamines	None
	Pipradrol	None
Neuropeptides	Vasopressin-like	None
	ACTH-like	None
	CCK-like	?
	Somatostatin-like	?
	Naloxone	?
Neurotransmitter enhancers	L-dopa	None
	THIP	None
	Tryptophan	None
	Alaproclate	None
	Choline	None
	Pilocarpine	None
	4-Aminopyridine	?
Miscellaneous	Gerovital H3	None
	Hyperbaric oxygen	None

"None" indicates that placebo-controlled trials involving a reasonable number of properly diagnosed patients have not shown useful benefit of the agent to the patients. "?" indicates that insufficient clinical data is currently available to assess efficacy. ACTH=adrenocorticotrophic hormone; CCK=cholecystokinin; THIP=tetrahydroisoxazolopyridinone.

Novel approaches to the drug treatment of Alzheimer's disease

It has widely been assumed that Alzheimer's disease was an almost inevitable consequence of ageing. Recent evidence however suggests that this may not be the case as the brain of the very old person not suffering from the disease does not show the widespread neuronal loss which characterizes the disease. It is well established that, like other chronic conditions such as heart disease, the development of Alzheimer's disease can be influenced by both genetic and environmental factors. As has already been mentioned some of these conditions such as the possession of certain gene variants, can greatly accelerate the onset of the disease whereas others such as the presence of oestrogens and certain anti-inflammatory or anti-oxidant drugs can have a protective effect.

Among the possible culprits that cause Alzheimer's disease the following have received considerable attention in recent years:

1. Inflammatory changes possibly associated with a disorder of immune regulation in the brain.
2. The deposition of the neurotoxic protein beta-amyloid.
3. Excessive phosphorylation of tau protein in neurons.
4. Possession of a variant of the cholesterol carrying protein apolipoprotein E_4 that may inhibit neuronal growth and thereby affect neuronal communication.
5. The mutation of two recently discovered proteins called *presilins* whose functions are still uncertain.

Attempts to reduce the neurodegenerative changes by means of drugs that counteract the effects of some of these pathological changes has so far met with only limited success. Some of the approaches which have been used will be briefly discussed.

Trophic factors

It is well established that nerve growth factors play a key role in the development of the mammalian brain, but the function of such factors in the adult brain is far from certain. Nevertheless, it has been postulated that the degeneration of the cholinergic neurons of the forebrain in patients with Alzheimer's disease could be partly attributable to a dysfunction of nerve growth factors. However, it seems unlikely that this could be due to a defect in their production, as there is evidence that the concentrations of growth factors are unchanged in Alzheimer's disease. Experimental studies have shown that infusion of nerve growth factors prevents the death of cholinergic cells in the basal forebrain following fimbria-fornix transection, and that growth factors are produced by peripheral nerves in adult animals following injury. Thus there would appear to be indirect evidence to suggest that nerve growth factors may be of importance in preventing premature neuronal degeneration. The major problem appears to lie in discovering the means whereby endogenous growth factor synthesis may be stimulated or how exogenous growth factors may be specifically targeted to selective brain regions in patients at an early stage of dementia.

There has also been interest in the role of gangliosides in enhancing neuronal differentiation, plasticity and repair, and experimental studies have shown that parenterally administered G_{M1} ganglioside can prevent retrograde degeneration of cholinergic cells in the rat basal forebrain. The clinical value of such findings is still uncertain.

Experimental studies have suggested that *glutamate* may also act as a trophic factor under some conditions. Thus neuronal sprouting has been shown to be enhanced by glutamate, but the glutamate concentration required to achieve this effect *in vitro* was found to be very critical and followed a "U-shaped" dose–response curve; the higher doses of glutamate caused cell death. Whether partial glutamate agonists may be more suitable as trophic factors remains to be seen.

When considering trophic factors it is also important to assess the potential of *brain tissue transplants* in the treatment of Alzheimer's disease. This approach is analogous to the use of fetal adrenal tissue transplants in the treatment of Parkinson's disease. So far experimental studies have shown that fetal cholinergic tissue can improve the behaviour of both young and aged rats with a lesion of the forebrain cholinergic system. Whether this is relevant to Alzheimer's disease, in which there are extensive changes in many neurotransmitters together with the global shrinkage of brain tissue, is presently uncertain.

Other approaches

Benzodiazepine receptor agonists are known to cause amnesia, whereas those drugs which act as *inverse agonists on the benzodiazepine receptor* exert promnestic properties, at least under experimental conditions. Attempts are therefore being made to develop inverse agonists with cognitive-enhancing properties. ZK 93426 is a benzodiazepine inverse agonist which has similar cognitive-enhancing effects in human volunteers to drugs that facilitate central cholinergic transmission, and experimental evidence suggests that ZK 93426 facilitates acetylcholine release. In this respect this inverse agonist resembles some of the centrally acting *angiotensin-converting enzyme inhibitors*, such as captopril, which have been shown to exhibit cognitive-enhancing properties in experimental studies, possibly by stimulating acetylcholine release.

Despite the numerous animal studies in which *neuropeptides* (analogues of adrenocorticotrophic hormone, vasopressin, cholecystokinin, beta-endorphin) have been shown to have potent and reproducible effects in facilitating learning and memory, there is to date no convincing evidence to suggest that these drugs are of any therapeutic benefit to patients with Alzheimer's disease.

Latest developments

The ultimate goal in the development of drugs to treat Alzheimer's disease is to prevent the degenerative changes that are responsible for the memory loss and the other symptoms of the disease. The detection of the massive destruction of cholinergic neurons in the brain of the Alzheimer patient over a decade ago prompted efforts to develop drugs that could improve central cholinergic function. The discovery of tacrine, a centrally acting anti-cholinesterase with an additional complex action on biogenic amines and excitatory amino acid transmitter function, helped to substantiate the hypothesis that a defect in central cholinergic function was of primary importance in treating the disease. Because of the potential hepatotoxicity of tacrine, together with the high frequency of gastrointestinal side effects, many pharmaceutical companies have developed anti-cholinesterases or cholinomimetic drugs that are largely devoid of secondary effects of other neurotransmitter systems. However, it is now generally realized that enhancing central cholinergic function can only partly compensate for the changes occurring in the brain of the patient with Alzheimer's disease. Unlike Parkinson's disease, where the lesion is primarily focused on dopaminergic neurons in the basal ganglia, in Alzheimer's disease there is a major loss of glutamate, serotonin, dopamine and various neuropeptide-containing neurons in addition to those synthesizing acetylcholine. This has led to novel strategies in drug development in an attempt to correct some of the non-cholinergic deficits that may be involved in the behavioural changes occurring in Alzheimer's disease. Table 13.4 summarizes some of these novel approaches to drug development.

The ampakines are a group of compounds that facilitate transmission by stimulating the AMPA glutamate receptors (see p. 61). The AMPA receptor is believed to play a major role in long-term potentiation, a physiological process that is important in memory formation. Experimental studies in aged rats have already shown that the ampakines can reverse age-associated memory loss but their activity in Alzheimer's patients has yet to be determined.

Another approach has been based on the epidemiological finding that oestrogens, anti-oxidants and anti-inflammatory drugs might delay the onset of Alzheimer's disease. Of the drugs undergoing studies under the auspices of the Alzheimer's Disease Co-operative Study in the USA, particular attention is being given to the anti-oxidant vitamin E and the monoamine oxidase-B (MAO-B) inhibitor deprenyl (selegeline) which has been widely used as an adjunct to L-dopa therapy in the treatment of Parkinson's disease. In addition to its MAO-B inhibitory effects, deprenyl has also been shown to act as an anti-oxidant. The rationale for studying such drugs is based on the belief that reactive oxygen-free radicals are produced in excessive amounts

Table 13.4.   Putative agents for the treatment of Alzheimer's disease

Example	Pharmacological activity	Possible mechanism of action
Tacrine, physostigmine, etc.	Acetylcholinesterase inhibitor	Compensate for the loss of acetylcholine due to destruction of cholinergic neurons
Cholinomimetics	Muscarinic receptor agonists	
Ampakines	Enhance activity at the AMPA-glutamate receptor	Improve memory by facilitating long-term potentiation
Non-steroidal anti-inflammatory drugs; prednisone and glucocorticoids	Anti-inflammatory action	Prevent inflammatory changes in brain
Vitamin E: deprenyl	Anti-oxidants	Protects brain from free-radical damage
Oestrogens		Promotes neuronal survival
Nerve growth factor and related peptides	Maintain cholinergic (and other) neurons	Promotes neuronal survival
Protease inhibitors	Reduce beta-amyloid formation	Prevents neuronal loss due to neurotoxicity of beta-amyloid
Cholesterol lowering drugs	Lower brain APOE$_4$ concentration	Prevents APOE$_4$ neurotoxicity
Calcium channel blockers	Inhibit excessive calcium flux into neurons	Reduce calcium-dependent neurotoxicity

in the ageing brain and that this process is particularly prominent in the brain of the Alzheimer's patient. Furthermore, there is evidence that excessive production of free radicals is linked to the neurotoxic effects of beta-amyloid which is prominently found in degenerative nerve terminals in the brain of the Alzheimer's patient.

In cell culture, it has been found that beta-amyloid can increase the synthesis of hydrogen peroxide and free hydroxyl radicals which can act directly on neuronal membranes and thereby damage the integrity of the cell. The neurotoxicity of beta-amyloid can be prevented, at least *in vitro*, by the addition of anti-oxidants including vitamin E. Whether the prophylactic administration of such anti-oxidants will delay the degenerative changes that precede Alzheimer's disease in those patients who are predisposed to the disease is unknown.

The possible beneficial effects of non-steroidal anti-inflammatory drugs in the treatment of the disease arose from a series of epidemiological studies carried out by McGeer and colleagues in Vancouver who showed that drugs such as aspirin, ibuprofen and naproxen sodium given to patients with chronic arthritis, have protective effects against Alzheimer's disease. The reduction in the number of patients with Alzheimer's disease varied between 50 and 75%.

A major problem in interpreting the results of this epidemiological data relates to the poor penetration of the blood–brain barrier by most of the non-steroidal anti-inflammatory drugs in common use. It is also possible that those who are predisposed to chronic arthritis are genetically less at risk from Alzheimer's disease. Nevertheless there is histological evidence to show that the plaques in the brain of the Alzheimer's patient are surrounded by macrophages that produce various cytokines and prostaglandins which gives a rational basis for the use of anti-inflammatory drugs as potential neuroprotective agents. Whether anti-inflammatory steroids such as prednisone, which more readily penetrate the blood–brain barrier, are more effective than aspirin-like drugs remains to be seen.

The oestrogens have also been shown to have a neuroprotective effect against the neurodegenerative changes seen in Alzheimer's disease. Many years ago it was shown that oestrogen promotes the growth of axons and dendrites in the developing mammalian brain. More recently, it has been shown that oestrogens also have a similar effect on neurons from adult mammals that had been damaged experimentally. It is now known that many of the nerve cell types that are damaged in Alzheimer's disease contain receptors for both oestrogens and nerve growth factor. Thus it has been postulated that oestrogens may have a co-operative role to play with nerve growth factor and other neurotrophic peptides to assist in neuronal growth and repair. The neuroprotective role of the oestrogens may be an explanation for the change in vulnerability of women to Alzheimer's disease following the menopause. It is possible that neuronal vulnerability may increase once the protective effect of the oestrogens decreases following the menopause.

Future directions in the development of drugs to treat Alzheimer's disease involves the administration of nerve growth factor, or similar peptides, to prevent the premature degeneration of cholinergic neurons. Such peptides have already been shown to improve learning and memory in aged rats. However, it is unlikely that nerve growth factor itself will be a useful drug as, being a high molecular weight protein, it does not readily cross the blood–brain barrier. No doubt progress will be made when a synthetic peptide is produced which has high affinity for the nerve growth factor receptor and that easily penetrates the blood–brain barrier.

Other approaches involve the development of drugs that target the specific proteins believed to be causally related to Alzheimer's disease. One strategy is to prevent the formation of beta-amyloid by inhibiting the protease that releases the amyloid from the amyloid precursor protein. Alternatively drugs may be developed that prevent the beta-amyloid from aggregating into its abnormal (and less soluble) neurotoxic state. Other approaches involve developing drugs to lower the concentration of $APOE_4$ in the brain, possibly by use of cholesterol lowering agents, or to reduce the hyperphosphorylation of tau protein.

Finally, it may be possible to reduce the excessive influx of calcium into neurons which may be a contributing factor to cell death in Alzheimer's disease. It is known that the density of calcium channels is increased three-fold in the neurons of aged rats in comparison to younger animals. Such changes are correlated with memory and learning deficits in the animals. Thus the use of centrally acting calcium channel inhibitory drugs might have a neuroprotective role to play. Which, if any, of these approaches will lead to drugs that are both effective and safe in slowing the decline in neurodegeneration remains to be proven.

In CONCLUSION, despite the very limited advances that have been made in developing drugs that are of real benefit to the patient with Alzheimer's disease, there have been some developments which may ultimately lead to this goal. The discovery of the defect in the forebrain cholinergic system has led to a treatment strategy which, although limited in its clinical value, raises the prospect of rational drug development.

Another important research strategy concerns the reasons why brain cells die prematurely in patients with Alzheimer's disease. Is this due to a genetically programmed change in the chemistry of the neurofibrillary tangles? One possible approach to this question would involve studying the nature of the cross-linking of the proteins that compose these filaments. It is not without interest that a dominant mutation has recently been described in a nematode worm that results in a toxic gene product causing degeneration of specific neurons in the adult. Could such a toxic gene product also be responsible for selective neuronal degeneration in patients prone to Alzheimer's disease?

A third approach involves studies on the way neurotrophic factors affect the functioning and viability of brain cells. The finding that the synthesis of the neuropeptide somatostatin is defective in Alzheimer's disease lends added impetus to the assessment of the role of brain peptides which may have neuromodulatory and/or trophic functions.

Other strategies include detailed studies of the changes in brain carbohydrate metabolism in ageing and how this may differ in patients with Alzheimer's disease. Changes in the composition and biophysical properties of neuronal membranes may also be of crucial importance in regulating the cytosolic free calcium, which could affect cellular homeostasis.

Finally, there is an increasing need to evaluate the importance of environmental toxins in the pathology of Alzheimer's disease. There has been much interest lately in the role of aluminium as a causative factor, while the studies of dementia associated with the acquired immunodeficiency syndrome have focused attention on the effects of slow viruses in causing brain cell death.

The systematic study of Alzheimer's disease commenced only relatively recently, despite the fact that Alois Alzheimer described the disease over 90 years ago. In the last decade our knowledge of the disease and of its possible aetiology has advanced from almost total ignorance to the stage where it is possible to develop therapeutic strategies. Perhaps we should be optimistic that the next decade will enable early diagnosis of this devastating disease to be followed by effective symptomatic treatment and attenuation of the inevitable destruction of the brain.

Stroke

Brain injury from stroke is a major public health problem in most industrialized countries in the world. For example, in the United States over 0.5 million cases of stroke occur annually, the incidence of stroke doubles approximately each decade over the age of 45 and occurs in up to 2% in those over 75. Frequently, stroke causes major disability with the patient having difficulty in communication, ambulation and movement, or in reasoning. Fortunately, the incidence and severity of stroke has been reduced in many countries by the introduction of preventative measures aimed at controlling hypertension, hypercholesterolaemia, smoking and by the use of anticoagulants in high risk groups.

Ischaemic stroke commonly occurs due to the occlusion of blood vessels which perfuse the brain by the occurrence of a blood clot that originates from the heart or an atherosclerotic arterial plaque. To date, most therapeutic strategies have failed to prevent cerebral infarction but currently a number of experimental studies in animal models of stroke have led to the development of potential agents that can reduce infarct size. Some of these experimental approaches will now be considered.

Pathophysiology of brain infarction

The brain is uniquely vulnerable to the effects of energy deprivation. Metabolically the brain is largely dependent on oxygen and glucose to maintain normal physiological activity. Oxidative metabolism results in the formation of high energy phosphate compounds of which adenosine triphosphate (ATP) is the most important. A primary function of ATP is directed towards maintaining and restoring ionic gradients related to synaptic transmission and the action potential.

Excitatory transmitters such as glutamate utilize much of the energy demand of the brain and it is well established that excessive activation of central excitatory amino acid receptors may be neurotoxic even in the

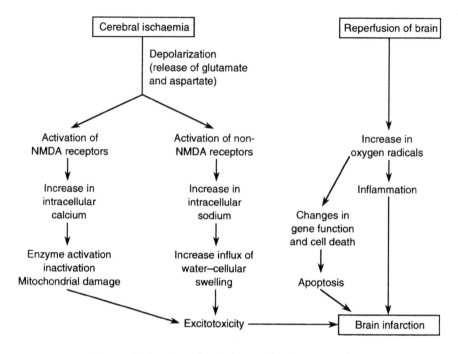

Figure 13.2. Cascade of changes leading to stroke.

presence of normal glucose and oxygen. This type of neurotoxic damage is termed excitotoxicity and may also be involved in other neurodegenerative processes such as Alzheimer's and Huntington's disease.

In brain ischaemia, the excessive stimulation of glutamate receptors causes a marked increase in intracellular calcium activated enzymes (such as the proteases, kinases, phospholipases and endonucleases) which promote neuronal and glial cell death. In addition, free radicals are produced by the damaged mitochondria and by the reaction of molecular oxygen with iron released from protein binding sites by proteases, acidosis and oxygenases. The cascade of changes which occurs following cerebral ischaemia is illustrated in Figure 13.2.

Because it is necessary for the stroke patient to receive prompt treatment before brain cell death occurs, any useful drug must be effective even when there is considerable time lapse (often several hours) between the occurrence of the stroke and the onset of treatment. The term "therapeutic window" refers to the critical time of intervention between the onset of the ischaemia and occurrence of brain infarction. Some of the drugs that have been developed and shown to be effective in the treatment of various animal

Table 13.5. Some drugs in development for the treatment of acute stroke

Action	Drug
Block glutamate receptors	Cerestat, dextrorphan, remacemide – NMDA receptor channel blockers Eliprodil, selfotel – NMDA receptor agonists
Free radical scavengers	Tirilazad (for subarachnoid haemorrhage and head trauma) Pergorgotein (for trauma)
Anticoagulants and thrombolysis enhancers	Prourokinase, arvin, alteplase, orgaron, streptokinase
Anti-inflammatory agents	Enlimomab (blocks adhesion of white blood cells)
Voltage-gated channel blockers	Lubeluzole, riluzole, fosphenytoin (sodium channel blockers) Nimodipine, lifarizine (calcium channel blockers)
Potentiates inhibitory neurotransmission	Chlormethiazole (potentiates GABA)

models of stroke, are listed in Table 13.5. It should be emphasized that none of these drugs is currently marketed for the treatment of stroke. All have been developed on animal models and recent positron emission tomography and magnetic resonance imaging studies have shown that the therapeutic window may be much more variable and prolonged in man than in such models. Only extensive double-blind clinical trials (estimated to require 600–2000 patients to demonstrate statistical reliability) will demonstrate which, if any, of these drugs is therapeutically useful.

Pharmacological strategies for the treatment of stroke

Drugs blocking glutamate receptors

NMDA receptor antagonists or channel blockers such as phencyclidine or dizocilpine reduce the size of focal ischaemia in many animal models of stroke but are less effective in models of global ischaemia that simulate the conditions following cardiac arrest. Theoretically the NMDA receptor ion channel antagonists may be advantageous in the treatment of acute stroke when the high glutamate concentration in the synapse is more likely to stimulate ion channel openings. Those drugs that modulate the NMDA receptors via an action on the polyamine or glycine sites (for example eliprodil) promote the NMDA ion channel opening and may be useful as neuroprotective agents in those patients liable to suffer from stroke. Some non-NMDA receptor antagonists have also been found to be neuroprotective in animal models of focal and global ischaemia. For example, compounds such as CNQX have been shown to be effective in animal models of global ischaemia.

Free radical scavengers

Oxygen-free radicals are highly reactive molecules that damage lipids, nucleic acids, carbohydrates and proteins thereby contributing to excitotoxic-induced neuronal death. In addition, free radicals can contribute to increased permeability of the blood–brain barrier, to brain oedema and to the movement of macrophages into the ischaemic zone. The gaseous neuro-transmitter nitric oxide contributes to cell death by combining with superoxide to form the highly reactive peroxynitrite anion. Two drugs are undergoing clinical trial at present, tiriliazad and pergorgotein, for the treatment of head trauma.

Thrombolysis and anticoagulants

Heparin-like anticoagulants such as nadroparin have been found to be useful in some clinical trials in stroke patients as have streptokinase-like drugs which dissolve the fibrin matrix of blood clots.

Anti-inflammatory agents

White blood cells readily traverse the blood–brain barrier 12–24 hours after ischaemia and contribute to the excessive production of oxygen-free radicals. Eventually the infarcted zone becomes infiltrated with lymphocytes, polymorphs and macrophages. The cytokines released from the macro-phages contribute to the injury of the vessel walls and to the consequent oedema, haemorrhage and necrosis. Thus the function of the anti-inflammatory agents is to reduce the initial adhesion of the white blood cells and thereby limit the extent of the inflammatory response.

Voltage-dependent channel blockers

The release of neurotransmitters is triggered by the opening of the calcium channels in the neuronal membrane which results from the depolarization of the neuron. The conventional calcium channel blockers (e.g. nimodipine) block the L-channels only and therefore do not affect those calcium channels necessary for neurotransmitter release. Nevertheless, the L-channel blockers may prevent excess calcium influx into the cytoplasmic and mitochrondrial compartments which may assist in preventing stroke in those patients at risk from vasospasm following subarachnoid haemorrhage. In addition to a variety of N-channel blocking compounds which are still largely experi-mental, drugs such as lamotrigine (an anti-epileptic drug which also modulates NMDA receptors), lubeluzole, rolizole and fosphenytoin have been shown to be effective in reducing ion flux through the sodium channel in the neuron and thereby attenuate neurotransmitter release.

In CONCLUSION, the future drug treatment of stroke will probably depend on a combination of both neuroprotection (e.g. hypothermia, glutamate receptor antagonists, free radical scavengers, etc.) with thrombolysis which attempts to re-establish normal blood flow. Such treatments may help to expand the window between the initial ischaemic episode and brain damage. Whether any of the drugs mentioned here will ultimately be of any value in the prevention and/or treatment of stroke is still a matter of conjecture.

14 Psychopharmacology of Drugs of Abuse

Introduction

Mankind has always shown a surprising ingenuity for finding drugs which have a pleasurable effect. Alcohol in its various forms is perhaps the oldest drug to be used for its effects on the brain, closely followed by various naturally occurring hallucinogens from fungi which have long been known to be an important component of religious ritual in many societies. Other such drugs, some of which have therapeutic uses, include the opioid analgesics such as morphine, cannabis, cocaine (until recently in a relatively crude form extracted from the leaf of the Andean coca plant) and the milder stimulants caffeine and nicotine. The use of extracts of opium, coca leaves and khat, a plant growing in some Middle Eastern countries that contains several stimulant components, has social importance in some non-industrialized societies where such substances are commonly used as social alternatives to alcohol and also have a role in counteracting hunger and fatigue. Most societies in which these drugs are used recognize their potential dangers to health should they be consumed to excess. Thus both the non-medical use of drugs and the related problem of drug abuse have been widely recognized since antiquity.

The term *drug abuse* refers to the use of any drug in a manner which is at variance with the approved use in that particular culture. Thus the term refers to socially disappproved use and is not descriptive of a particular pattern of abuse. For example, chewing the leaves of *Catha edulis*, or khat, is socially acceptable in the Yemen and other Middle Eastern countries, where there is little evidence that, within the confines of that culture, it is abused or that it causes major health problems. In most European countries, however, its use is illegal and it is treated as a criminal offence to be in possession of this substance. Conversely, alcohol is a major health hazard in most industrialized countries where it is socially accepted, but is banned in many Muslim countries with dire consequences for those transgressing the ban.

Non-medical drug use is a term covering the occasional use of alcohol to the regular use of the opioid analgesics. This term includes the occasional

275

recreational use of licit and illicit drugs for their pleasurable effects (e.g. the use of amphetamines, cannabis, etc.).

Drug dependence is defined as a syndrome in which the individual continues to take the drug because of the pleasurable effect which is derived from it. This behaviour occurs despite the adverse social or medical consequences which it may have; the dependent individual thus needs to continue taking the drug for his or her continued well-being. Often the dose of the drug must be increased to maintain its desired effect. This leads to a change in the behaviour of the dependent individual which varies from a mild desire to obtain the drug to a craving or compulsion. With some drugs of abuse, for example the opioids, physical and psychological dependence on the drug may occur when the life-style of the individual becomes dominated by the need to secure further supplies of the drug.

The term *addiction* has so many meanings that it should no longer be used. When used, it suggests that the individual is severely dependent on a drug of abuse.

Three factors are generally involved in drug dependence. Firstly, *tolerance* often occurs whereby an increasing amount of the drug must be administered to obtain the required pharmacological effect. Tolerance may occur as a result of the drug being more rapidly metabolized, so-called *metabolic tolerance*, or may be due to a drug-induced insensitivity of the receptors upon which it acts within the brain, termed *tissue tolerance*. Thus tolerance should be considered to be a general phenomenon that is not restricted to drugs of abuse. For example, tolerance is known to develop to anticholinergic agents. Regarding drugs of abuse, tissue tolerance commonly occurs to the opioids, ethanol and sedatives of the benzodiazepine type. Tolerance does not develop to all drugs of abuse, however. Thus cocaine and the amphetamines maintain their stimulant and euphoriant effects for a prolonged period of administration without any need to appreciably increase the dose.

Physical dependence is the term used to describe the phenomenon in which abnormal behavioural and autonomic symptoms occur when the drug is abruptly withdrawn or its effects are terminated by the administration of a specific antagonist. Most drugs of abuse produce some measure of physical dependence (e.g. the opioids, sedatives, ethanol), but the symptoms are relatively mild following the abrupt withdrawal of cannabis, the psychostimulants and cocaine. The nature of the *withdrawal symptoms* depends upon the neurotransmitter systems that are the target of the drug. Cocaine and the amphetamines alleviate fatigue, cause anorexia and elevate mood; withdrawal therefore results in a feeling of fatigue, hyperphagia and depression. Abrupt withdrawal from sedatives such as barbiturates or following high doses of benzodiazepines can be associated with anxiety, insomnia and spontaneous seizures. It must be emphasized that the relationship between tolerance, physical dependence and compulsive drug use is complex and depends both on the category of drug and the personality of the abuser. For example, it appears that the majority of patients prescribed benzodiazepines for periods of many months only experience relatively minor withdrawal symptoms when the drugs are abruptly stopped. Others, however, experience severe anxiety states and have extreme difficulty in stopping the drugs.

Psychological dependence occurs with most drugs of abuse. Such drugs produce an immediate pleasurable effect and, following their continuous administration, the individual experiences dysphoria and intense craving should the drug be abruptly stopped. Many drugs of abuse cause both physical and psychological dependence.

Cross-dependence arises when a drug can suppress the symptoms of withdrawal due to another drug. For example, the effects of ethanol withdrawal can be suppressed by the administration of a benzodiazepine. As both drugs enhance transmission involving gamma-aminobutyric acid (GABA), albeit by different mechanisms, a benzodiazepine can prevent the withdrawal symptoms that arise following the abrupt cessation of ethanol administration. However, cross-tolerance and cross-dependence can only occur between drugs with a similar mechanism of action at the cellular level. For example, benzodiazepines cannot suppress the effects of morphine withdrawal.

The criteria for diagnosing drug and alcohol dependence, as recommended by the American Psychiatric Association, are shown in Table 14.1.

Mechanisms of drug dependence

All drugs of dependence cause changes in mood which the individual finds pleasing. The change in mood is usually euphoric but can also be a reduction in a dysphoric state. At the cellular level, these changes are brought about by the drugs of dependence mimicking the actions of endogenous transmitters or neuromodulatory peptides.

Most drugs of abuse that cause an elevation of mood that is the basis of a positive reinforcement bring about the release of dopamine. This action applies to most classes of drugs of abuse with the possible exception of the benzodiazepines and barbiturates. For example, in experimental studies it has been shown that nicotine, alcohol and cocaine release dopamine either in the nucleus accumbens or prefrontal cortex. This release of dopamine may either be direct (as for example, by cocaine and the amphetamines) or indirect (whereby the opiates inhibit the firing of the GABAergic neurons that tonically inhibit dopamine release). These mood elevating effects may be prevented by the administration of neuroleptics that block the D_1 or D_2

Table 14.1.   Criteria for diagnosis of drug or alcohol dependence

---

Any three of the following are sufficient for the diagnosis.

1. The substance is often taken in larger amounts or over a longer period than the person intended.
2. Persistent desire or one or more unsuccessful efforts to cut down or control substance use.
3. A great deal of time spent in activities necessary to get the substance, taking the substance, or recovering from its effects.
4. Frequent intoxication or withdrawal symptoms when expected to fulfil major role obligations at work, school, or home, or when substance use is physically hazardous.
5. Important social, occupational, or recreational activities given up or reduced because of substance use.
6. Continued substance use despite knowledge of having a persistent or recurrent social, psychological, or physical problem that is caused or exacerbated by the use of the substance.
7. Marked tolerance, i.e. the need for markedly increased amounts of the substance to achieve intoxication or a desired effect, or markedly diminished effect with continued use of the same amount of substance.
8. Characteristic withdrawal symptoms, depending on the individual drug, upon stopping its use.
9. Substance often taken to relieve or avoid withdrawal symptoms.

---

receptors. It is of interest that some studies have shown that genetic polymorphism of the D_2 receptor is strongly linked to drug abuse thereby suggesting that an abnormality of dopaminergic function may be an important predisposing factor. Once the drug of abuse is abruptly discontinued, dopamine release decreases below the normal rate which may help to explain the "crash" which those dependent on the stimulants describe; similar effects are seen after nicotine, opioid and alcohol withdrawal. In addition, many of the symptoms of delirium tremens may be associated with dopaminergic hyperactivity in the prefrontal region of the brain while chronic dysregulation of the dopaminergic system in detoxified alcoholics has been indicated by the decreased number of dopamine uptake sites as revealed by single photon emission computed tomography (SPECT) studies. Thus hyperactivity of the dopaminergic system in both limbic and mesocortical areas of the brain would appear to be of crucial importance in causing dependence on most classes of drugs of abuse.

Despite the clinical evidence that links the hyperactivity of the dopaminergic system to the positive reinforcing effects of many different classes of drugs of abuse, there is in addition clear evidence that other neurotransmitter systems also play an important role. It is known, for example, that opioid withdrawal is associated with a profound change in *noradrenergic activity*. Excessive sympathetic activity is known to be associated with abrupt opiate withdrawal, and a similar state accounts for many of the features of alcohol withdrawal including anxiety, tremor, sweating and hypertension. The relationship between opioid withdrawal and increased sympathetic activity may help to explain why the alpha$_2$ adrenoceptor agonist clonidine can attenuate many of the symptoms of opiate withdrawal although it cannot protect against the seizures which often accompany alcohol withdrawal. Similar changes in central noradrenergic function may also be involved in the symptom of stimulation withdrawal.

Serotonin may also play an important role in drug dependence. It is known from experimental studies that serotonin plays an important role in appetite, impulsivity and craving. Those alcoholic patients with a criminal history have a reduced turnover of brain serotonin possibly due to a defect in the gene controlling the rate-limiting step in the synthesis of this transmitter by tryptophan hydroxylase. This subgroup of alcoholics shows an abnormal response to the 5-hydroxytryptamine (5-HT$_2$) receptor agonist m-chlorophenyl piperazine (mCPP) which usually causes anxiety, but in this group of alcoholics causes craving for alcohol. In recent clinical studies, it has been shown that the selective serotonin reuptake inhibitors (SSRIs), by enhancing central serotonergic function, can reduce voluntary alcohol consumption in heavy social drinkers and extend the period of remission in those alcoholics that have undergone alcohol detoxification. Thus a malfunctioning serotonergic system may play an important role in predisposing to drug abuse while drugs such as the SSRIs may have an important role to play in the rehabilitation of some types of drug dependence (for example, alcoholics).

The main excitatory and inhibitory neurotransmitters in the brain are the closely related amino acids *glutamate* and *GABA*. Alcohol and the barbiturates modulate the GABA receptor sites but also antagonize some of the glutamate receptors. Following the chronic use of alcohol and the barbiturates there is a compensatory increase in the number of glutamate receptors which may contribute to the hyperexcitability that occurs following the abrupt withdrawal of these drugs. This might account for the brain damage that occurs in heavy social drinkers and alcoholics.

Changes in *glutamate receptor* function may also account for some aspects of opioid dependence. For example, tolerance to opioids can be attenuated by co-treatment with the N-methyl-D-aspartate (NMDA) receptor antagonist dizoclipine (MK-801). As NMDA receptors are probably involved in long-term potentiation, the physiological basis of memory and learning, it seems possible that such glutamate antagonists may have an important role to play in the reconditioning of the drug-dependent patient. The anti-alcohol drug acamprostate is thought to act in this way.

Besides the benzodiazepines which appear to owe their dependence to excessive facilitation of GABAergic activity, it is also known that the *cannabinoids* appear to bring about their dependence-producing effects by activating specific receptors in the brain. The endogenous ligand for the receptor is probably an anandamide, an ethanolamide derivative of arachidonic acid. The central cannabinoid receptor is a G protein coupled receptor, it is widely distributed in the brain with moderate densities in the cortex and hippocampus and high concentrations in the cerebellum. It has been hypothesized that the adverse effects of the cannabinoids on memory and learning may be due to their suppression of hippocampal activity. The link with the dopaminergic system may be associated with the high density of canniboid receptors that occur in the dopamine-rich nucleus accumbens; the cannabinoids have been shown to enhance dopamine release in this region of the brain.

Lastly, changes in the functioning of some types of *calcium-channels*, may also play a role in drug dependence. It is known that the L type calcium channel is affected by alcohol and some other drugs of abuse; alcohol reduces calcium entry through the L type channels and an abrupt withdrawal leads to the dramatic influx of calcium with the consequent enhanced neurotransmitter function. Calcium channel antagonists of the dihydropyridine type may be particularly useful in attenuating the effects of alcohol withdrawal.

Which brain regions are involved in drug dependence?

Experimental studies show that the primary neuronal circuit involved in drug dependence is the dopaminergic tract that projects from the ventral tegmental area through the nucleus accumbens to the prefrontal cortex. Such studies show that stimulants such as cocaine enhance dopaminergic activity at the terminal region (prefrontal cortex), whereas the opioids enhance dopaminergic function by increasing the activity of the ventral tegmental area of the nucleus accumbens (cell body region).

In summary:

1. Stimulants – cocaine, amphetamines – increase dopaminergic activity in prefrontal cortex.
2. Opioids, stimulants, ethanol, nicotine – increase dopaminergic activity in nucleus accumbens.
3. Opioids, ethanol – increase dopaminergic activity in ventral tegmental area.

Brain regions involved in dependence

Evidence in favour of the dopamine hypothesis of dependence is derived from studies in which the direct administration of these drugs into these dopamine-rich areas has a reinforcing effect on the behaviour of the animals as shown by increased self-administration of the drug. Furthermore, withdrawal of these drugs leads to reduced dopaminergic activity in these regions. The aversive effects of some drugs, for example, the kappa opioid receptor antagonist nor-binaltorphine, inhibit dopamine release when injected into the ventral tegmental-nucleus accumbens area.

Other brain regions that are important in the dependence-producing effects of these drugs include the globus pallidus (a dopamine-rich region of the basal ganglia) and the amygdala. Both of these regions receive projections from the nucleus accumbens. In addition, the noradrenergic cell bodies of the locus ceruleus and the serotonergic cell body region of the raphé also play an important role and serve to link the dopaminergic, noradrenergic and serotonergic systems in different aspects of drug abuse. Whether these regions are equally important in man is presently unclear, but the use of positron emission tomography (PET) and SPECT imaging methods (using ^{18}Fglucose and ^{99m}Tc HMPAO respectively) may help to validate this possibility.

In CONCLUSION, it is clear that major advances have been made in the neurobiological basis of drug dependence in recent years with the application of such techniques as *in vitro* dialysis and drug self-administration studies in animals. The application of neuroimaging techniques in both man and animals now offers the possibility of a clearer understanding of the action of these drugs in the conscious state which may help in the development of more specific treatments (for example, using potential agonists that act on the specific receptors that are instrumental in drug reinforcement or withdrawal) for drug dependence. Table 14.2 summarizes the mechanisms of action of many of the commonly used drugs of abuse and how, at least theoretically, they may be treated.

Sedative drugs of abuse

Ethanol, the barbiturates and the benzodiazepines are included in this group, all of which facilitate GABAergic activity.

Psychopharmacology of alcohol

Introduction

Alcohol is the most important drug of dependence in all industrialized countries and the clinical and social problems that arise from its widespread abuse are legion. In the United States the total annual economic costs of alcoholism and its related disorders has been estimated to be approximately $80 billion, and this does not include the human cost which is impossible to quantify.

Table 14.2. Drugs of abuse and how their effects may be treated

Mechanism involved	Main neurotransmitter affected	Potential treatment
Action on endogenous receptors for endogenous ligands		
Opioids	Endorphins, enkephalins	Partial agonists (e.g. buprenorphine) Antagonists (e.g. naltrexone)
Alcohol	GABA, endorphins	Partial agonists (e.g. bretazenil) Opiate antagonists (e.g. naltrexone)
Benzodiazepines	GABA	Partial agonists (e.g. bretazenil) Antagonists (e.g. flumazenil)
Nicotine	Acetylcholine	Antagonists (? mecamylamine)
Cannabinoids	? Anandamide	Antagonists (e.g. SR 141716A)
LSD and related hallu- cinogens	5-HT	5-HT$_2$ receptor antagonists (e.g. ritanserin)
Increasing the release of endogenous neurotransmitters		
Cocaine	Dopamine	D$_2$ receptor antagonist* Antagonist of the uptake site (e.g. SSRI)
Solvents	? Noradrenaline	? Receptor antagonists
Antagonizing the action of natural transmitters		
Alcohol	Glutamate	NMDA antagonists (e.g. dizocilpine)
Barbiturates	Glutamate	AMPA antagonists (e.g. 2,3- benzodiazepines such as GYKI 52466) and some dihydroquirioxalines such as CNQX)

*Most typical (e.g. haloperidol) and atypical (e.g. sulpiride, tiapride, risperidone) neuroleptics have a high affinity for D2 receptors.

The *Diagnostic and Statistical Manual of Mental Disorders* of the American Psychiatric Association (DSM–IV) defines *alcohol abuse* as a condition whereby the social life of the individual is impaired for at least 1 month as a result of alcohol. *Alcoholism* is defined as the occurrence of tolerance and physical dependence that results from prolonged alcohol abuse. It has been calculated that alcoholism now rivals heart disease and cancer as the major health problem in industrialized countries, with 9% of adult males and 5% of females currently at risk. In lifetime prevalence rates, alcoholism now ranks first of all psychiatric disorders. However, it is not yet possible to identify any biological, psychological, social or cultural variable which is predictive of alcohol abuse or alcoholism.

There is some epidemiological evidence to show that alcoholism shows a *familial predisposition*. Thus the incidence of the illness is four times greater in the offspring of alcoholics, and the rate amongst identical twins is greater than amongst non-identical twins. There are many animal studies which also show that some inbred strains have an increased sensitivity to the effects of alcohol and have a greater alcohol intake when placed in a free choice situation. From the numerous animal and human studies it has been concluded that alcoholism is a polygenic and multifactorial problem in which genetic factors contribute to the risk of developing the illness.

Recent epidemiological evidence shows that very moderate alcohol consumption, amounting to under three units per day in the case of the adult male and two units in the female (one unit being equivalent to about 0.25 litres of beer, one glass of wine, etc.), may protect the individual against myocardial infarction. However, regular consumption of alcohol above 21 units per week for the male and 14 units for the female predisposes the individual to brain, liver, heart and gastrointestinal tract malfunction. Additional health problems arise as a consequence of multiple drug abuse, particularly of tobacco, minor tranquillizers, sedatives and caffeine, which many alcoholics exhibit.

Pharmacokinetic aspects

Alcohol is readily absorbed from an empty gastrointestinal tract, the rate of absorption being impeded by food. It is widely distributed throughout the body according to the water content of the tissue, easily penetrating both the blood–brain and the placental barriers. More than 90% of the drug is oxidized in the liver to carbon dioxide and water by alcohol dehydrogenase and aldehyde dehydrogenase, while the remainder is excreted unchanged through the lungs, skin and kidneys. The rate of oxidation is dependent on the degree of tolerance of the individual, the non-tolerant person oxidizing approximately 10–15 ml of absolute alcohol per hour.

The daily intake of one or two units of alcohol rapidly leads to a level of tolerance which is not as extensive as that observed following the administration of any of the opiates and is readily lost after a few days of abstinence. Psychological tolerance to alcohol develops at a faster rate than metabolic tolerance. Thus death from alcohol overdose can occur in a psychologically tolerant individual following only a moderate increase in alcohol intake above that normally consumed. A "reverse tolerance" has also been described whereby an alcoholic may become intoxicated, aggressive and antisocial following a small quantity of alcohol. This occurs in those individuals who have brain or liver damage and therefore show an enhanced sensitivity to the disinhibiting actions of the drug or have a decreased metabolism. Cross-tolerance also readily occurs between alcohol and other central depressants such as the benzodiazepines and the barbiturates.

Mode of action

Meyer in 1901 was the first to suggest that alcohol acted like a general anaesthetic by dissolving into cell membranes and thereby disrupting the lipid network that comprises the cell wall. It is now known that, at pharmacologically relevant concentrations in the range of 25–100 mM, alcohol increases the fluidity of cell membranes following its acute administration, these changes paralleling the sedative effects of the drug. This suggests that alcohol produces its effects in a relatively non-specific manner, but it is now known that the nerve membrane is structurally and functionally heterogeneous and that specific regions of the membrane are more sensitive to the disordering effects of the drug than other regions. Thus alcohol may affect the calcium flux across the nerve membrane or, by disrupting the phosphatidylinositol system intracellularly, may affect the intraneuronal availability of calcium. This could have a profound effect upon neurotransmitter release. Thus, while there is little evidence to suggest that alcohol produces its pharmacological effects via a specific "alcohol receptor", some lipids do show a particular vulnerability to the disorganizing effects of the drug. For example, alcohol selectively inhibits type B monoamine oxidase and not type A in human platelets and brain; similarly it inhibits sodium/potassium dependent adenosine triphosphatase (Na^+/K^+-ATPase) in the neuronal membrane but not in the glial membrane. With regard to its effect on neurotransmitter function, alcohol increases adenylate cyclase activity possibly via the membrane-bound G protein complex. The effect of alcohol on the secondary messenger system appears to depend on its location; the noradrenaline-linked cyclase in the cortex seems to be directly affected by the drug, whereas the dopamine-linked enzyme in the basal ganglia appears to be altered by a combination of changes in the membrane fluidity together with those in the G protein cyclase complex.

As alcohol has pronounced sedative properties, it is not surprising to find that it facilitates central inhibitory transmission. It has been shown that alcohol has a direct effect on the portion of the GABA-benzodiazepine complex that controls the chloride ion channel. In clinical studies it has recently been shown that such inhibitory effects may be reversed by some partial inverse benzodiazepine receptor agonists, but their development as therapeutic agents has been discontinued because they do not reverse other detrimental effects of alcohol on brain function.

Alcohol tolerance has been explained in terms of the adaptational changes in lipids in the nerve membranes. Thus acute alcohol administration is associated with enhanced membrane fluidity due to the disordering effects of the drug, whereas after chronic administration the membranes become more rigid due to an increased replacement of the unsaturated by saturated fatty acids. Nevertheless, it seems unlikely that such changes are due to a single type of lipid, it being more likely that different populations of lipids within the nerve membrane show adaptational changes at different rates.

Another approach to elucidating the biochemical mechanisms associated with tolerance in animals has been to use specific neurotoxins to lesion the noradrenergic and serotonergic systems. Thus lesions of the central noradrenergic system block the development of both environmentally dependent and independent tolerance. *Environmentally dependent tolerance* is the situation in which tolerance to alcohol develops more rapidly when the drug is consumed or administered in the same environment. Lesions of the serotonergic system are associated only with a block of environmentally linked tolerance. The results of such studies suggest that tolerance is a phenomenon which can be separated from the development of physical dependence and may not therefore be a part of a unitary mechanism for all drugs of abuse.

With regard to the neurotransmitter correlates of alcohol withdrawal and dependence, there is evidence of decreased GABA-benzodiazepine receptor function following chronic alcohol administration which may be causally related to dependence. Changes in the number of muscarinic receptors in the cortex and hippocampus have been reported to occur in alcohol-dependent animals which return to control levels following withdrawal, but the precise significance of this is unknown. Recently experimental studies have suggested that alcohol may reduce NMDA receptor function following acute administration. However, following withdrawal of alcohol the functioning of these receptors is enhanced.

In CONCLUSION, while there is no evidence that alcohol produces its effects via a specific "alcohol receptor", it does have specific effects on central neurotransmission as a result of subtle changes in lipid function both within the nerve membrane and in subcellular particles.

Pharmacological effects

Central nervous system. Like anaesthetics, alcohol initially causes stimulation when blood concentrations are below 0.1%. This effect is largely ascribed to a suppression of inhibitory pathways that modulate cortical activity, thereby causing a release of cortical activity (so-called cortical disinhibition). The behavioural consequences of this are garrulousness, expansiveness, emotional lability and inhibition of self-control. As the blood and brain alcohol level rises, more general states of anaesthesia become apparent, leading ultimately to respiratory depression and death.

A low dose of alcohol may reduce an existing anxiety state, but larger quantities are liable to precipitate anxiety. Alcohol appears to have a narrow and variable therapeutic "window" as an anxiolytic and therefore it is not possible to predict if a given quantity of alcohol will cause or alleviate anxiety. In addition, alcohol lowers the seizure threshold, which could predispose epileptics to a fit, and convulsions may arise as a result of the abrupt withdrawal of the drug from an alcoholic. Alcohol disturbs the sleep pattern by decreasing rapid eye movement (REM) sleep and increasing that of stage 4 sleep, these effects being particularly evident during alcohol intoxication. As the effects of the drug decline, REM sleep increases, leading to nightmares. A dose-related memory impairment is well established and has been attributed to the drug suppressing hippocampal function.

Liver and cardiovascular system.   The liver is the primary organ involved in the oxidation of alcohol, alcohol dehydrogenase initiating the first step in the oxidation process by converting alcohol to acetaldehyde and hydrogen ions. Under normal circumstances, acetaldehyde is then rapidly oxidized to carbon dioxide and water by aldehyde dehydrogenase. However, in the case of a reduction in aldehyde dehydrogenase activity, acetaldehyde accumulates and can inhibit protein synthesis in the hepatocytes, thereby accentuating liver damage. Furthermore, the excess protons increase the conversion of pyruvate, formed from the metabolism of glucose by the glycolytic pathway, to lactate. This conversion, coupled with the low blood glucose level resulting from a low carbohydrate diet in alcoholics, appears to be a major cause of hypoglycaemia. Lactic acidosis also impairs the renal excretion of uric acid thereby leading to hyperuricaemia and gout.

The excess of hydrogen ions formed from the oxidation of alcohol by alcohol dehydrogenase also facilitates the synthesis of saturated fatty acids which accumulate in the liver. This can lead to fatty liver, reduced liver function and further damage to the accumulation of acetaldehyde and hydrogen ions.

The ability of alcohol to mobilize fat from extrahepatic stores, combined with the increased synthesis of saturated fatty acids, leads to hyperlipidaemia and a predisposition to atherosclerosis. Thus heavy alcohol consumption predisposes the individual to heart disease.

A heavy intake of alcohol, by adversely affecting hepatic protein synthesis, is often associated with jaundice due to the accumulation of bilirubin. Chronic relapsing pancreatitis is associated with an alcohol intake of over 20 units per day. Impaired prothrombin and fibrinogen formation and reduced transferrin synthesis, which impedes the uptake of iron from the diet, are added complications.

Steroid metabolism in the liver may be enhanced, which, in the case of the male, leads to an increase in the oestrone and androstenedione plasma concentrations. The established reduction in circulating testosterone levels is probably accounted for by direct damage to the Leydig cells of the testes by the drug. The consequence of the fall in the testosterone concentration is loss of libido, infertility and a change in the distribution of body hair. The increase in circulating oestrogens in the male leads to gynaecomastia. Finally, hepatic coma intervenes when sufficient hepatocytes are destroyed.

Many drugs increase their own rate of metabolism by *inducing hepatic microsomal enzyme activity*. The effect of alcohol on the cytochrome P450 system, which is commonly involved in the oxidation of drugs by the liver, depends on the duration of alcohol abuse and the resulting functional state of the liver. In the alcoholic with a significant degree of hepatic impairment, the anticoagulants, most psychotropic drugs which are metabolized by the liver, non-steroidal anti-inflammatory drugs, etc. are likely to produce an enhanced pharmacological response providing they are absorbed from the gastrointestinal tract!

Gastrointestinal tract and endocrine system. Alcohol stimulates gastric secretion and, if taken to excess, particularly in the absence of food, gastric hypersecretion, erosive gastritis and eventually atrophic gastritis can occur. Hypersecretion of pancreatic enzymes also occurs; when the pancreatic ducts become blocked with proteinaceous material pancreatic insufficiency arises, which contributes to the malabsorption syndrome.

Drugs interacting with alcohol

Disulfiram ("Antabuse") is sometimes used to assist the detoxified alcoholic to remain temperate. The rationale behind the use of disulfiram is that it inhibits liver aldehyde dehydrogenase. Any alcohol consumed will lead to an elevation in blood acetaldehyde levels and the aversive toxic effects of acetaldehyde will become apparent. These include nausea, vomiting and gastrointestinal distress. It should be noted that other drugs which may be given for other medical conditions can also inhibit liver aldehyde dehydrogenase and can cause the "Antabuse" reaction. These include the sulphonylurea antihyperglycaemics and the antibacterial agents metronidazole and furazolidone.

It must be emphasized that alcohol will potentiate the action of any drug that has a sedative effect.

Fetal alcohol syndrome.   Physicians have known for over 50 years that alcohol can severely damage the developing fetus. *Fetal alcohol syndrome*, a constellation of physical and CNS abnormalities, is a major preventable cause of mental retardation in industrialized countries. However, the precise mechanism whereby the toxic effects of alcohol affect the developing brain is still the subject of debate. Nevertheless experimental studies have recently shown that the equivalent of 1–3 units of alcohol daily can cause molecular changes in the developing brain that profoundly affect both learning and memory. It would appear that one of the cellular adhesion molecules (the Li protein) is extremely sensitive to the effects of alcohol. This adhesion molecule brings about a cascade of neurochemical changes in the developing brain that affect neuronal migration. It would appear that even moderate doses of alcohol significantly decreases the adhesiveness to the Li protein. This effect of alcohol appears to be specific for the Li protein as alcohol does not affect the structurally related neuronal cell adhesion molecules (N-CAMs). How the changes in cellular adhesion molecules are linked to the defect in hippocampal function that underlies learning and memory is unknown. Experimental studies have clearly shown that the offspring of rats exposed to the equivalent of 2–3 units of alcohol per day show difficulty in learning complex tasks even though they can perform easy novel tasks as well as the control animals. This defect in hippocampal plasticity is associated with a marked reduction in long-term potentiation probably due to a reduction in glutamate release.

How these experimental changes relate to fetal alcohol syndrome is still a matter of conjecture. Only about 6% of children born to women who drank heavily during pregnancy develop the classical signs of fetal alcohol syndrome. This suggests that genetic predisposition as well as environmental factors play a crucial role. However, the results of the experimental studies do suggest that even modest drinking during the critical first trimester of pregnancy could have long-lasting effects on the developing brain. Heavy smoking during pregnancy appears to enhance the fetal toxicity of alcohol.

Anxiolytics and sedatives

The pharmacological properties of these drugs are discussed elsewhere in this book and therefore only their propensity to cause physical and psychological dependence will be considered here. Due to their lack of efficacy, and particularly because of their toxicity, barbiturates should never be used as anxiolytic or sedative drugs. For this reason, emphasis will be placed on the benzodiazepines, which are not only effective but also relatively safe. Nevertheless, problems have arisen regarding their ability to cause dependence and therefore this aspect of their pharmacology must be considered.

The benzodiazepines are the most widely used drugs for the management of insomnia, anxiety, muscle spasticity and seizures. Approximately 12% of the adult population in the United States use such drugs on more than one occasion during a year for the treatment of insomnia or anxiety, approximately 2.4% of adults have taken such drugs for a period of 4 months or longer. Figures for European countries vary, some being higher and some lower than those reported in the United States, but in all cases detailed studies of the prescribing of benzodiazepines show that they are being used appropriately in both the United States and in most European countries. Despite this, there has been an increased concern over the dependence potential of these drugs following their therapeutic use which has led to restrictions on their prescription and the recognition of the need to limit their period of administration to approximately 6 weeks in most cases.

Drugs of abuse are characterized by their *reinforcing* effects on behaviour, a term which refers to their relative efficacy in maintaining the pleasurable effect for which they are taken. In practice, this may be assessed by determining their value for illicit use. In the case of the benzodiazepines the "street value" is low and there is little evidence that they are widely used illicitly. In eight clinical studies in which the reinforcing effects of diazepam, chlordiazepoxide and triazolam were compared with pentobarbitone, the barbiturate was consistently shown to have a greater abuse potential. In other studies, lorazepam and diazepam were found to have greater reinforcing properties than chlordiazepoxide, oxazepam and halazepam. It is clear from such studies that there is no direct correlation between the elimination half-life of the drug and the potential for abuse. Among the barbiturates, pentobarbitone and secobarbitone (quinalbarbitone) were found to have a greater abuse potential than phenobarbitone.

Physical dependence

Repeated administration of either sedative or anxiolytic drugs may result in dependence which, on abrupt termination, may cause withdrawal effects such as severe anxiety, insomnia, agitation, anorexia, nausea, vomiting, hypersensitivity to light and sound, and tremor. In extreme cases depersonalization, hallucinations, delusions, grand mal seizures and rarely death can occur. Such severe withdrawal effects are only observed following prolonged exposure to high doses of these drugs. Qualitatively similar effects have been reported with the barbiturates, but the severity and freqency of the effects appears to be greater than with the benzodiazepines. Furthermore, unlike the benzodiazepines, the withdrawal effects appear to be closely correlated to the blood levels of the drugs prior to withdrawal.

Following high therapeutic doses of a benzodiazepine (e.g. 60–120 mg diazepam daily or the equivalent) for 6 months, abrupt termination of the drug leads to severe withdrawal effects which may persist for up to 6 weeks. In general it appears that abrupt withdrawal from high doses of benzodiazepines is associated with a lower frequency of severe symptoms such as seizures and delirium than occurs with the barbiturates. This may be related to the slower rate of elimination of the benzodiazepines compared with the barbiturates.

At *therapeutic doses*, benzodiazepines have also been known to produce dependence following prolonged treatment. Withdrawal effects include anxiety, insomnia, irritability, tremor, headache and gastrointestinal irritation, and a wide variety of perceptual changes, including paraesthesia and hypersensitivity to light and sound, have been reported. Following abrupt drug withdrawal, such symptoms may occur within 1–10 days depending on the half-life of the drug, and the effects may persist for between 1 and 6 months. Approximately 45% of patients on long-term treatment experience some withdrawal effects, but most will be slight; such withdrawal effects have rarely been reported to occur after only 4–6 weeks' administration. In general, while some studies have suggested that there is a relationship between the half-life of the drug and the severity of the withdrawal effects, the drugs with the shorter half-lives being more prone to cause more severe withdrawal effects, more recent studies have suggested that there are intrinsic differences between the benzodiazepines that render some more likely to cause such effects.

One factor which must be considered when assessing the dependence propensity of the benzodiazepines is the possibility that *re-occurrence* of the original symptoms of anxiety or insomnia may arise as a consequence of abruptly terminating the drug. Symptoms such as anxiety, insomnia, gastrointestinal upset, hypervigilance, etc. are associated with anxiety states for which benzodiazepines are usually given. As they may also arise when a benzodiazepine is abruptly withdrawn, it is sometimes difficult to decide whether they represent a re-occurrence of the illness or are a reflection of the patient's dependence on the drug. In contrast, *rebound* occurs when the severity of the symptoms is increased relative to the initial untreated state or the symptoms differ from those occurring initially. Such symptoms may include hypersensitivity to sound, hallucinations and depersonalization. Clearly many patients on therapeutic doses of benzodiazepines show a recurrence of their symptoms which cannot be attributed to a true withdrawal effect. The major problem now exists of determining to what extent true dependence on the benzodiazepines occurs following a therapeutic dose and to what extent other factors, such as abuse of other drugs, including alcohol, and personality, predispose the patient to benzodiazepine dependence.

Opioid analgesics as drugs of abuse

Introduction

The medical use of opium as a pain-relieving drug dates back to the third century. Arab physicians used extracts of the oriental poppy to treat diarrhoea and are believed to have introduced it to the Far East. However, because of its erratic absorption from the gastrointestinal tract, its use as an effective analgesic only became possible with the introduction of the hypodermic syringe in the middle of the last century. Opium is obtained from the dried juice of the seed capsule of the oriental poppy, *Papaver somniferum*. The dried juice contains up to 17% morphine and 4% codeine by weight as well as other non-addictive alkaloids that lack analgesic activity such as noscapine, papaverine and thebaine. Papaveretum is a standardized preparation of opium containing 50% morphine.

The term *opioid* is used to designate a group of drugs that have opium-like, or morphine-like, properties. The term *opiate analgesic* is often used as an alternative. The opioids produce their pharmacological effects by interacting with a closely related group of peptide receptors, thereby suggesting that endogenous opioid-like peptides exist, which presumably have a physiological function. The term *narcotic analgesic* is now obsolete; it was formerly used to describe potent opiate analgesics which had sedative properties.

In recent years there has been a major research effort, so far without success, to produce potent, centrally acting analgesics that do not have an abuse potential. The discovery of various types of opioid receptor which may have different effects on central neurotransmitter function may ultimately lead to the development of such a drug. In the meantime, the most widely used opioids, for example morphine, heroin (also called diamorphine or diacetylmorphine) and codeine, are therapeutically effective but are liable to be abused and are dependence producing. The structure of some of the morphine-like analgesics, and their antagonists, is shown in Figure 14.1.

Substitution of an allyl group on the nitrogen atom of morphine produces drugs which act as antagonists, reversing the analgesia, euphoria and respiratory depressant effects of agonists such as morphine and heroin. Other structural analogues of morphine, such as nalorphine, act as partial agonists. When nalorphine, for example, is injected into an animal, it will produce analgesia, etc. but will also counteract such an effect of morphine if this pure agonist is given concurrently.

All the opioids exert their pharmacological effects by binding to specific receptors located in the brain and on peripheral organs. The seminal studies of Kosterlitz and Hughes in the 1970s clearly demonstrated the relationship between opioid receptor occupancy and the ability of a drug to inhibit

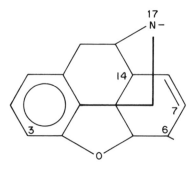

Drug	Chemical groups inserted in positions		
	3	6	17
Morphine	-OH	-OH	-CH$_3$
Heroin	-OCOCH$_3$	-OCOCH$_3$	-CH$_3$
Levorphanol*	-OH	-H	-CH$_3$
Levallorphan*	-OH	-H	-CH$_2$CH=CH$_2$
Codeine	-OCH$_3$	-OH	-CH$_3$
Hydrocodone†	-OCH$_3$	=O	-CH$_3$
Nalorphine	-OH	-OH	-CH CH=CH$_2$
Naloxone†	-OH	=O	-CH CH=CH$_2$
Naltrexone†	-OH	=O	-CH$_2$—◁
Buprenorphine*	-OH	-OCH$_3$	-CH$_2$—◁
Butorphanol*†	-OH	-H	-CH$_2$—⬡

* OH group added to position 14 of molecule.

† Oxygen bridge in molecule is missing.

* Etheno bridge inserted between positions 6 and 14 of rings;
  hydroxy, trimethyl propyl substitution on position 7.

Figure 14.1. Chemical structure of some opiate analgesics and their antagonists.

electrically stimulated contractions of the guinea-pig ileum *in vitro*. Later
studies showed that the opiates have a high affinity for specific binding sites
in the brain and gastrointestinal tract which are both saturable and
stereospecific. However, there does not appear to be a direct relationship
between the affinity of an agonist for the central opioid receptors and its
analgesic potency. This can be partly explained by the relative lack of
accessibility of many opiates to the brain due to their low lipophilicity, but
other factors such as the differences in their affinity for the various types of

Tyr-Gly-Gly-Phe-Leu-OH
Leucine enkephalin

Tyr-Gly-Gly-Phe-Met-OH
Methionine enkephalin

Tyr-Gly-Gly-Phe-Met-Thr-Ser-Glu-Lys-Ser-Gln-Thr-Pro-Leu-Val-Thr-Leu-Phe
γ-Endorphin

Tyr-Gly-Gly-Phe-Met-Thr-Ser-Glu-Lys-Ser-Gln-Thr-Pro-Leu-Val-Thr
α-Endorphin

Tyr-Gly-Gly-Phe-Met-Thr-Ser-Glu-Lys-Ser-Gln-Thr-Pro-Leu-Val-Thr-Leu-Phe-
Lys-Asn-Ala-Ile-Ile-Lys-Asn-Ala-Tyr-Lys-Lys-Gly-Glu-OH
β-Endorphin

Figure 14.2.   Structure of some opioid peptides.

opioid receptors must also be considered. Ligand binding studies, subcellular fractionation to determine the location of the receptors at the cellular level, and the application of histochemical and immunocytochemical techniques to map the distribution of the receptors in the brain have now enabled a detailed assessment to be made of their distribution, and possible function, in man and other mammals.

The highest concentration of opioid receptors appears to be in the sensory, limbic and hypothalamic regions of the brain, with particularly high concentrations being found in the amygdala and the periaqueductal grey matter. The importance of the receptors in these regions was evaluated by applying morphine to these sites by microinjection. Injection of morphine into the periaqueductal grey matter was found to be associated with analgesia, retrograde amnesia resulted when the drug was applied to the amygdala, and hyperactivity occurred when it was injected into the basal ganglia. The high density of opioid receptors in the spinal cord, particularly the substantia gelatinosa, an area highly innervated by peripheral type C fibres, accounts for the spinal analgesia which many opiates produce.

Actions of opioids on opioid receptors

The first endogenous ligands for the opioid receptors were isolated by Kosterlitz and Hughes in the mid-1970s and were found to be the pentapeptides *methionine* and *leucine enkephalin* (met- and leu-enkephalin). The structure of these, and related peptides which also act as endogenous ligands for these receptors, is shown in Figure 14.2.

Two further families of opioid peptides have since been isolated namely the *endorphins* and the *dynorphins*. Each family of peptides is derived from a distinct precursor polypeptide; these have been identified as proenkephalin

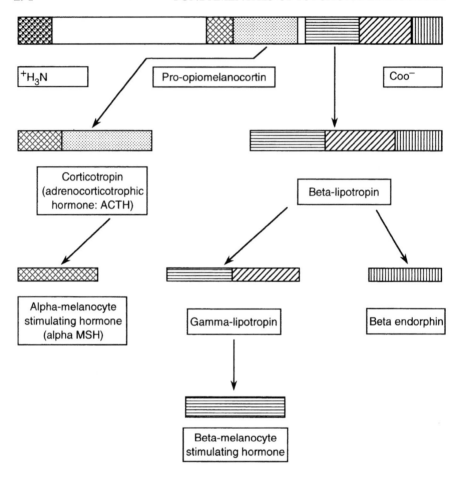

Figure 14.3. Pro-opiomelanocortin and its relationship to beta-endorphin and other
neuroactive peptides.

(from which met- and leu-enkephalin are derived), pro-opiomelanocortin
(which gives rise to alpha and gamma melanocyte-stimulating hormone,
adrenocorticotrophic hormone, beta-lipotrophin and met-enkephalin) and
pro-dynorphin which produces alpha- and beta-neoendorphins and leu-
enkephalin. Figure 14.3 illustrates the relationship between various
neuropeptides which are derived from pro-opiomelanocortin. Detailed
binding studies in the brain and peripheral tissues have now established
that these various opioids interact with different types of receptors that have
been designated *mu, kappa* and *delta* receptors. The synthetic opioid

Table 14.3. Effects of some opiate agonists and antagonists on opioid receptors in mammalian brain

Opiate agonist or antagonist	Receptor type		
	Mu	Delta	Kappa
Morphine	++	+	+
Butorphanol	−	0	++
Pentazocine	−	0	++
Buprenorphine	+/−	0	−
Naloxone	−	−	−
Nalorphine	−	0	+

Potency of agonist or antagonist shown as + and − respectively.
0=inadequate data available; +/−=partial agonist.

compound N-allylnormetazocine (SKF 10047) has been shown to preferentially bind to another class of receptor termed the *sigma* receptor, but it is now recognized that this category of opioid receptor is not directly associated with the pharmacological activity of the opioid analgesics (see Chapter 18 for a discussion of the possible functional significance of sigma receptors). In addition to the opioid peptides which occur in the mammalian brain, it is now evident that morphine, codeine and related benzomorphans occur naturally in trace amounts in the brain in a conjugated form, usually bound to brain proteins. The significance of these substances to brain function is unclear.

All opioids produce their effects by activating one or more of the three types of receptors. Thus analgesia involves the activation of the mu receptors that are located mainly at supraspinal sites and kappa receptors occurring in the spinal cord; delta receptors may also be involved but their relative contribution is unclear. Nevertheless, the actions of the opioids on these receptors is complex as there is evidence that the same substance may act either as a full agonist, a partial agonist or as an antagonist at different sites within the brain.

In man, the changes that result from the activation of different receptors have been inferred from clinical observation and from extrapolation from studies on animals. A summary of the interaction of morphine and a number of synthetic opioids on the three main receptor types is given in Table 14.3.

To add a further complication to the understanding of ways in which the opioids act, it now appears that the mu receptors may be further subdivided into mu_1 and mu_2 subtypes, the former being high affinity receptors that mediate supraspinal analgesia, while the latter are of relatively low affinity and are involved in respiratory depression and in the gastrointestinal effects of the agonists.

Certain benzomorphan analgesics related to pentazocine selectively bind to kappa receptors in the spinal cord, thereby producing analgesia. This analgesia still occurs in animals that have been made tolerant to the analgesic effects of morphine, suggesting that there is a distinct separation between the functional effects of these receptor subtypes. The kappa agonists produce dysphoria, rather than the euphoria caused by morphine-like drugs, and occasionally psychotomimetic effects such as disorientation and depersonalization. The precise role of the delta receptors in man is uncertain, as specific agonists have not yet been developed which cross the blood–brain barrier. The structure of pentazocine and some other opiates is shown in Figure 14.4.

The *mechanism of action* of opioids at their receptor sites is complex and still incompletely understood. However, the receptors all share a number of characteristics. Thus they all facilitate inhibitory transmission in the brain and gastrointestinal tract, and appear to be located presynaptically, where they function as heteroreceptors. Furthermore, they all appear to be coupled to guanine nucleotide binding regulatory proteins (G proteins) and thereby regulate the transmembrane signalling systems. In this way the opioid receptors can regulate adenylate cyclase, the phosphatidylinositol system, the ion channels, etc. There is evidence that the mu and delta receptors appear to operate via potassium channels and the adenylate cyclase system, while kappa receptors inhibit voltage-dependent calcium channels.

Pharmacological properties

Opioid analgesics include morphine, heroin, pethidine, methadone, codeine, dihydrocodeine, dextropropoxyphene, pentazocine, phenazocine, levorphanol and buprenorphine. The principal antagonist in clinical use is naloxone.

All agonists in this therapeutic group increase tolerance to painful stimuli, which is their main clinical application. They tend to subdue dull, persistent pain rather than sharp pain, but this difference is to some extent dose-dependent. The major difference between the non-opioid analgesics such as aspirin and the opiates is that the former reduce the perception of peripherally mediated pain by reducing the synthesis of local hormones that activate the pain fibres, whereas the latter attenuate the affective reaction to pain without altering the perception of pain. This clearly suggests that the site of action of the opiate analgesics is in the central nervous system.

Euphoria is a common side effect of most opiates following their chronic use, and undoubtedly this effect contributes to their dependence-producing tendency. It may also play an important part in modifying the response of the patient to chronic pain. Many opiates also produce sedation, particularly after acute administration.

The opiates reduce anxiety, possibly due to their sedative effect, and also induce nausea and vomiting. These effects are more marked after acute

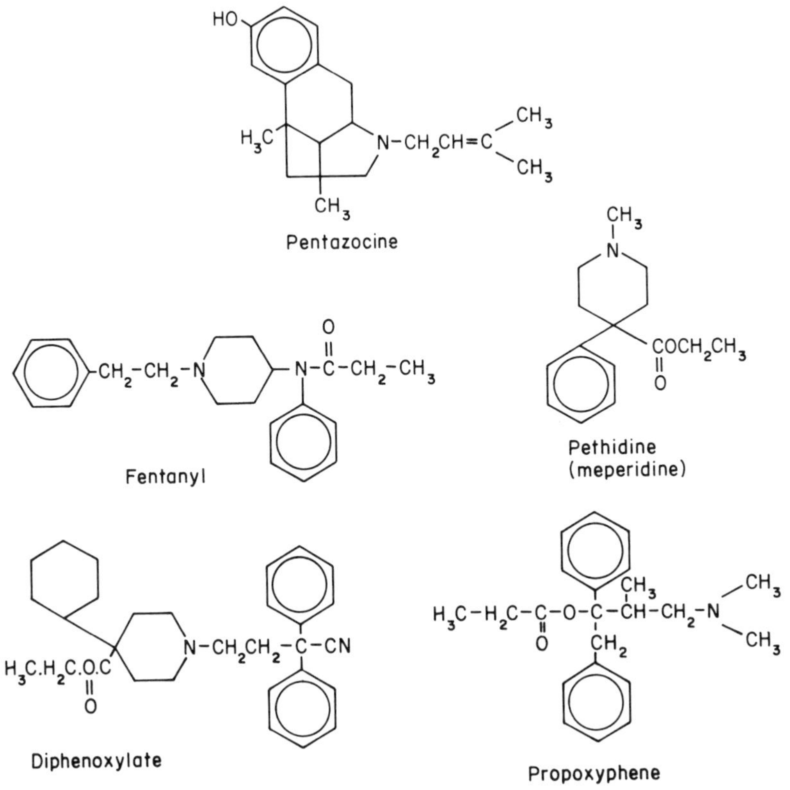

Figure 14.4. Chemical structure of some non-morphine type opiates. Pentazocine is an example of a synthetic opioid analgesic which acts as a partial agonist at mu receptors. Cyclazocine and phenazocine are structural analogues of pentazocine with qualitatively similar profiles. Fentanyl is a full agonist at mu receptors, is approximately 80 times more potent than morphine and is used as an anaesthetic–analgesic agent. Pethidine (merperidine in the USA) is also a full agonist at mu receptors but has one-tenth of the potency of morphine. It is commonly used in obstetrics but, like morphine, is liable to produce respiratory depression. Diphenoxylate is used as an antidiarrhoeal agent, usually in combination with atropine. Usual therapeutic doses are devoid of opiate-like activity but high doses show typical morphine-like effects. Propoxyphene (dextropropoxyphene), a structural analogue of methadone, acts as an agonist on mu receptors with a potency of one-half to two-thirds of that of codeine. It is used therapeutically for mild to moderate pain which is not alleviated by aspirin-like drugs.

administration. The emetic action is due to their stimulation of the chemoreceptor trigger zone in the medulla, an effect that has been ascribed to an activation of dopamine receptors. The emetic effect is particularly pronounced in the case of the non-analgesic analogue of morphine, apomorphine, which has been used experimentally in the past in the treatment of parkinsonism and in inducing emesis following a drug overdose.

The opiates cause constipation by inducing spasm of the stomach and intestines, presumably via the stimulation of opioid receptors in the myenteric plexus leading to a reduction in the release of acetylcholine. This property is often used therapeutically for the symptomatic relief of diarrhoea. Biliary colic and severe epigastric pain can occur due to contraction of the sphincter of Oddi and the resulting increase in pressure in the biliary ducts.

One of the serious complications of the use of the opiate analgesics, even at therapeutic doses, is respiratory depression, an effect which is further complicated by the ability of these drugs to decrease the sensitivity of the respiratory centre to carbon dioxide. The administration of oxygen to a patient whose respiration has been depressed by the opiates is therefore counterproductive and may lead to total respiratory paralysis.

Many opiate analgesics are effective cough suppressants (also called antitussives), although codeine and dihydrocodeine are generally restricted for this purpose. As there is a dissociation between the antitussive and analgesic actions of the opiate, dextromethorphan and noscapine are now commonly used as cough suppressants because of their efficacy and lack of dependence-producing properties.

Miosis is a characteristic symptom of opiate administration and, while tolerance develops to many of the pharmacological effects of this class of drugs, tolerance to the miotic effects only occurs at a much slower rate. Miosis is due to an excitatory action on the autonomic segment of the nucleus of the oculomotor nerve, an effect attributed to the stimulation of the mu receptors. In general it would appear that the actions of morphine and its analogues on the brain, spinal cord and gastrointestinal tract are due to stimulation of the mu receptors.

Tolerance and dependence

An acute dose of 100–200 mg of morphine, or its equivalent, in the non-tolerant adult can lead to respiratory depression, coma and death. In the tolerant individual, single doses of more than 10 times this amount can have little visible effect. The development of tolerance to the opiates does not appear to be due to enhanced metabolism (metabolic tolerance) but is probably due to opioid receptor insensitivity (tissue tolerance). The dependent individual therefore ultimately requires high doses of the opiate to prevent the occurrence of withdrawal effects.

Cross-tolerance occurs between all opiates that act primarily via the mu receptors. This is the basis of the methadone substitution therapy which is commonly used during withdrawal in individuals who are dependent on heroin or morphine; methadone is used because of its relatively long half-life (about 12 hours) and its ease of administration in an oral form. Cross-tolerance does not occur between the opiates and other classes of dependence-producing drugs such as the barbiturates, alcohol or the amphetamines, as these act via different mechanisms.

A sudden reduction in plasma opiate levels, or the administration of an opiate antagonist such as naloxone, leads to *withdrawal symptoms*. These include restlessness, craving, lacrimation, perspiration, fever, chills, vomiting, joint pain, piloerection and mydriasis. These effects are maximal 2–3 days after the abrupt withdrawal of heroin, morphine or related drugs, but slower in onset and less severe in the cases of drugs like methadone which have a longer half-life and whose tissue concentration therefore decreases more slowly.

Endogenous opioids and the pain response

It has long been known that stress can elevate the pain threshold. In rodents this may be quantified by measuring the increase in the pain threshold following prolonged unavoidable foot-shock. The pain threshold has also been shown to increase under conditions of environmental stress in man. Such effects have been attributed to a rise in opioid peptides in the cerebrospinal fluid (CSF). Conversely, in chronic pain syndromes, the CSF concentration of the endorphins decreases.

While the physiological basis of acupuncture is incompletely understood, it is now apparent that the endogenous opioid systems are activated by such techniques. Furthermore, when acupuncture is simulated in animals, there is a decrease in the pain response to noxious peripheral stimuli which can be reversed by naloxone.

From such studies, it may be concluded that physical stress leads to an activation of endogenous opioid systems that raise the pain threshold. The euphoriant effect of physical exercise (jogging, squash, etc.) may also be attributed to the effects of these opioids.

The discovery that the opioid peptides cause analgesia and have antitussive and antidiarrhoeal effects led to the widespread search for synthetic peptides that could be administered orally but that would not have the dependence-producing effects of morphine and related drugs. Synthetic peptides modelled on the endogenous opioids have been synthesized which have longer half-lives than the endogenous substances and which are resistant to the enkephalinases which rapidly degrade the endogenous opioids. Unfortunately, to date all of the experimental and clinical studies have been disappointing, as it has been found that morphine-dependent animals show cross-tolerance with all such compounds. It is established that the endogenous opioid peptides have a range of affinities for the different types of opioid receptor. Some met-enkephalin derivatives, for example, show affinity for mu and delta receptors, whereas other peptides derived from pro-enkephalin show a preference for the delta sites only. All peptides from pro-dynorphin act predominantly on kappa sites, while beta-endorphin behaves like the enkephalins and shows selectivity for the mu and delta sites. Perhaps it may be possible to use this diversity and selectivity of action to develop new synthetic opiates in the future that will have therapeutic advantages over morphine and its analogues which, in one form or another, have been used by mankind for over 2000 years.

Psychostimulants as drugs of abuse

The subjective effects of all the psychostimulants depend on the personality of the individual, the environment in which they are administered, the dose of the drug and the route of administration. For example, moderate doses of D-amphetamine (10–20 mg) in a normal person will produce euphoria, a sense of increased energy and alertness, anorexia, insomnia and an improvement in the conduct of repetitive tasks. Some individuals become anxious, irritable and talkative. As the dose of amphetamine is increased, these symptoms become more marked and the influence of the environment less pronounced.

The psychostimulants include the amphetamines, such as methamphetamine, and the amphetamine-like drugs phenmetrazine, methylphenidate and diethylpropion. Naturally occurring psychostimulants include cocaine, cathinone and related compounds. The shrub khat, from Yemen and other Middle Eastern countries, contains the stimulant (−)-cathinone which has properties similar to the synthetic psychostimulants. The main difference between cocaine and the amphetamine-like drugs lies in its shorter duration of action, the half-life for cocaine being about 50 minutes while that of amphetamine is 10 hours.

Cocaine

Cocaine is a major alkaloidal component from the Andean bush *Erythroxylum coca*. Leaves of this plant are chewed by Andean Indians to decrease the feeling of hunger and fatigue; there is little evidence that dependence is caused by this means of administration. A major health problem arises, however, when cocaine is used in industrialized countries.

Thus in the United States over 20 million are estimated to use the drug either by nasal ("snorting") administration, injection of the salts or smoking the free alkaloid ("crack").

Because of its widespread abuse, particularly in the United States, detailed studies have recently been undertaken on the pattern of abuse of cocaine. Some 20% of those experimenting with the drug go on to become regular users (i.e. psychologically dependent). Once dependent, the individual may administer the drug as frequently as every 15 minutes for up to 12 hours at a time. The initial social effects, such as increased energy and motivation, are positive, but eventually the individual becomes asocial and preoccupied with the drug-induced euphoria. Severe psychological and social impairment finally intervenes. The consequence of long-term abuse is unclear, but it does seem that individuals taking cocaine by the intranasal route may recover without progressing to other forms of drug abuse.

Mechanisms of action

The *reinforcing* (i.e. dependence-producing) effects of cocaine are thought to result from its ability to inhibit the reuptake of dopamine and to thereby increase dopaminergic activity, particularly in the ventral tegmental area and the nucleus accumbens, enhancing the activity of the dopaminergic system in the mesolimbic areas of the brain. By contrast, the stimulant amphetamines such as D-amphetamine and methamphetamine release dopamine from most brain regions. These drugs also inhibit the reuptake of all biogenic amines, but the effects on the noradrenergic and serotonergic systems do not appear to be directly associated with the dependence potential of the drugs. *Fenfluramine* is an amphetamine that selectively stimulates the release of 5-hydroxytryptamine (5-HT) and lacks dependence and stimulant properties. This drug is used as an anorexiant, a property which it shares with the stimulant amphetamines. The structure of some of these stimulants is shown in Figure 14.5.

Toxicity

Cocaine

The most serious toxic effects of cocaine involve changes in the cardiovascular system. These include cardiac arrhythmias, myocardial ischaemia and infarction, and cerebrovascular spasm, all of which can be largely explained by the facilitation of the action of catecholamines on the cardiovascular system. Another explanation of the cardiotoxicity of cocaine lies in the direct vasoconstrictive properties of its major metabolite norcocaine. It seems unlikely that the vasoconstrictor effects of cocaine are due to a reduction in sodium flux across the cardiac cell wall as all local anaesthetics block sodium channels but only cocaine causes vasoconstriction.

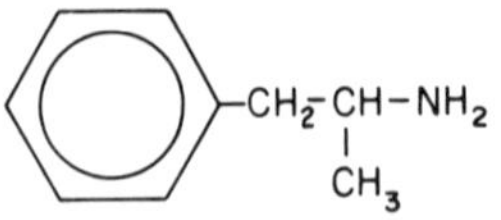

Amphetamine

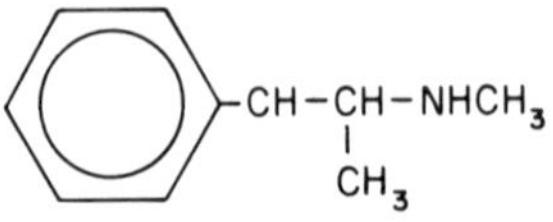

Methamphetamine

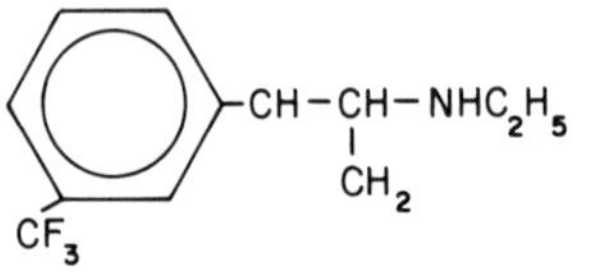

Fenfluramine

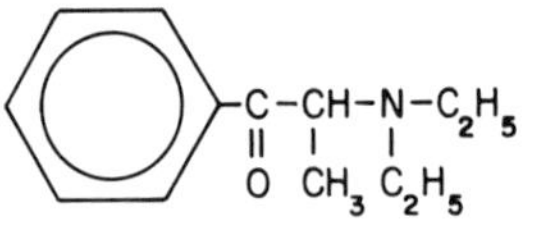

Diethylpropion

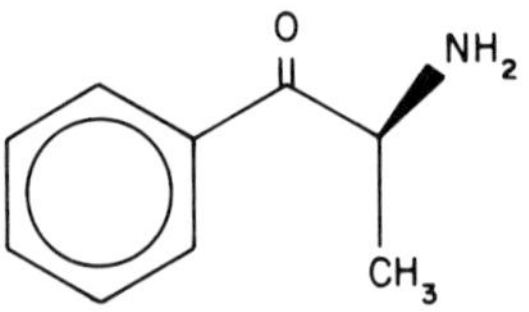

Cathinone
(one of the active ingredients of khat)

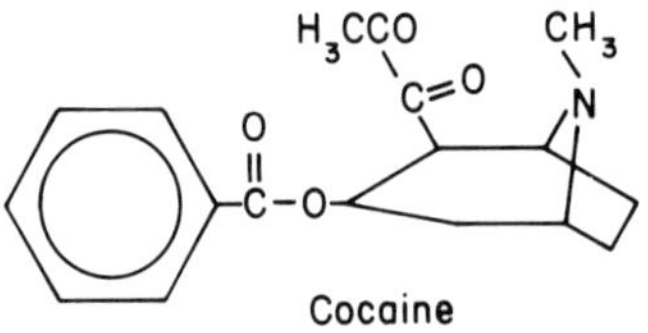

Cocaine

Figure 14.5. Chemical structure of some centrally acting stimulants.

It has been estimated that about 20% of those dying of cocaine overdose show myocarditis on autopsy. It has been established that cocaine increases the release of adrenal catecholamines and sensitizes the cardiac adrenoceptors to their action; dopamine appears to have little direct action on the heart and therefore is unlikely to be involved.

Seizures, possibly due to the local anaesthetic effects of drug at toxic doses, can occur, particularly in those predisposed to epilepsy. Although such toxic and often fatal effects occur more frequently after intravenous and inhalational administration, nasal administration has also been reported to result in such toxicity even in young apparently healthy individuals. There is a poor correlation between the euphoriant effects of cocaine and its cardiotoxicity, so that an individual who uses the euphoriant effects of the drug to regulate the dose may be unaware of the cardiovascular toxicity.

Anxiety and panic attacks may be associated with high doses of cocaine. These effects may be associated with paranoid ideation, visual and tactile hallucinations (called formication) and visual pseudo-hallucinations (seeing "snow lights"). Similar effects have been reported after abuse of the amphetamines which, in addition, may be associated with increasing stereotyped behaviour and a full psychotic episode (auditory, visual and tactile hallucinations often unassociated with cardiovascular symptoms) which may be difficult to differentiate from paranoid schizophrenia. This is the basis for using amphetamine as a model for schizophrenia both in animals and human volunteers. These central effects of high doses of cocaine and the amphetamines may be suppressed by the administration of neuroleptics.

Amphetamines

The toxicity following the administration of high doses of these drugs arises as a consequence of the release of catecholamines from peripheral and central sympathetic neurons combined with their reduced metabolism due to the reduction in their reuptake. The cardiotoxicity is similar to that described for cocaine, in which the sympathetic drive to the heart is increased. There is now evidence that high chronic doses of the amphetamines can cause a degeneration of dopaminergic neurons, possibly due to the formation of an endogenous neurotoxin, 6-hydroxydopamine. The amphetamines are weak inhibitors of monoamine oxidase type B, which may limit the oxidative deamination of such a metabolite and thereby lead to its accumulation. The pronounced anhedonia seen after chronic amphetamine abuse may be ascribed to a degeneration of dopaminergic neurons in the mesolimbic region of the brain.

Acute intoxication with amphetamine is associated with tremor, confusion, irritability, hallucinations and paranoid behaviour; hypertension and sweating, and occasionally cardiac arrhythmias, convulsions and death may occur. The cardiovascular effects of these stimulants may be treated by beta blockers, or by the combined alpha and beta blocker labetalol; calcium channel antagonists such as nifedipine may correct the arrhythmias, while intravenous diazepam is of value in attenuating any seizures.

Tolerance and dependence

Tolerance only develops to some of the effects of cocaine, for example the euphoric "rush" following intravenous administration and some of the cardiovascular effects, and the degree of tolerance is limited. Most long-term users require increasing amounts of the drug to produce the same subjective effects to those experienced initially when taking the drug.

Amphetamine users also develop a tolerance to some of the central effects, such as the euphoria and anorexia, which may lead to escalation of the dose; this may be partly ascribed to enhanced excretion of the drug. Cross-tolerance occurs between the psychostimulants.

Reverse tolerance, or sensitization, can occur with all the psychostimulants and may be partly related to enhanced striatal dopaminergic function. Such increased sensitivity to the effects of these drugs need not depend on the drugs being given daily. The stereotyped behaviour seen in amphetamine abusers may be attributed to the increased activity of the striatal dopaminergic system. *Kindling* may account for the reduction in the seizure threshold following chronic cocaine abuse. This phenomenon has been described elsewhere (see p. 219) and occurs when small, subconvulsive doses eventually give rise to spontaneous seizures.

Withdrawal effects following the abrupt termination of the administration of psychostimulants are associated with depression, anxiety and craving, followed by a general fatigue and disturbed sleep pattern. Hyperphagia and anhedonia are common. In general, the mood returns to normal after several days. There are no grossly observable signs of physical dependence following prolonged psychostimulant abuse.

The abuse potential of "designer" drugs

The term "designer drug" was first used to the United States to describe a synthetic opioid analogue that was sold to heroin addicts in California in 1980 as a very potent form of heroin (called "China white", and reputed to be 200 times more potent than morphine). Subsequently, the compound was identified as alpha-methylfentanyl, an analogue of the dissociation analgesic fentanyl. It has been estimated that this compound has caused over 100 deaths through overdose in California alone to date, the main danger being the narrow margin between the dose-producing euphoria and that leading to respiratory depression. Individuals using these fentanyl derivatives show all the features of opiate abuse.

Another synthetic heroin-like compound was sold to heroin-dependent individuals in California in 1982 as "new heroin", and was soon recognized to be a cause of Parkinson's disease in young people. Eventually it was discovered that "new heroin" contained pethidine together with a *N*-methyl-phenyl-tetrahydropyridine (MPTP) contaminant. It is now established that MPTP is converted to a neurotoxic metabolite, the 1-methyl-4-phenyl-pyridinium ion (MPP$^+$), by the action of monoamine oxidase type B in the substantia nigra which then acts as a neurotoxin and destroys the dopamine cell bodies. This produces an irreversible parkinsonism which is amenable to treatment with L-dopa (levodopa). Treatment of some species of animal with MPTP is now used to produce a model of the disease.

More recently, a number of amphetamine analogues have been introduced for illicit use. Of these, 3,4-methylenedioxymethamphetamine (MDMA), also known as "ecstasy" and "E", has been widely used for its stimulant properties. It has all the cardiotoxic and psychotoxic properties associated with the amphetamines. A close analogue of MDMA, 3,4-methylenedioxy-amphetamine (MDA), has the additional toxic property of causing the destruction of central serotonergic terminals, at least in experimental animals. In recent years MDMA has been the subject of widespread abuse among young people in many European countries. Its popularity is ascribed to its euphoric effect (a "love drug") and relative lack of the stimulant effect usually associated with D-amphetamine. As it is commonly used by young people attending discos, hyperthermia, dehydration and sudden circulatory collapse can occur under the influence of the drug. The long-term consequences of abusing a drug that is neurotoxic is presently unknown but studies in animals, including primates, should act as a warning of the possible detrimental effects of abusing this drug.

The structure of some of these "designer drugs", and their relationship to the amphetamines and opiates, is shown in Figure 14.6.

Hallucinogens

Many different classes of drugs can produce hallucinations when given in toxic doses (e.g. the anticholinergics atropine and hyoscine), but such symptoms are generally associated with confusion and lack of sensory clarity. As such, these hallucinations are a component of a toxic psychosis. True hallucinogens, also called *psychedelics* or *psychotomimetics*, produce their effects without causing changes in the level of consciousness. Such effects are usually associated with a heightened sensory awareness, but a diminished control of the incoming sensory impressions. Thus the individual frequently finds it impossible to differentiate between one sensory impression and another, thereby leading to a feeling of being "in union with mankind or the universe", a chemically induced equivalent of a religious experience.

The drugs usually included among the hallucinogens are either of the indolealkylamine type (like lysergic acid diethylamide; LSD), the pheny-lethylamine type (mescaline-like) or phenylisopropanolamine (ampheta-mine-like) type. Figure 14.7 gives the structure of some of the more common hallucinogens.

Another method of classification is based on criteria such as their subjective effects, the neurophysiological changes they produce and their

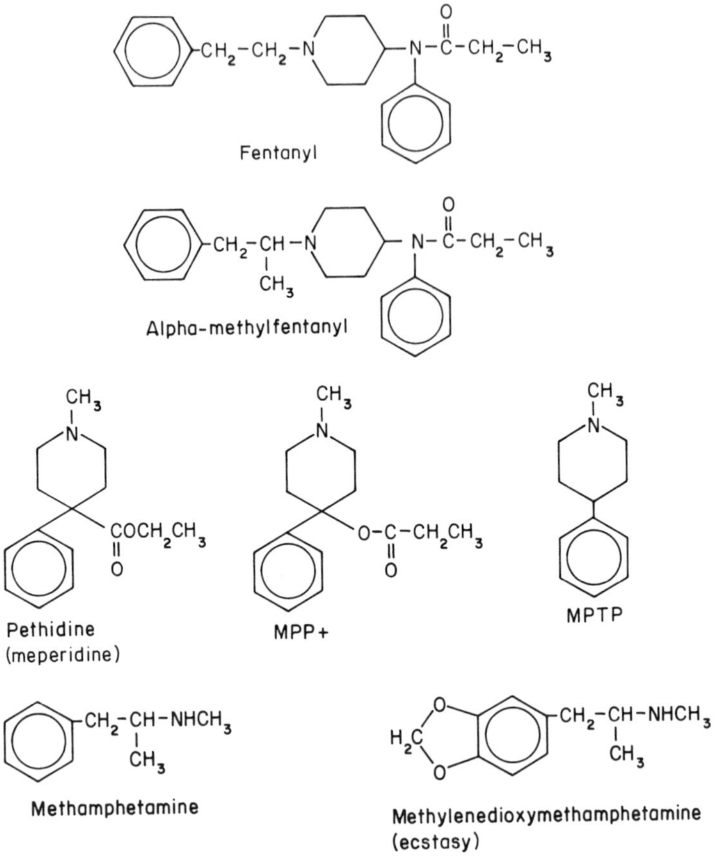

Figure 14.6. Chemical structure of some "designer" drugs of abuse and their relationship to the amphetamines and opiates. MPP$^+$=1-methyl-4-phenylpyridinium ion; MPTP=N-methyl-phenyl-tetrahydropyridine.

ability to cause cross-tolerance with members of the same or different chemical series. This has led to the classification into:

1. LSD-like, e.g. LSD, psilocybin and psilocin.
2. Dimethoxyamphetamine (DMA), dimethoxymethamphetamine (DOM), dimethyltryptamine (DMT) and related drugs.
3. Methylenedioxyamphetamine (MDA) and related drugs, which also have amphetamine-like properties.
4. Drugs which lack LSD effects but which are hallucinogenic, such as the cannabinoids (e.g. delta-9-tetrahydrocannabinol from cannabis), bufotenine and phencyclidine. These are dealt with later in this chapter.

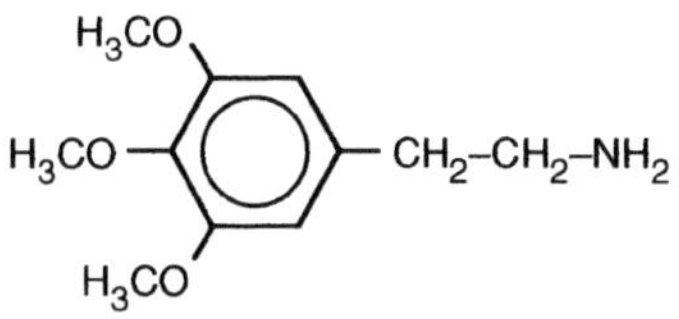

Mescaline*

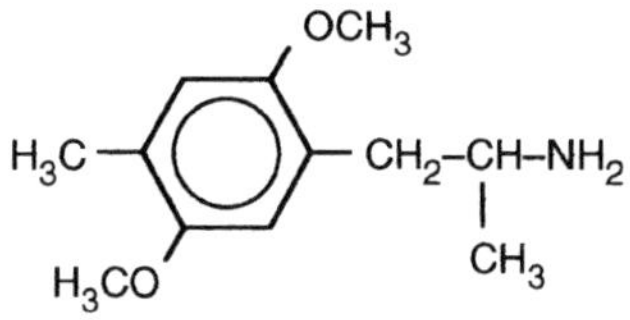

Dimethoxymethamphetamine (DOM, STP)

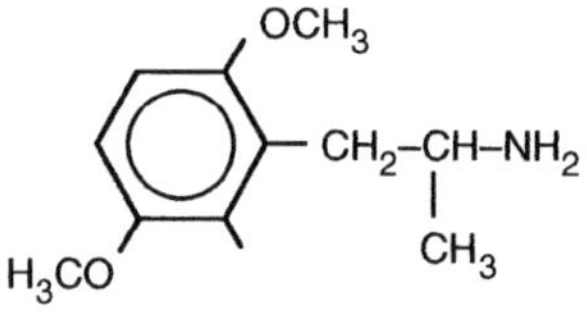

Dimethoxyamphetamine

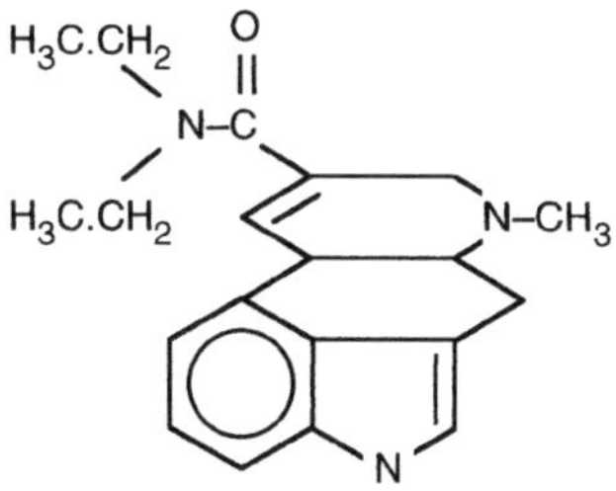

Lysergic acid diethylamide (LSD)

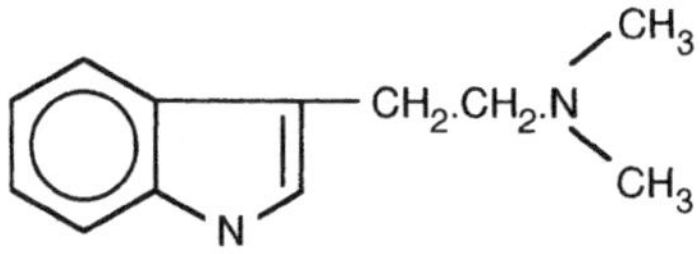

Dimethyltryptamine* (DMT)

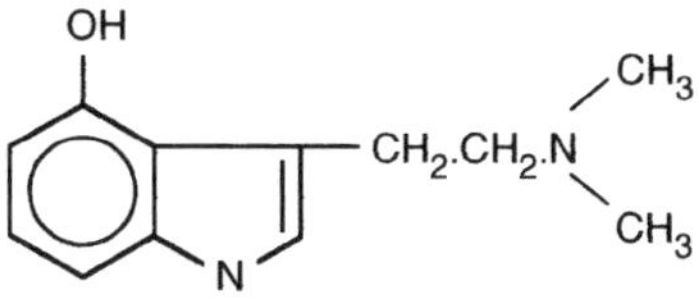

Psilocin*

Figure 14.7. Chemical structures of some naturally occurring (marked with an asterisk) and synthetic hallucinogens.

LSD was discovered accidentally by the Swiss chemist Hoffman in 1943 while he was trying to prepare oxytocic derivatives related to the ergot alkaloids. The profound visual hallucinations which LSD produced suggested that an understanding of the mechanism of action of such drugs may give some insight into the basis of psychotic disorders. Although drugs like LSD have had no lasting clinical application, they have been used illicitly for over two decades. However, since 1980, illicit use of LSD has declined, particularly in the United States.

Mechanism of action

Research into the action of the hallucinogens has largely concentrated on the serotonergic system following the seminal hypothesis of Wolley and Shaw in the 1950s that LSD blocked 5-HT receptors in the brain. It was subsequently found that the firing rate of dorsal raphé neurons was specifically attenuated by low doses of LSD applied systemically or microiontophoretically. It is now known that such drugs stimulate the presynaptic 5-HT receptors, thereby inhibiting the firing of the raphé neurons; similar effects can be produced by applying 5-HT. The net result is decreased activity of the 5-HT terminals in the forebrain. It would appear that the hallucinogens produce their effects by activating $5-HT_2$ receptors, effects which can be selectively blocked by the specific antagonist ritanserin. Most hallucinogens can also affect the activity of the locus ceruleus, again via the $5-HT_2$ receptors located on the noradrenergic cell bodies. These receptors are linked to the phosphatidylinositol secondary messenger system and it has been observed that drugs like LSD which have an effect on this system act more like partial than full agonists. The rapid development of tolerance to the hallucinogenic effects of LSD-like drugs has been related to the rapid desensitization of these receptors.

Pharmacological properties

Doses as low as 20–25 µg of LSD in the normal adult can produce pronounced effects on the brain with negligible changes in peripheral organs. Higher doses produce peripheral sympathomimetic effects such as pupillary dilatation, tachycardia, hypertension, hyperreflexia, tremor, nausea, piloerection and hyperthermia. With slightly higher doses, the euphoriant effects tend to predominate initially, closely followed by visual hallucinations and peripheral changes after 2–3 hours; auditory hallucinations are rare. The term synaesthesia is applied to the overlap of sensory impressions so that music is "seen" and colours "heard". This loss of sensory boundaries can be highly disturbing to the individual and can lead to severe anxiety and even panic. At this stage the mood is often labile. After 4–5 hours, should the effects of a "bad trip" not occur, the individual may become detached in their thinking and behaviour. Doses of LSD in the range 1–16 µg/kg are associated with an accentuation of all these effects which may last for 12 hours; the half-life of the drug is 3 hours. There is no evidence of long-term personality changes.

The pattern of effects of *other hallucinogens* is somewhat similar to LSD, but most are less potent and often must be inhaled or injected because of their poor oral absorption. With the hallucinogenic amphetamines such as DOM or MDA, low doses produce mild euphoria without hallucinations and enhanced self-awareness, while higher doses have LSD-like effects. These changes can be effectively blocked by selective 5-HT antagonists, suggesting that all hallucinogens act via a common serotonergic pathway.

Tolerance and dependence

Tolerance to the effects of LSD can occur after only three to four daily doses, presumably due to desensitization of the 5-HT$_2$ receptors; the cardiovascular system shows a much slower development of tolerance. Cross-tolerance occurs between LSD, mescaline and psilocybin, but not between this group and the amphetamine type of hallucinogens. This suggests that the latter must produce their effects by acting on other transmitter processes in addition to the 5-HT system.

Unlike other drugs of abuse, the hallucinogens do not produce a pattern of regular use. Abrupt withdrawal is not associated with any noticeable physical or psychological effects. The primary adverse effect of these drugs (a "bad trip") is associated with severe anxiety and panic which usually respond to anxiolytics. A recurrence of hallucinations even when the user is not taking the drug, termed a "flash-back", occurs in about 15% of former hallucinogen users. It is often precipitated by anxiety and may occur for several years following the last administration of a hallucinogen. In some individuals, the use of hallucinogens can precipitate a severe psychiatric disorder, such as depression or a schizophrenia-like psychosis.

Phencyclidine and related compounds

Phencyclidine was first developed as a dissociation anaesthetic in the 1950s, but its use was mainly confined to veterinary anaesthesia after it had been established that it caused delirium and hallucinations in patients. A closely related congener, *ketamine*, is however still used clinically as a dissociation anaesthetic as its psychotomimetic effects are minimal. Both drugs produce intense analgesia, amnesia and finally anaesthesia following their intravenous administration. Recovery from ketamine-induced anaesthesia is nevertheless often accompanied by nightmares and occasionally hallucinations, many patients also experiencing delirium and excitement.

Phencyclidine has been favoured as an illicit drug of abuse for some 20 years, but use appears to have declined recently due to the availability of relatively inexpensive cocaine. The drug has the street names of "PCP", "angel dust" and "crystal". The structure of phencyclidine and ketamine is shown in Figure 14.8.

Both phencyclidine and ketamine are arylcyclohexylamines with stimulant, depressant, hallucinogenic and analgesic properties. In man, small doses produce signs of intoxication as shown by staggering gait, slurred speech and nystagmus. Higher doses also cause sweating, a catatonic

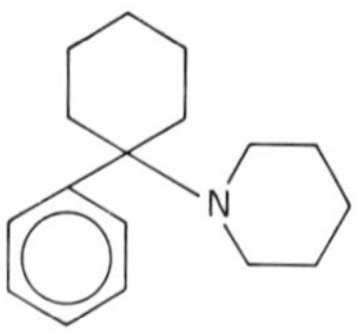

Phencyclidine

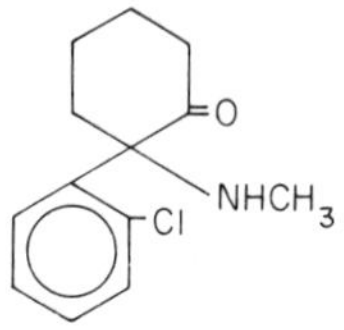

Ketamine

Figure 14.8. Chemical structure of the psychotomimetic compound phencyclidine and the structurally related dissociation anaesthetic ketamine.

rigidity and disorientation; drowsiness and apathy may also be apparent. Such a state is sometimes accompanied by physically aggressive behaviour. As such drugs are potent amnestic agents the individual is unaware of the violent acts on recovering from the effects of the drug. Increasing doses lead to anaesthesia and eventually coma. Heart rate and blood pressure are elevated and the individual shows hypersalivation, fever and a muscular rigidity. Convulsions may occur at high doses. The effects of a single dose may last for 4–6 hours; perceptual disturbances, disorientation and intense anxiety commonly occur.

Mode of action

Both phencyclidine and ketamine bind with high affinity to a number of receptors in the brain, but it is now accepted that the primary target is the ion channel located in the NMDA excitatory amino acid receptor complex.

Considerable attention is now being paid to the way in which phencyclidine and ketamine block the ion channel controlled by the NMDA receptor. This prevents the movement of calcium ions in particular into the cell which, in the case of the NMDA receptors situated in the hippocampus, inhibits long-term potentiation and thereby blocks memory formation. These drugs can also exhibit a neuroprotective effect against nerve cell damage arising from cerebral hypoxia. Such an action is of potential importance in the future development of drugs to prevent the brain damage that arises as a consequence of stroke.

The pronounced effects of phencyclidine on locomotor activity in both animals and man, and the psychotomimetic effects in man, may be a consequence of its facilitatory effects on dompaminergic transmission, particularly in the mesolimbic regions of the brain. This is unlikely to be due to a direct effect of the drug on dopamine receptors but is probably due to its action on NMDA heteroreceptors on dopaminergic terminals in these brain regions.

After chronic use, the drug appears to have an extended half-life of up to 3 days. This is due to the extensive enterohepatic circulation combined with the availability of its metabolites, some of which are pharmacologically active.

Tolerance and dependence

Tolerance to the effects of phencyclidine develops in both animals and man. A slight physical dependence has been reported in man characterized by a craving for the drug, persistent amnesia, slurred speech and difficulty in thinking, which may last for up to 1 year after having discontinued the drug. Severe personality changes have also been reported.

Cannabis and the cannabinoids

The hemp plant, *Cannabis sativa*, has been used commercially as a source of hemp for the manufacture of rope and sacking for well over 2000 years. The hemp seeds have also been used as a source of oil for animal feed and as a form of soap, while the leaves were first used in China because of the psychoactive ingredients they contained. From China, the use of hemp spread first to India and then to Europe via the Middle East in the 16th century.

All parts of the hemp plant contain psychoactive substances, some 60 active ingredients or cannabinoids having been isolated from the plant to date. In addition, over 300 non-cannabinoid compounds have been identified which do not appear to contribute to the psychoactive properties of the plant. The highest cannabinoid concentrations are found in the flowering heads.

There are three main types of cannabis preparation in use. *Herbal cannabis*, known variously as "grass", "pot", "joint" or marijuana, is prepared by collecting the flowering heads or the upper leaves of the plant, allowing them to dry and then removing the stems and stalks by rubbing the dried material. The resultant material is then rolled into cigarettes or placed in a pipe and smoked. The cannabinoid content of herbal cannabis varies according to the climate and growing conditions, but it can contain up to 8% of cannabinoids.

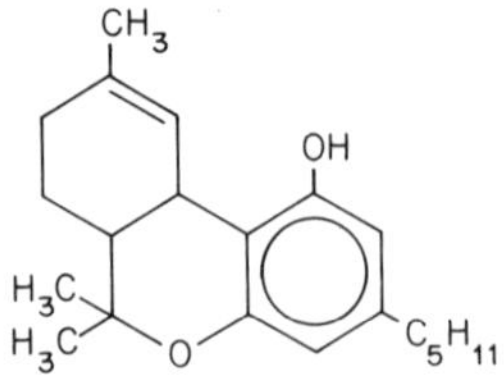

Figure 14.9. Chemical structure of delta-9-tetrahydrocannabinol (THC), the main psychoactive ingredient of the cannabis plant.

Cannabis resin, an exudate secreted from the hairs on the leaves of the plant, is also collected from the upper leaves and contains up to 14% of cannibinoids. The resinous material is powdered and usually compressed into a hard, brownish mass which darkens in the air as a result of oxidation. This form of the drug is known as "hash", "resin" or "charas".

The purest form of the drug produced for illicit use is *cannabis oil.* This is prepared by solvent extraction of the resin followed by further purification to produce an oil that contains up to 60% cannabinoids. Cannabis oil is generally added in small quantities to tobacco and smoked.

Cannabis in its various forms is still the most commonly used illicit drug in most countries. In the United States, more than 50% of young adults report the use of this drug on some occasion, but it would appear that its casual use has declined among young people in that country from 37% in 1978 to about 18% 10 years later. Despite statements from the advocates of its legalization, there is evidence that the smoke from the dried leaves contains potential carcinogens, together with carbon monoxide, and is therefore liable to adversely affect the respiratory and cardiovascular systems in a similar manner to tobacco.

The main active ingredients of cannabis are *cannabinol, cannabidiol* and several isomers of *tetrahydrocannabinol,* of which delta-9-tetrahydrocannabinol (THC) is probably responsible for most of the psychoactive effects of the various preparations. It is of interest to note that THC does not contain nitrogen in its three-membered ring system. The structure of THC is shown in Figure 14.9.

THC and related compounds are very lipophilic and therefore readily absorbed from the lung and gastrointestinal tract. The bioavailability of oral THC varies from 4 to 12% depending on the way in which it is delivered, whereas the availability of THC when smoked can be as high as 50%. Under optimal conditions this could mean that a 1 g cigarette could lead to the delivery of up to 10 mg of THC to the circulation. The plasma concentration peaks at about 10 minutes and the psychoactive effects reach a maximum after 20–30 minutes and last for about 2–3 hours. The time of peak effect and the duration of the pharmacological response is slower after oral administration.

THC is metabolized in the liver to form active metabolites which are further metabolized to inactive polar compounds; these are excreted in the urine. Some metabolites are excreted into the bile and then recycled via the enterohepatic circulation. Because of their high lipophilicity, most of the active metabolites are widely distributed in fat depots and the brain, from where they are only slowly eliminated. The half-life of elimination for many of the active metabolites has been calculated to be approximately 30 hours. Traces of the cannabinoids can be detected in the blood and urine of users for many days after the last administration. There is some evidence of metabolic tolerance occurring after chronic use of the drug. THC and related cannabinoids readily penetrate the placental barrier and may possibly detrimentally affect fetal development.

Mechanisms of action

The high lipophilicity of THC and related compounds implies that these drugs are widely distributed throughout the brain, particularly in the grey matter; they appear to be taken up into neurons rather than the glia. The precise mechanism of action of these drugs is unclear, despite the recent discovery of a specific THC receptor in the mammalian brain whose precise function is still being elucidated. There appear to be a number of high affinity binding sites in the brain and liver, but their characteristics do not appear to correlate well with the pharmacological properties of these drugs. The lipophilicity of THC also suggests that it may increase neuronal membrane fluidity, an action which it shares with alcohol; pharmacologically inactive cannabinoids do not apparently affect membrane fluidity. Unless it can be shown that THC has a regionally specific effect on neuronal membrane fluidity, it must be concluded that such an action is unlikely to be related to its pharmacological effects. The changes in prostenoid synthesis said to occur following THC administration may account for the suppression of the cellular and humoral response which has been reported in animals following chronic drug administration. The importance of this observation to the clinical situation is currently uncertain.

Tolerance and dependence

Regular use of cannabis can lead to an intake of THC which would be toxic to the naïve user. This suggests that tolerance develops. While there is some evidence that metabolic tolerance may arise, it would appear that tissue tolerance is the most likely explanation for the effects observed. Tolerance develops to the drug-induced changes in mood, tachycardia, hyperthermia and decrease in intraocular pressure. Tolerance also develops to the effects of THC on psychomotor performance and the electroencephalogram changes. *Cross-tolerance* occurs between THC and alcohol, at least in animal studies, but does not appear to occur between the cannabinoids and the psychotomimetics. The abrupt withdrawal of very high doses of THC from volunteers has been associated with some withdrawal effects (irritability, insomnia, weight loss, tremor, changed sleep profile, anorexia), suggesting that both physical and psychological dependence may occasionally arise.

Pharmacological effects

Smoking a cigarette containing 2% THC causes changes in the memory, motor co-ordination, cognition and sense of time, all of which are adversely affected. There is an enhanced sense of well-being and euphoria accompanied by a feeling of relaxation and sleepiness. The intensity of these effects depends to some extent upon the environment in which the drug is taken. The effect upon short-term memory and the impairment of the ability to undertake memory-dependent, goal-directed behaviour is called *temporal disintegration*. This is correlated with a tendency to confuse the past, present and future and to feel depersonalized. Such effects may last for several hours and may be intensified if the subject also consumes alcohol.

Higher doses of THC are associated with hallucinations, delusions and paranoid feelings; the sense of depersonalization also becomes more intense. High doses of THC can trigger a schizophrenic episode in predisposed individuals. In addition, "flashbacks" have been reported in those individuals who have been exposed to high doses of the drug.

Chronic cannabis users frequently exhibit the *"amotivational syndrome"* characterized by apathy, impaired judgement, memory defects and loss of interest in normal social pursuits. Whether chronic cannabis abuse leads to more permanent changes in brain function is uncertain, but it is known that chronic drug administration to animals results in permanent damage to the hippocampus. Regular use of cannabis by adolescents frequently predisposes such individuals to other types of drug abuse later. This may reflect the social pressures placed upon the individual rather than the pharmacological consequences of abusing cannabis as such.

The most consistent effects of THC on the cardiovascular system are tachycardia, increased systolic blood pressure and a reddening of the conjunctivae. As myocardial oxygen demand is increased, the chances of angina are enhanced in patients predisposed to this condition.

Pulmonary function is impaired in chronic cannabis smokers, despite the clear evidence that acute use of the drug results in a significant and long-lasting bronchodilatation. However, it should be noted that the tar produced by cannabis cigarettes is more carcinogenic than that obtained from normal cigarettes, so that the risks of lung cancer and heart disease are increased in chronic cannabis smokers.

There are conflicting reports on the effects of chronic high doses of THC on human sexual function, but there is some evidence that spermatogenesis and testosterone levels are decreased in such users. In women, a single cannabis cigarette can suppress luteinizing hormone release, so that lack of ovulation frequently occurs in women who abuse this drug. Lowered birth weight and increased chances of malformations have also been reported in the offspring of women who abuse THC during pregnancy. It is also possible that exposure to this drug *in utero* causes behavioural abnormalities in childhood.

There are two features of the cannabinoids which may ultimately be of therapeutic importance. THC is known to lower the intraocular pressure, which may be of possible benefit in the treatment of glaucoma. There is also evidence that THC is a moderately effective antiemetic agent. Such a discovery has led to the development of *nabilone*, a synthetic cannabinoid, as an antiemetic agent, but its use is limited because of the dysphoria, depersonalization, memory disturbance and other effects which are associated with the cannabinoids. Whether the bronchodilator action of THC will ever find therapeutic application in the treatment of asthma remains an open question.

Nicotine

This alkaloid was first isolated from the leaves of the tobacco plant *Nicotiana tabacum* in 1828 and the first pharmacological studies were initiated by Orfila some 15 years later. A closely related alkaloid lobeline was isolated from *Lobelia inflata* by the German chemist Wieland in 1915 and found to have a similar, although less potent, effect to nicotine.

Nicotine is of considerable medical significance not only because of its toxicity in high doses but also because of its propensity to cause dependence in those using the various forms of tobacco. The complex and often unpredictable actions of nicotine are due not only to its actions on a variety of neuroeffector and chemosensitive sites but also to its ability to both stimulate and desensitize receptors. For example, nicotine can increase the heart rate by exciting the sympathetic or paralysing the parasympathetic ganglia and, conversely, it can slow the heart rate by paralysing the sympathetic and stimulating the parasympathetic ganglia. In addition, due to its action on the medullary centres in the brain, together with its ability to act on the chemoreceptors of the carotid and aortic bodies, nicotine can raise or occasionally lower the heart rate. Additionally, nicotine can activate nicotinic receptors in the adrenal medulla and facilitate the release of adrenaline. As a consequence both the heart rate and the blood pressure will increase. In the brain, nicotine has a marked stimulant action particularly in the naïve smoker. This can lead to tremors and, in high doses, to convulsions. Stimulation of the brain is usually followed by depression and, in high doses, death may result from respiratory failure due to central paralysis and peripheral blockade of the intercostal muscles. Stimulation of respiration is a prominent action of nicotine in low doses due to the reflex excitation of the chemoreceptors in the carotid and aortic bodies. Both nicotine and lobeline induce vomiting by both central and peripheral actions. The central component of vomiting is due to the direct stimulation of the chemoreceptor trigger zone in the area postrema of the medulla oblongata. In addition, nicotine activates vagal and spinal afferent nerves that form the sensory input of the reflex pathways in the act of vomiting.

Poisoning from nicotine may occur from the accidental ingestion of insecticide sprays in which nicotine is the active ingredient or from the over use of tobacco products. The acute fatal dose of nicotine in the adult has been estimated to be about 60 mg; cigarettes contain betwen 1 and 2% of nicotine. The gastric absorption of nicotine taken orally is delayed by slow gastric emptying so that vomiting caused by the central effects of the initially absorbed fraction generally removes much of the tobacco that remains in the gastrointestinal tract. Clearly this generally protects the individual from the acute lethal effects of the drug. The onset of symptoms of acute nicotine poisoning is rapid and includes nausea, salivation, abdominal pain, vomiting, diarrhoea, headache, dizziness, disturbances of vision and hearing, mental confusion and muscle weakness. Changes in the cardiovascular system follow leading to collapse and terminal convulsions. Death results from respiratory failure. Treatment of nicotine poisoning consists of inducing vomiting or gastric lavage; any remaining nicotine is removed by activated charcoal.

Nicotine as a drug of abuse: because of the reinforcing properties of nicotine, smoking cigarettes is the most common cause of preventable premature death in most countries of the world. The dependence produced by cigarette smoking is very persistent. Thus although over 80% of smokers express a desire to stop the habit, only about 35% attempt to stop each year and fewer than 5% are successful. While there are many casual users of alcohol, few individuals smoke tobacco in a small enough quantity (estimated to be a maximum of 5 cigarettes a day) to avoid dependence. Nicotine is absorbed readily through the skin, mucous membranes and through the lungs. Once absorbed through the lungs the stimulant effect on the brain becomes apparent in about 7 seconds. Thus each puff of a cigarette produces some degree of reinforcement and therefore the average smoker on 20 cigarettes a day will reinforce the habit approximately 200 times, assuming that there are 10 puffs per cigarette.

The dependence-producing effects of nicotine, as with most drugs of dependence, is associated with an activation of the mesocortical and mesolimbic dopaminergic systems in the brain. In experimental studies in rodents it has been found that injection of pharmacologically relevant doses of nicotine results in an increased release of dopamine in these brain regions, the nucleus accumbens being the most affected. It is also known that nicotine causes the release of endogenous opioids and glucocorticoids which may contribute to both the dependence-producing effect of the drug and to the adrenocortical activating effect.

As with most other drugs of dependence, tolerance to nicotine develops rapidly. The term *negative reinforcement* refers to the benefits obtained when an unpleasant state is reversed. In dependent smokers, it has been shown that the urge to smoke correlates with low blood nicotine concentrations which may be associated with the beginning of withdrawal symptoms. Thus smokers smoke in order to achieve the reward of the stimulant effects of nicotine but also to avoid the unpleasant effects of nicotine withdrawal. The nicotine withdrawal syndrome consists of the following symptoms.

1. Irritability, impatience, hostility, anxiety.
2. Dysphoric or depressed mood.
3. Difficulty in concentrating.
4. Restlessness.
5. Decreased heart rate.
6. Increased appetite and weight gain.

Pharmacological treatment of nicotine dependence mainly consists of using either nicotine chewing-gum or the nicotine patch. It has been shown that these methods of drug delivery maintain fairly constant plasma concentrations of nicotine and do not produce the rapid rise in the tissue concentration which is characteristic of cigarette smoking. Experimental studies show that the abrupt rise in the brain concentration is correlated with a rapid release of dopamine in mesocortical regions of the brain. Thus cigarette smokers can transfer their dependence to the chewing-gum or patch method of delivery and then gradually reduce their daily intake of the drug over a period of days or weeks. This method is analogous to withdrawing an opioid-dependent person by substituting methadone for the shorter half-life opioid. In double-blind clinical trials, considerable success has been achieved in treating nicotine dependence by the substitution of nicotine patches or chewing-gum. Other methods that have been tried with limited success involve the use of clonidine, which reduces noradrenaline release and may therefore reduce some of the central stimulant effects of nicotine, and the opioid antagonist naloxone which produces a small but significant decrease in craving presumably by blocking the effects of endogenously increased opioids.

Caffeine

Theophylline, caffeine and theobromine are three closely related alkaloids that occur in a number of plants such as *Thea sinensis*, the leaves of which are used to make tea, *Theobroma cacao*, the plant from which cocoa and chocolate are made, and *Coffea arabica* from which coffee is derived. Cola flavoured drinks usually contain considerable quantities of caffeine which is derived from the nuts of *Cola acumulata*.

The stimulant properties of caffeine and the related methylxanthines has been well known for centuries. In addition, these drugs have several therapeutic actions due to their ability to relax bronchial smooth muscle, stimulate cardiac muscle and cause diuresis through their action on the kidney. Only the stimulant properties of caffeine as an example of the methylxanthines will be considered here.

The pharmacological action of the methylxanthines may be considered under five main headings.

1. They inhibit intracellular phosphodiesterases and thereby prevent the breakdown of cyclic AMP which acts as a second messenger in many neurotransmitter systems.
2. They directly increase intracellular calcium concentrations and thereby increase calcium-mediated neurotransmitter release.
3. They indirectly affect intracellular calcium by causing membrane hyperpolarization.
4. By uncoupling intracellular calcium from normal metabolic processes, the free calcium enhances muscle contractility.
5. The methylxanthines block the activity of adenosine receptors. It is generally accepted that the antagonism of adenosine receptors is the most likely explanation for the stimulant effects of these drugs and occurs at drug concentrations that are consumed in caffeine-containing beverages. Conversely, the concentrations of caffeine and related drugs that are required to produce the biochemical effects listed under items 1 to 4 above only occur when toxic doses of the xanthines are administered.

The purine nucleotide adenosine occurs widely throughout the nervous system and in the cardiovascular system and is released from nerves following depolarization. Adenosine acts as a neuromodulator in that it alters the physiological response to other neurotransmitters that may be released concurrently. In addition, adenosine does have direct inhibitory actions on nervous tissue by increasing potassium conductance. Its main modulatory effects are on acetylcholine, noradrenaline and dopamine; in addition it can depress the release of the excitatory amino acid glutamate.

Adenosine produces its physiological effects by activating three classes of adenosine receptor, termed A_1, A_2 and A_3. The A_1 receptors are coupled to the G protein that inhibits adenylate cyclase but they are also responsible for the increase in potassium currents and the suppression of neurotransmitter release. Clearly many of the pharmacological actions of caffeine are due to an inhibition of both these and the A_2 receptors; the latter are also G protein linked but stimulate adenyl cyclase activity. At present, little is known about the physiological properties of the A_3 receptors. Experimental studies have shown that selective agonists of the A_1 receptors have anticonvulsant, antinociceptive and neuroprotective properties.

Those ingesting caffeine or caffeine-containing beverages usually experience less drowsiness, less fatigue and an ability to think more rapidly. Like other stimulants such as the amphetamines, those taking moderate doses of caffeine can excel in repetitive tasks. As the intake of caffeine increases so the signs of progressive central nervous system stimulation occur leading to anxiety, nervousness, insomnia and tremors. At still higher doses, focal and generalized convulsions occur; occasionally such seizures are refractory to the therapeutic effects of anticonvulsants. Patients with panic disorder are particularly sensitive to the adverse effects of all methylxanthines, including caffeine. Indeed excessive caffeine intake by patients taking conventional neuroleptics and antidepressants which have significant anticholinergic side effects may be partly to relieve the thirst caused by such drugs and also as an attempt to counteract their sedative side effects. The adverse effect of a high caffeine intake on the response of psychiatric patients to neuroleptic medication is seldom recognized even though there are several studies showing that a significant improvement in the response of schizophrenic patients to their medication occurred when decaffeinated beverages were substituted for those containing caffeine; this improvement was reversed when caffeinated beverages were reintroduced. Thus the identification of caffeine abuse, particularly in psychiatric patients, could be of considerable importance both for accurate diagnosis and for the design of effective treatment. The most frequently encountered situations where caffeine abuse may occur can be summarized as follows.

1. Caffeine abuse may be misdiagnosed as an anxiety disorder thereby resulting in additional anxiolytics being prescribed rather than reducing the daily caffeine intake of the patient.
2. Caffeine can cause agitation and hyposomnia which can lead to misdiagnosis of depression.
3. High caffeine intake has been reported to exacerbate psychosis.
4. Caffeine may be a complicating factor in anorexia.
5. Caffeine may interact with other drugs given concurrently to a psychiatric patient. It is well established that the methylxanthines are largely metabolized in the liver by a process of demethylation and oxidation. This process is largely due to the action of the cytochrome P 450 1A2 isoenzyme (see p.80) that also metabolizes warfarin, propranolol, clozapine and many of the tricyclic antidepressants. The SSRI antidepressant fluvoxamine inhibits this isozyme. Thus the possibility arises that significant competition can occur between any of these drugs

given concurrently with caffeine. As it has been calculated that there is a four-fold variation in the elimination half-life of the methylxanthines, the effect of such interactions in a psychiatric patient could be considerable.

Both caffeine and theobromine are potent CNS stimulants whereas theobromine is virtually inactive as a stimulant in the doses usually consumed. Low doses (one or two cups of tea for example) of caffeine reduces drowsiness and fatigue but as the dose of caffeine is increased CNS stimulation becomes more apparent leading to nervousness, anxiety, restlessness, insomnia, tremors and hyperaesthesia. At toxic doses, focal and generalized convulsions are likely to occur. The stimulant effect on respiration appears to be due to the sensitization of the medullary centre of the brain to carbon dioxide.

There is experimental and clinical evidence to show that low doses of the methylxanthines, such as 2 mg of theophylline, can rapidly reverse the narcotic effect of 100 mg morphine given intravenously; the methylxanthines can also antagonize the analgesic effects of opioids in animals. The antagonistic action of drugs such as caffeine and theophylline on the analgesic effect of opioids appears to be due to a block of adenosine receptors as there is evidence that adenosine is also involved in the analgesic effect of the opioids.

Over-indulgence in caffeine-containing beverages can lead to psychic dependence. Very occasionally an individual may show extreme sensitivity even to a single cup of coffee which may be associated with an abnormal metabolism of the drug in that individual. It is perhaps more important to advise those patients with a peptic ulcer to limit their caffeine intake. This recommendation should also include decaffeinated beverages which, like caffeine, also enhance the secretion of gastrin and acid.

In CONCLUSION both experimental and clinical studies indicated that caffeine and related methylxanthines are mild stimulants that can cause psychic dependence if consumed in large doses. However, there is little evidence to suggest that caffeine is as dependence-producing as nicotine or alcohol, the two other legally available drugs of dependence. Because of the possibility of drug interactions occurring between caffeine and several classes of psychotropic drugs, the prescribing psychiatrist should be aware of the possibility that the poor response of a patient to a particular neuroleptic or antidepressant may be due to a caffeine-dependent interaction involving the liver microsomal system.

15 Paediatric Psychopharmacology

Introduction

When any psychotropic drug is to be given to either a very young or an elderly patient, the general rule is to start with the lowest dose that is therapeutically beneficial in contrast to the standard dose that would be given to a young adult. There are a number of reasons for this practice. The rates of drug absorption, metabolism and distribution differ. In the case of the young child and aged person, hepatic microsomal enzyme metabolism, which is largely responsible for the metabolism of psychotropic drugs, is suboptimal. In the elderly patient, the cardiac output and renal perfusion rates are substantially decreased, even in the physically healthy person. There is also evidence that tissue sensitivity to many psychotropic drugs is altered at the extremes of age. Thus the general rule is to start at the lowest possible dose and, if necessary, increase the dose slowly until optimal therapeutic benefit is achieved.

In the treatment of psychiatric disorders of children, the clinician is faced with a problem which is less apparent in the adult patient. In adult psychiatry, the diagnosis of the condition assists in ensuring optimal treatment. For example, the treatment of the symptoms of anxiety will depend on the underlying condition with which the anxiety is associated. Thus the type of drug used will depend, for example, on whether the patient is an anxious schizophrenic, an anxious depressive or a patient with panic disorder. As psychiatric diagnosis of childhood disorders is at a more elementary stage than it is in adult psychiatry, the diagnostic approach to treatment still leaves much to be desired. This chapter will therefore be confined to a discussion of those disorders of childhood for which there seems to be reasonable agreement over diagnosis and treatment.

Hyperactivity disorders

The term "attention deficit disorder with hyperactivity" is included in the *Diagnostic and Statistical Manual of Mental Disorders* of the American Psychiatric Association (DSM–IV) to characterize children who show overactivity, impulsivity, poor attention span and a multiplicity of conduct and learning disorders. These symptoms are not generally associated with an abnormal electroencephalogram, obvious neurological defects or abnormal psychometric tests. Drugs used in the treatment of the hyperactivity disorders include psychostimulants, neuroleptics and tricyclic antidepressants.

D-amphetamine was first used by Bradley in 1937 to treat hyperactive children and, since that time, *stimulants* have been the drugs of choice. In Europe, methylphenidate is most frequently used, but other stimulants for which there is evidence of efficacy include D-amphetamine and magnesium pemoline. The short-term usefulness of these agents has been demonstrated in several controlled studies, and they have been shown to be particularly useful in attenuating hyperactivity, impulsivity and short attention span. The success rate for such drugs has been calculated to be as high as 90%, and it is claimed that the general social behaviour of the child returns to normal. However, there is evidence that the improvement in attention does not necessarily lead to the acquisition of specific skills such as reading or mathematics or to an improvement of memory.

While there is clinical evidence that appropriate doses of methylphenidate and D-amphetamine are equally and rapidly effective in the treatment of hyperactivity disorders, magnesium pemoline appears to take up to 2 weeks before it becomes optimally effective. There is no direct relationship between the plasma drug levels of the psychostimulants and their therapeutic effects. The general pharmacological properties of the psychostimulants are covered elsewhere (see p. 303).

The *side effects* of the psychostimulants are predictable. Anorexia and a delay in the onset of sleep occur in approximately 30% of children on moderate doses of the drugs. Rarely mood changes may occur, but tend to diminish with continuing treatment. Both D-amphetamine and methylphenidate decrease weight gain and body growth, but D-amphetamine appears to have the most potent growth-inhibiting effect out of the psychostimulants in common use. As rebound acceleration in growth occurs once the drugs are discontinued, "drug holidays" are generally recommended.

There is some controversy regarding the duration of treatment with psychostimulants. Nevertheless, it would generally appear that treatment should continue until normal behaviour is maintained following drug withdrawal. Studies on adolescents and adults who had hyperactivity disorders in childhood suggests that while the symptoms may diminish with age, they can persist into adulthood. Furthermore, psychostimulants may be effective in adolescents with hyperactivity disorder.

Total refractoriness to psychostimulants is uncommon, but should this occur neuroleptics or antidepressants may be considered as alternatives. The *neuroleptics* chlorpromazine and thioridazine have been shown to be beneficial in the treatment of hyperactivity, but are less effective in treating distractibility. Drowsiness is the most common side effect with these drugs. As with all neuroleptics, the clinician must be aware that a potential long-term side effect is tardive dyskinesia.

Tricyclic antidepressants have been shown to be superior to placebo in the treatment of brain-damaged hyperactive children, their beneficial effects being greater in those children showing electroencephalographic and neurological abnormalities than in those in whom such defects are absent.

Behavioural techniques have also been applied to the treatment of hyperactivity disorder but, while such an approach may be useful, clinical evidence suggests that a drug such as methylphenidate is superior.

Affective disorders of childhood and adolescence

There is much controversy regarding the occurrence of major depressive disorder in prepubertal children. However, several studies in both the United States and Britain have suggested that depressive disorder does exist, although the frequency appears to be lower than in adolescents. There is endocrinological evidence, based on the hypersecretion of cortisol and an abnormal growth hormone response to insulin-induced hypoglycaemia, to suggest that children with major depressive disorder show similar endocrine abnormalities to those of adolescents and adults. However, the number of patients in these studies is small and clearly more thorough investigations must be undertaken before any conclusion may be reached.

Regarding the drug treatment of depression in children, there is so far a paucity of good clinical trials to show that antidepressants are effective. Several small studies suggest that daily doses of up to 5 mg/kg of imipramine may be beneficial, but there is no data to show whether other types of antidepressant medication are effective. The side effects and toxicity of tricyclic antidepressants are legion and have been discussed in detail elsewhere.

Manic disorders would appear to be extremely rare in young children and only single case reports have appeared in the clinical literature. They are more common in adolescence but not as frequent as among adults. Some authorities have argued that the extent of mania among adolescents is underestimated and that many patients have been misdiagnosed as schizophrenics. Regarding treatment, lithium would appear to be the drug of choice. Since children and adolescents appear to have a higher lithium renal clearance than adults, it is occasionally necessary to give the drug in a higher oral dose than would be usual for the adult. Apart from the possible detrimental effect of lithium on bone growth in children, the monitoring of the young patient should follow the same procedures as outlined for the adult.

Anxiety disorders

The DSM–IV classifies anxiety disorders in children into four categories, namely social anxiety, overanxious disorder, phobias and separation anxiety. Only separation anxiety, a fear of losing a loved one or a close attachment, has been reasonably well studied from the point of view of drug treatment. School phobia is perhaps the most severe form of separation anxiety and there are several trials to show that imipramine, in daily doses of up to 5 mg/kg, is effective. Many patients require drug treatment for at least 6 to 8 weeks before an optimal response is achieved. Frequently, children remain symptom free after a 3–4 month course of treatment. In addition to the usual anticholinergic effects of imipramine, it should be noted that children are often susceptible to withdrawal symptoms such as nausea and gastro-intestinal spasm. This may be reduced if the drug is slowly withdrawn over a 2-week period.

Obsessive–compulsive disorders

These occur only rarely in children but more frequently in adolescents. There have been no extensive studies of drug treatments of this condition in young patients, but anecdotal reports suggest that tricyclic antidepressants such as clomipramine and amitriptyline may be as effective as they are in adults.

Pervasive development disorders

These include impaired social and emotional functioning as well as the persistence of bizarre behaviours, extreme rage and mood changes. They differ from infantile autism in that they occur after 30 months of age and may be distinguished from childhood schizophrenia by the absence of delusions, hallucinations and formal thought disorder. These conditions appear to respond quite well to relatively high doses of neuroleptics (chlorpromazine, thioridazine, haloperidol and fluphenazine). Neuroleptics combined with behavioural therapy appear to be the best treatment for such disorders. It should be remembered that stereotypies, mannerisms and tics are often found in children with developmental disorders and these may recur upon drug withdrawal. These behaviours should not be confused with drug-induced tardive dyskinesia.

Aggression and conduct disorders

Aggression is a symptom of many disorders in childhood (e.g. depression, hyperactivity disorder, mental retardation) and therefore a thorough psychiatric assessment should be made before drug treatment is considered. Drugs that may be used to treat aggressive disorders in children and adolescents include lithium (for autistic and mentally retarded children) and the neuroleptics. It should be noted that, despite the effectiveness of neuroleptics in the treatment of aggression in children and adolescents, the occurrence of drowsiness, weight gain, dermatosis and extrapyramidal side effects means that these drugs should be used only when other approaches have failed. Withdrawal symptoms, with or without dyskinetic movements, may occur more frequently in the younger patient than in the adult.

There would appear to be general agreement that the anxiolytic benzodiazepines have no place in the treatment of psychiatric conditions in children, even though benzodiazepines such as clonazepam are clearly beneficial in some types of childhood epilepsy. This is probably due to the behaviourally disinhibiting effect of these drugs, which appears to be more pronounced in children than adults.

Nocturnal enuresis

Of the psychotropic drugs which have received some prominence in Europe for the treatment of *nocturnal enuresis*, imipramine is widely accepted as the drug of choice for this condition. While the precise cause of this condition is uncertain, it would appear that the beneficial effects of this drug are not due to its anticholinergic action.

Infantile autism

It is now widely accepted that infantile autism is a heterogeneous behavioural syndrome. Three major studies suggest that a familial clustering of cognitive and/or language problems exist in siblings and families of autistic children. There is a suggestion that the fragile X chromosome may be linked to this syndrome, a frequency of 5–29% having been reported to occur in male patients. Other factors that have been suggested as contributing to this condition include pre- and perinatal insults to the developing brain. This may be associated with the electroencephalographic abnormalities and the gross structural changes in the brain found in recent brain imaging studies in autistic patients. Neurochemical abnormalities in the body fluids of autistic patients have also been reported. These include hyperserotonaemia in about

30% of the cases, a raised concentration of homovanillic acid in the cerebrospinal fluid and a decrease in the concentration of plasma opioids that correlates with self-mutilation.

A dysfunction in the hypothalamic–pituitary axis has also been reported, which is reflected in a prolonged growth hormone response to insulin-induced hypoglycaemia and a blunted prolactin response to a 5-hydroxytryptophan challenge. The blunted prolactin response may be indicative of a malfunctioning central serotonergic system.

Based on these findings, the 5-hydroxytryptamine (5-HT) releasing agent fenfluramine has been used to treat autism. While preliminary results of these studies seem promising, fenfluramine has been shown to have adverse effects on discrimination learning, and concern has been raised that the depletion of 5-HT caused by the drug may be irreversible. Dopamine receptor antagonists, particularly haloperidol have been found to be effective in treating many of the behavioural symptoms of autism, while preliminary studies suggest that the opiate antagonist naltrexone decreases the aggressiveness and stereotypies, and increases the socialization, of young autistic children.

In SUMMARY, the relatively small number of psychotropic drugs which have been used for the treatment of psychiatric diseases in children and adolescents reflects the diagnostic uncertainty regarding the clinical status of the patients, the lower frequency of established psychiatric disorders in these groups of patients and, as a consequence, the paucity of good clinical trials in which the efficacy of drug treatments may be established. Nevertheless, there is good evidence that psychostimulants, particularly methylphenidate, are of value in the treatment of hyperkinetic disorders, while conventional neuroleptics and tricyclic antidepressants may have an application in the treatment of a diverse group of disorders ranging from depression to separation anxiety and aggression. In view of the well-established side effects and toxicity of such drugs, it is to be hoped that they will soon be superseded by safer drugs whose efficacy has already been established in adult patients.

16 Geriatric Psychopharmacology

Introduction

The elderly person is likely to experience many socioeconomic, emotional and physiological changes which will have a major bearing on psychotropic drug treatment. Such a population is therefore more likely to be exposed to more types of drug treatment than younger age groups.

It has been found that the vast majority of elderly patients being treated for a psychiatric disorder also have at least one physical disorder that requires medication; 80% of all elderly patients in the United States have at least one chronic physical illness. Thus the elderly are the most likely group to experience adverse drug reactions and interactions. Studies show that patients over the age of 70 years have approximately twice as many adverse drug reactions as those under 50 years.

Another problem which particularly affects the elderly population concerns compliance with prescribed medication. Factors such as impaired vision, making it difficult for the patient to recognize the various medications, hearing, manual dexterity and cognition all contribute to the non-compliance. Perhaps one of the most important factors that governs non-compliance is the increased frequency and severity of the side effects that occur with most types of medication in the elderly. This may be illustrated by the tricyclic antidepressants and phenothiazine neuroleptics, both these classes of drugs having pronounced antimuscarinic activity even in the physically healthy young patient. In the elderly there is evidence of excessive sensitivity to the anticholinergic effects of drugs. This is compounded by the decline in cognitive function which accompanies ageing. Thus one must anticipate that the patient compliance for any psychotropic drug with pronounced anticholinergic and sedative side effects will be low.

Another problem which can compromise compliance concerns the hypotensive actions of many psychotropic drugs (e.g. tricyclic antidepressants, phenothiazine neuroleptics). Due to the alpha$_1$ receptor antagonistic action of these drugs, they are likely to cause severe orthostatic hypotension in some elderly patients. This can cause patients to fall and damage themselves. The increased sensitivity of the elderly to the sedative effects of drugs is also well known. As hypnotics and anxiolytics are frequently administered to the elderly, the sedative effects of these drugs can be minimized by using drugs that have a short to medium half-life. There seems little justification for using the long half-life sedative hypnotics in the elderly patient.

Dementia

The pathological and clinical features of the various types of dementia have been the subject of detailed discussion elsewhere in this book (see Chapter 13). A variety of conditions that occur in the elderly must be differentiated from true dementia. Delirium, for example, is associated with an alteration in the level of consciousness, disordered thinking and fluctuating cognitive impairment. Such a delirious state can occur for a variety of reasons, including inadequately treated diabetes, hyperparathyroidism or hepatic encephalopathy. Dementia must also be distinguished from psychosis, in which the patient shows impairment of thinking but not impairment of memory. The term "pseudo-dementia" is often used to describe a depressive episode in which the patient presents with abnormalities of mood, appetite and sleep disturbance with cognitive dysfunction which is directly caused by the depression. The cognitive deficits usually resolve with treatment of the underlying condition. Finally cerebrovascular disease (as exemplified by multi-infarct dementia, which is the second most common cause of dementia) or carotid occlusion may be associated with episodic memory loss. It is therefore important to diagnose correctly the cause of the memory and cognitive impairment so that appropriate treatment may be given. Should the results of clinical and neurological investigation clearly establish the existence of Alzheimer's disease, drug treatment will be of little benefit to the patient!

Depression

A disturbance in the sleep pattern is a common symptom of depression but changes in the sleep pattern also occur as a consequence of ageing. Once depression has been diagnosed, there are several types of antidepressants which may be given. Because of their potent anticholinergic side effects, there seems little merit in prescribing the older tricyclic antidepressants (e.g. amitriptyline, imipramine) to such patients. There is now sufficient evidence to suggest that sedative antidepressants such as mianserin or trazodone given at night reduce the likelihood that the patient will require a sedative hypnotic. For the more retarded elderly patient, a non-sedative antidepressant such as lofepramine or one of the new 5-hydroxytryptamine (5-HT) reuptake inhibitor antidepressants (e.g. fluoxetine, fluvoxamine or sertraline) may be used.

The side effects and cardiotoxicity of the tricyclic antidepressants have been discussed in detail elsewhere in this volume and, while there is ample evidence of their therapeutic efficacy, it seems difficult to justify their use, particularly in a group of patients who are most vulnerable to their detrimental side effects. Of the newer antidepressants, the reversible inhibitors of monoamine oxidase type A such as moclobemide may also be of value in the elderly depressed patient, particularly in those patients who fail to respond to the amine uptake inhibitor type of antidepressant. It should also be remembered that electroconvulsive shock therapy (ECT) is a safe and effective treatment for severe depression in all patients, including the elderly.

Psychosis

A variety of psychotic conditions occur in the elderly, but it is important to remember that an elderly person who develops agitation, paranoid ideation or delusions may be suffering from a drug-induced delirium. The most common causes of such a condition are drugs that have potent central muscarinic-blocking properties, such as the antiparkinsonian agents, antihistamines, tricyclic antidepressants and antipsychotics. Withholding all psychotropic drug medication for a few days may be the most judicious management for this type of toxic psychosis.

Agitation and aggression are often symptoms of advanced Alzheimer's disease and high potency neuroleptics such as haloperidol may be of value in such patients. Such drugs would also appear to be the best tolerated in the elderly schizophrenic patient. Drugs such as chlorpromazine and thioridazine are more likely to produce hypotension, cardiac abnormalities and excessive sedation in the elderly patient, and side effects are, of course, a problem with the high potency neuroleptics in the elderly; centrally acting anticholinergic agents that are used to reverse some of the symptoms of parkinsonism in such patients should be used as little as possible and in the lowest possible doses.

Mania can occur in any age group. Acute manic episodes in the elderly may best be managed with high potency neuroleptics. The use of *lithium* is not contraindicated in the elderly provided renal clearance is reasonably normal. The dose administered should be carefully monitored, as the half-life of the drug is increased in the elderly to 36–48 hours in comparison to about 24 hours in the young adult. The serum lithium concentration in the elderly should be maintained at about 0.5 mEq/litre. It is essential to ensure that the elderly patient is not on a salt-restricted diet before starting lithium therapy.

The side effects and toxicity of lithium have been discussed in detail elsewhere (see p. 146 *et seq.*), and, apart from an increase in the frequency of confusional states in the elderly patient, the same adverse effects can be expected as in the younger patient.

Anxiety and insomnia

Most psychotropic drugs are highly lipophilic, and the increased fat to lean body mass ratio and the decreased metabolism and excretion in the elderly patient mean that the half-lives of most psychotropic drugs are increased. The benzodiazepine anxiolytics and hypnotics are no exception. Following a single dose of chlordiazepoxide, diazepam or flurazepam, the time for elimination of the parent compounds and their active metabolites can be as long as 72 hours. For this reason, it is now general practice to administer a short-acting benzodiazepine (e.g. oxazepam, alprazolam or temazepam) only as needed and for as short a period as possible. Such drugs should only be used for a period not exceeding 6 weeks. Supportive psychotherapy, either as an adjunct to drug therapy or as an alternative, has an important role to play in treating mild anxiety states in the elderly.

Insomnia is a common complaint in the elderly. As people age they require less sleep, and a variety of physical ailments to which the elderly are subject can cause a change in the sleep pattern (e.g. cerebral atherosclerosis, heart disease, decreased pulmonary function), as can depression. Providing sedative hypnotics are warranted, the judicious use of short half-life benzodiazepines such as temazepam, triazolam, oxazepam and alprazolam for a period not exceeding 1–2 months may be appropriate. Because of their side effects, there would appear to be little merit in using chloral hydrate or related drugs in the treatment of insomnia in the elderly. It should be noted that even benzodiazepines which have a relatively short half-life are likely to cause excessive day-time sedation. The side effects and dependence potential of the anxiolytics and sedative hypnotics have been covered elsewhere in this volume (Chapter 8).

In addition to the benzodiazepines, there may be a role for the non-benzodiazepine drugs such as buspirone and zopiclone in the treatment of anxiety and insomnia in the elderly. Both drugs appear to be well tolerated in younger populations of patients, but it is essential to await the outcome of properly conducted trials of these drugs on a substantial number of elderly patients before any conclusions may be drawn regarding their value as alternatives to the benzodiazepines.

In SUMMARY, it can be seen that the types of psychotropic drug medication that may be used in the elderly are essentially similar to those used in the younger adult patient. The main difference lies in the reduction in distribution, metabolism and elimination of the drugs, which necessitates their administration in lower doses initially followed by a slower escalation of the dose until optimal benefit is obtained. Side effects, particularly anticholinergic effects, are more pronounced in the elderly and can contribute to poor compliance. Clearly the use of the older psychotropic medications, such as the tricyclic antidepressants and less potent neuroleptics, should be avoided in elderly patients whenever possible.

17 The Iznter-relationship Between Psychopharmacology and Psychoneuroimmunology

The background

The adverse effects of stress and depression, the effects of bereavement, unemployment and social isolation on mental and physical health have been known since antiquity. Aristotle advised physicians, "Just as you ought not to attempt to cure eyes without head or head without body, so you should not treat body without soul." One of the fathers of modern medicine put it more scientifically in the 19th century when he recommended that when attempting to predict health outcomes from tuberculosis in patients, it is just as important to know what is going on in a man's head as it is in his chest.

These are two of the numerous examples, largely anecdotal, that document the complex and intimate connection between the mind and the body. In the past 20 years this has given rise to a new science of psychoneuroimmunology that is devoted to the study of the inter-relationship between the brain, behaviour and the immune system. Interest in this area of neuroscience has undoubtedly been due to the impact of acquired immune deficiency syndrome (AIDS) in which it has been estimated that at least 10% of these patients will develop mood, behavioural, cognitive and memory changes before they develop somatic signs of the illness. Similarly, studies have shown that 6 months before patients with pancreatic cancer develop clinical signs of the disease, a significant proportion develop depression. Such observations suggest that not only does the brain influence the immune system by way of the endocrine and efferent neuronal pathways but also that products of immune cell activity, such as the cytokines, play a role in modifying human behaviour by directly modulating central neurotransmitter pathways.

Basic structure of the immune system

It is not the purpose of this short introduction to psychoneuroimmunology to give a comprehensive view of the immune system, and readers are referred to the key references cited at the end of the book.

Most of the cells comprising the immune system can be divided into one of two categories depending on the targets of their action. Thus the immune cells are either primed to eliminate specific pathogens or to respond to any type of cell that is not recognized as being a normal body component. The first category of cells comprises the different types of lymphocytes which are divided into the B-lymphocytes (B cells) that are responsible for antibody production, and the T-lymphocytes (T cells) that directly phagocytose pathogens or release specific biologically active proteins, the cytokines, that regulate the activity of other cells in the immune system. Both T and B cells respond in a highly specific manner when attacking pathogens. In addition to these specific immune cells, there are phagocytic cells, such as the monocytes and neutrophils, that respond to any cell type or foreign molecule that is not recognized as being a normal constituent of the body.

The phagocytic cells such as the monocytes and neutrophils are basically scavenger white blood cells that ingest invading bacteria or viruses. Some of the monocytes also enter the tissues where they become macrophages. They can also provide signals enabling T cells to respond more efficiently to the pathogen. In this situation the antigen becomes attached to the monocyte membrane which is then presented to a T-lymphocyte together with the cytokine interleukin-1 (IL-1). This initiates a further activation of T-lymphocytes. Monocytes also produce mediators of inflammation, the complement proteins, which help to create a hostile environment for foreign organisms. In addition to complement proteins other mediators of the immune response including histamine (which acts as a local hormone to cause capillary dilatation), the prostglandins and leukotrienes which act to initiate and terminate the activities of the macrophages and T cells.

Lymphocytes are derived from bone marrow but whereas some of the cells remain in the bone marrow until they reach maturity (the B cells), others migrate early in their development to the thymus gland to become T cells. Thus B and T cells learn to distinguish between the normal constituent cells of the body and foreign objects, due to the presence of specific memory cells which are under genetic control. B and T cells circulate throughout the vascular system before concentrating in lymphoid tissue (spleen and lymph nodes) where they remain inactive until stimulated by specific antigens. Because of the specificity of function imparted on the T and B cells by the memory cells, the lymphocytes are highly selective in responding to relatively few antigens. The main properties of the immune cells that are altered in psychiatric illnesses are summarized in Table 17.1.

T cells exist in several different forms. Thus the T-helper cells (Th cells) play a regulatory role by facilitating the antibody production by B cells and also activate the macrophages. Other types of T cells can directly attack pathogens or normal cells that have been infected with a virus or bacterium for example. These are the cytotoxic T cells, or natural killer cells (NKCs).

Table 17.1. The main properties of the immune cells that are altered in psychiatric illnesses

Natural killer cells (NKCs)	Recognize changes on cell-membrane virus-infected and cancer cells and destroy the cells. NKCs bind to surfaces of target cells and inject cytotoxic molecules into the cell membrane, destroying the cells. There are several types of cells that have NKC activity
Phagocytes	Two major classes of WBCs are involved in removing invading microorganisms by a process of phagocytosis. These are polymorphonuclear leukocytes and mononuclear phagocytes, or monocytes. In tissues, monocytes differentiate into macrophages and, in the brain, into microglia
T and B lymphocytes	Produced by lymphoid tissue. Lymphocytes represent about 20% of the WBCs in adults; they have a long life span (sometimes several years). They probably serve as memory cells for the immune system. These mononuclear cells may be small, agranular structures (T and B cells) or large, granular cells (NKCs). Different types of T cells may only be differentiated by their cell-surface markers (CD markers — clusters of differentiation). CD markers are identified using labelling antibodies

Not only can such cells destroy pathogens but they also secrete such cytokines as IL-1 which have a key role to play in orchestrating the immune system both peripherally and in the brain. The immunoglobulins (the most important in man being IgM, IgG, IgE, IgD and IgA), are produced following the activation of B cells by specific antigens.

Fever and sleep are important events which assist recovery following an infection by helping to destroy heat-sensitive foreign microorganisms. One of the key promoters of sleep and fever following an infection is IL-1. This cytokine can penetrate some areas of the blood–brain barrier and raise the temperature "set point" in the hypothalamus thereby producing a fever. Similarly Il-1 promotes slow-wave sleep and thereby facilitates tissue repair due to the secretion or growth hormone during that sleep phase. In addition to facilitating tissue repair, growth hormone can also boost the immune system. Whereas the precise mechanism whereby the cytokines can enter the brain and initiate subtle changes in brain function is uncertain, CNS changes initiated by peripherally produced IL-1 (and also by the microglial cells within the brain) provides convincing evidence that the immune system directly impacts upon the brain.

The endocrine immune relationship

One of the major pathways whereby the central nervous system regulates the immune system is via the hypothalamic–pituitary–adrenal (HPA) axis. Various neurotransmitters (e.g. serotonin, noradrenaline, acetylcholine) regulate the secretion of corticotropin releasing factor (CRF) which controls the release of adrenocorticotrophic hormone (ACTH) from the anterior pituitary. ACTH directly activates the adrenal cortex to produce glucocorticoids (e.g. cortisol). Following the rise in the plasma concentration of the glucocorticoids, a negative feedback mechanism normally operates to block the further release of ACTH from the pituitary. In depression, however, there would appear to be an insensitivity of the central glucocorticoid receptors to this feedback regulation. As a consequence, the plasma concentration remains elevated and cannot be easily suppressed by a potent synthetic glucocorticoid such as dexamethasone. This forms the basis of the dexamethasone suppression test (DST) which is often used as a biological marker of depression.

T cells are particularly sensitive to the inhibitory effects of the glucocorticoids. In particular, the nascent T cells which represent about 90% of all T cells in the thymus gland, are very sensitive to the inhibitory effects of these steroids; high steroid concentrations can also prematurely induce the migration of T cells from the thymus to other immune tissues. This leads to a decrease in the size of the thymus gland. It should be emphasized that the effects of the glucocorticoids on the immune system are biphasic; in high concentrations they suppress major components of the immune system whereas in low concentration they activate it. In addition to glucocorticoid receptors, T cells also contain receptors for prolactin and growth hormones which suggests ways in which the endocrine system can directly affect the immune system.

The adrenal gland secretes glucocorticoids in a pulsatile rhythmical way with the highest plasma concentrations being reached during the day. It has been shown that the lowest plasma concentration of the glucocorticoids coincides with the time at which the lymphocytes respond most actively to antigens. As the hypersecretion of cortisol is a characteristic feature of depression and other psychiatric conditions, it is perhaps not surprising to find that components of the immune system are also abnormal in this condition.

Anatomical links between the brain and the immune system

What is the mechanism whereby the nervous system can influence the immune system? Two major routes serve to link the brain with the immune system. The first is via the HPA axis, already referred to. The second is via the autonomic nervous system.

It has been known for over 20 years that there were adrenoceptors on T cells, B cells and macrophages. In addition, noradrenergic fibres directly innervate the bone marrow, thymus, spleen, lymph nodes and virtually all other immune organs. These sympathetic nerve terminals not only release noradrenaline but also possibly neuropeptides as well. There is evidence that many sympathetic nerve terminals innervating the immune organs make direct contact with the parenchyma, ending adjacent to the cells of the immune system. In the spleen for example, the sympathetic terminals penetrate the areas that contain a high density of helper T cells and also cytotoxic and suppressor T cells. Electron microscopic evidence suggests that the sympathetic nerve terminals can form direct physical contact with T-lymphocytes and macrophages.

The functional connection between the peripheral sympathetic system and the immune system can be illustrated by the changes which take place in ageing. It is known that in the aged animal, the sympathetic innervation of the spleen is dramatically reduced. This appears to be associated with deficiencies in T cell function and in cellular immunity. At the cellular level, immunosenescence is associated with a change in responsiveness of the immune cells and in their ability to regulate the beta adrenoceptors on their cell surfaces. Such changes appear to shift the metabolism of the sympathetic nervous system to a state that encourages apoptosis (or programmed cell death) possibly by inducing an increase in the production of cytotoxic metabolites. Experimental evidence suggest that the monoamine oxidase-B (MAO-B) inhibitor deprenyl (selegiline) can reduce these neurodegenerative changes in the peripheral sympathetic system and lead to the restoration of sympathetic innervation of the spleen.

Figure 17.1 summarizes the inter-relationship between the nervous system and the immune system.

Stress and the immune system

All forms of stress result in the activation of the pituitary–adrenal axis, with a consequent rise in circulating catecholamines and glucocorticoid hormones from the adrenal gland. The secretion of ACTH from the pituitary gland, which is controlled by hypothalamic CRF, triggers the secretion of adrenal glucocorticoids, while stress-induced activation of the sympathetic system is responsible for the catecholamine secretion. It is now apparent that ACTH secretion can also be increased by thymic peptides (such as thymopoietin), while interleukin-1 (IL-alpha), a product of macrophage activity, has been shown to regulate ACTH secretion.

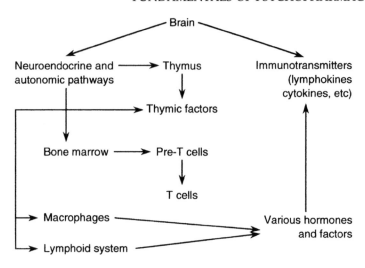

Figure 17.1. Summary of the pathways postulated to be involved in the interaction between the nervous and immune systems.

Such events show how the immune, endocrine and central nervous systems are integrated in their responses to any form of stress. It is well established that physical or psychosocial stress causes increased secretions of prolactin, growth hormones, thyroid, and gonadal hormones, in addition to ACTH. Endogenous opioids are secreted under such conditions and function as immunomodulators, while also elevating the pain threshold. Receptors for such hormones exist on immunocompetent cells, along with receptors for catecholamines, serotonin and acetylcholine.

In addition to the regulatory effects of the nervous system on the immune system, there is now convincing evidence that the immune system can influence brain function. Thus changes in the activity of specific nuclei in the hypothalamus of the rat have been described following the formation of antibodies to specific antigen challenges. Alterations in electrical activity appear to be linked to specific decreases in noradrenaline concentrations in these nuclei. Changes in the activity of the serotonergic neurons in the hippocampus also occur shortly after the occurrence of the immune response. These findings illustrate how the immune system, presumably via the release of immunoregulatory peptides (also called immunotransmitters) such as interleukins from macrophages, can influence the activity of the hypothalamic–pituitary axis and also higher centres of the brain (such as the hippocampus), which are involved in short-term memory processing. The triad of inter-relationships between the brain, endocrine and immune systems is illustrated in Figure 17.2.

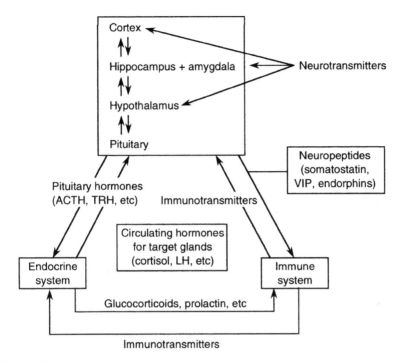

Figure 17.2.   Inter-relationship between the brain and the immune and endocrine systems.

Immune system in affective disorders

Susceptibility to bacterial and viral infections, and to the establishment of tumours, is reported to arise more frequently in those who are depressed than in those who are not. An analysis of the immune systems of those suffering the severe psychological stress of bereavement has shown that the activity of those immune cells that are fundamentally involved in the host defence against infections (e.g. NKCs and T-lymphocytes) is dramatically reduced. Such an effect can occur following chronic and subchronic stress.

The past 20 years have witnessed a broad interest in the role of the hypothalamic–pituitary–adrenal axis in the psychobiology of affective disorders. In depressed patients, increases in serum cortisol are frequently reported in addition to disruptions of circadian patterns of cortisol secretion and an insensitivity of cortisol secretion to suppression by glucocorticoids such as dexamethasone.

One consequence of hypercortisolaemia is a suppression of immune function. As impaired immune responses have been frequently reported in depressed patients, it has been suggested that the reduction in immune function is primarily a reflection of hypercortisolaemia. However, it would appear that the immune changes are not a direct reflection of such an event. For example, studies of the T cell response to mitogen stimulation *in vitro* have shown that the suppression of T cell replication occurred in all depressed patients independently of their plasma cortisol concentrations. Other studies have shown that the number of T cells is decreased in ambulatory depressed patients but not in those with other types of major psychiatric illness, such as schizophrenia. While the precise cause of the decreased T cell function is unclear, it would appear that peptides such as endogenous opioids, neurotensin, vasoactive intestinal peptide, substance P and somatostatin, are causally involved. It has been speculated that such peptides depress T cell function via their action on the hypothalamic–hypophysial pathway.

In addition to a suppression of T cell and NKC activity in depressed patients, changes have also been found to occur in the activity of neutrophils and monocytes. Thus, recent studies have shown the activity of monocytes is enhanced, and that of neutrophils decreased, in untreated depressed patients. On recovery, the activity of the phagocytes returns to control values suggesting the changes are state, rather than trait, markers of depression. Such changes in phagocytosis are qualitatively different from those found in patients with schizophrenia, mania, anxiety states, alcoholism or Alzheimer's disease. One possible explanation for the changes in neutrophil and monocyte activity lies in the elevation of prostaglandin concentrations in the plasma of depressed patients. As some of the prostaglandins have been shown experimentally to inhibit the release of noradrenaline from central neurons, it may be speculated that brain cyclo-oxygenase (the enzyme synthesizing the prostaglandins from arachidonic acid) may play an important role in linking central amine neurotransmission with the action of cytokines and other immunomodulators.

There is convincing evidence that immunoregulation is partly mediated by the peripheral and central sympathetic systems and that prostaglandins can modulate central neurotransmitter release, possibly by modifying the passage of calcium into neurons. It is also known that drugs that are therapeutically effective in treating depression (such as monoamine oxidase inhibitors, tricyclic antidepressants and lithium) can inhibit the synthesis of prostaglandins. Monocytes are an important source of IL-1 and prostaglandins, and as the activity of these cells is enhanced in depressed patients, it may be hypothesized that they play an important role in elevating peripheral and, due to the activity of the microglia in the brain, central immuno-transmitters.

Clearly, more detailed studies must be undertaken to validate this hypothesis, but these preliminary findings link proven neurotransmitter

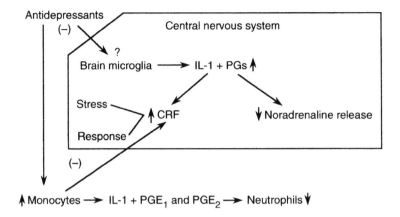

Figure 17.3. Possible changes in immune function and the brain in depression.

changes in depressed patients with the delays in onset of action of antidepressants and the changes in cellular immunity. Figure 17.3 summarizes the possible links between depression and changes in some aspects of the immune system.

It now seems probable that specific disturbances occur in the immune system in psychiatric illness that are not artefacts of non-specific stress factor, institutionalization or medication. The known effects of the neuroendocrine system on the immune response, and the recent evidence that receptor sites for neurotransmitters and neuroendocrine factors occur on lymphocytes and macrophages, support the hypothesis that immunological abnormalities may assist in precipitating the symptoms of anxiety and depression, commonly symptoms of major affective disorders. The next step in research is to define more precisely which specific immune factors are involved.

Changes in the immune system in schizophrenia

Evidence suggesting an abnormality in immune function in those subject to severe stress or suffering from depression largely relates to an abnormality in function. Such abnormalities do not appear to occur in schizophrenia. Possibly because of its well-established genetic component, many aspects of the immune system would appear to be deranged in schizophrenic patients. Thus abnormalities in the concentration of serum immunoglobulins and deficiencies in immune responsiveness have been reported to occur in such patients.

Several investigators have reported a generalized increase in the immunoglobulins in both acute and chronic stages of schizophrenia, although not all investigators have been able to confirm this. There is some evidence that antibrain antibodies which could selectively destroy specific types of brain cells, have been detected in schizophrenic patients. Some years ago, a factor was isolated from the serum of schizophrenic patients that produced catatonia and an abnormal electroencephalographic pattern when injected intravenously into monkeys or human volunteers; the electroencephalogram changes were similar to those seen in schizophrenic patients. The serum protein causing these abnormalities was termed taraxein. These findings were confimed by some researchers but not by those who used a more reliable radioimmunoassay method. However, in an extensive study of antibrain antibodies in 69 schizophrenics and 58 controls, it has been shown that if antibrain antibodies play any role in psychiatric disorders, they are non-specific and only present in a small percentage of patients.

Allergic reactions entail disordered immune functioning, and controversy exists regarding allergies to various food substances and the incidence of schizophrenia. Some studies have suggested that schizophrenics have an increased incidence of allergies in childhood, especially involving an intolerance to wheat gluten. However, there are few adequately controlled studies to show that food allergies play any role in the aetiology of schizophrenia and, to date, there is little unequivocal evidence to support the view that allergies play a causal role in this illness.

There is evidence to suggest that there are at least two genetically determined components in those at risk from schizophrenia. One of these components facilitates a decrease in suppressor cells, while the other promotes the accumulation or antithymic immunoglobulins. The consequences of the resultant imbalance between the helper and suppressor mechanism which arises from these immune malfunctions are the occurrence of specific antitissue antibodies, the formation of which is normally controlled by a balance between helper and suppressor T cell mechanisms.

There have been several suggestions whereby the negative symptoms of schizophrenia could represent an autoimmune encephalitis-like syndrome in which a viral infection, for example, could initiate an autoimmune response against dopaminergic pathways. One possibility is that dopamine receptor stimulating antibodies could be produced as part of the pathological processes that have a high affinity for the dopamine autoreceptors and thereby decrease the release of the neurotransmitter in specific dopaminergic pathways. However, it must be emphasized that the clinical data upon which many of these speculations are based have been obtained from patients on prolonged treatment with neuroleptics. These drugs are known to modify the immune system which could increase the subsequent vulnerability of the patient to viral infections.

It may be speculated that an inherited primary defect in the immune system could initiate schizophrenia by stimulating the production of antibrain antibodies or by increasing the vulnerability of the patient to a viral infection. Alternatively, a primary defect in central neurotransmitter metabolism, possibly involving dopamine, may cause the immune abnormalities which have been described. In this case it may be argued that the immune changes are an epiphenomenon of the disease and not necessarily the primary cause.

In CONCLUSION, it seems probable that some disturbances in immune function do occur in mental illness and are not artefacts of medication or the effects of institutionalization. The known effects of the neuroendocrine system on the immune response and the recent evidence that receptor sites for neurotransmitters and neuroendocrine factor occur on lymphocytes and macrophages, support the hypothesis that immunological abnormalities may assist in precipitating the symptoms of anxiety, depression and schizophrenia. Nevertheless, the nature of specific immunological disturbances which underlie these diseases remains elusive.

18   Possible Function and Therapeutic Role of Sigma Receptors

Introduction

The sigma opiate receptor was originally proposed by the American neuropharmacologist William R. Martin as the site that mediates the psychotomimetic and stimulatory effects of cyclazocine, pentazocine, N-allyl normetazocine (SKF 10047) and related opiates in humans and dogs. However, there is now considerable evidence to suggest that these effects are not mediated by opioid receptors. Many of the opiates that have psychotomimetic properties also bind with a high affinity of phencyclidine (PCP) receptor sites situated in the channel of the N-methyl-D-aspartate (NMDA) receptor. It now appears from electrophysiological, biochemical, anatomical and molecular studies that there are two distinct sites that bind opioid analgesics that have an affinity for sigma receptors. One site is on the PCP receptor situated in the NMDA receptor. The other sigma site is defined as non-opioid, non-dopaminergic and shows a high affinity for haloperidol and N-allyl normetazocine. Using a highly selective ligand for sigma-receptors such as ditolyguanidine (DTG), it has now been possible to separate sigma receptors into two major types. Sigma-1 receptors are the main neuronal type and exhibit a high affinity for centrally acting antitussive and anticonvulsant drugs. The other site has a low affinity for most sigma ligands except DTG and haloperidol. This site is found in the red nucleus and cerebellum (as well as many other brain regions) where it may mediate the motor (dystonic) effects of different types of sigma ligand. Biochemically the sigma-1 and sigma-2 receptors may also be distinguished by the nature of the second messenger to which they are attached. Thus the sigma-1 receptors appear to be linked to guanylyl nucleotide binding proteins (G proteins) whereas the sigma-2 sites are not and may bring about their physiological effects by modulating K^+ channels.

Sigma receptors and psychosis

Some 20 years ago, Martin and coworkers proposed that the psychotomimetic effects of pentazocine and related opiate analgesics was due to their effect on sigma receptors. It is now known that the sigma receptors are quite distinct from PCP, opioid, serotonin and dopamine receptors. However, many psychotropic drugs that bind to dopamine, serotonin and PCP receptors also have a high affinity for sigma receptors. For example, haloperidol and the novel benzamide neuroleptic remoxipride bind with high affinity for both D_2 and sigma receptors. Nevertheless, there are many potent neuroleptics that have a negligible affinity for sigma receptors and conversely, many sigma ligands that do not apparently have any neuroleptic activity, but it remains a possibility that there could be an involvement of sigma receptors in the pathology of schizophrenia. Thus receptor autoradiographic studies of post-mortem schizophrenic brain have demonstrated a significant reduction of sigma binding sites in the frontal cortex, amygdala and hippocampus without any significant change in the density of PCP binding sites. Therefore, the evidence linking a malfunctional sigma receptor system to schizophrenia, or the use of selective sigma receptor ligands as putative neuroleptics, is inconclusive.

Sigma receptors and the immune and endocrine systems

Experimental evidence suggests that sigma receptors play an important role in regulating and integrating both immune and endocrine functions. In experimental studies, it has been shown that the selective sigma ligand N-allyl-normetazocine stimulates the hypothalamic–pituitary–adrenal axis but suppresses luteinizing hormone and prolactin secretion. A high density of sigma receptors has been identified on human leucocytes and in the rat spleen, testis, ovary and adrenal gland. In human leucocytes it has also been shown that sigma receptors are involved in the second signalling mechanisms that are essential for cellular activation. In addition, sigma receptors have been identified on human and rat T and B cells. There is experimental evidence to show that the suppression of T cell replication, and enhanced activity of monocyte phagocytosis, that occurs in some rodent models of depression, can be effectively reversed by the chronic administration of selective sigma ligands such as igmesine. This suggests that such compounds may be of benefit in correcting the diverse immune and possibly endocrine defects that characterize depression.

Clinical implications

Schizophrenia

Following the discovery that some antipsychotic drugs bind to sigma receptors, the suggestion arose that sigma receptors may be involved in schizophrenia and in the mode of action of antipsychotic drugs. Support for this hypothesis arose from the observation that the density of sigma receptors was dramatically reduced in several brain regions of post-mortem brains from schizophrenic patients. Such changes appeared to be restricted to the sigma receptor and did not involve the NMDA receptor or the PCP receptor. Whether such findings implicate alterations in sigma receptor function in schizophrenia is uncertain as it is possible that the changes in the density of these receptors is a function of the duration of treatment with neuroleptics. Support for the possible involvement of sigma receptors in schizophrenia, and in the action of antipsychotic drugs comes from the observation that haloperidol had a high affinity for these receptors in rat brain. Furthermore rimcazole, a putative neuroleptic, was found to have a high affinity for sigma receptors with little action on dopamine receptors. Several other sigma-selective ligands were also developed as possible neuroleptics. Unfortunately, despite convincing pre-clinical data showing that many of the sigma-selective ligands were active in animal models predictive of antipsychotic activity, none proved to have efficacy in clinical trials. It would therefore seem that the sigma ligands so far developed are unlikely to become the novel neuroleptics of the future.

Movement disorders

The most common symptomatic dystonias result from the administration of neuroleptics and occur as acute dystonic reactions or as tardive dyskinesia. The dystonias are disorders that involve sustained, involuntary muscle contractions and abnormal posture which interferes with normal motor function. Dystonias can be focal, as in the case of torticollis in which the neck involuntarily rotates, or they may be progressive and generalized as in torsion dystonia in which the body slowly becomes contorted. Torsian dystonia is familial and recent studies have identified a defective gene which may be responsible.

Acute dystonic reactions occurring following the administration of potent neuroleptics are reported primarily in young men and usually develop shortly after the start of therapy. By contrast, tardive dystonia occurs following chronic neuroleptic treatments; as with tardive dyskinesia, symptoms often begin after the abrupt withdrawal of the neuroleptic. Although less severe than acute dystonic reactions, tardive dystonia is frequently permanent and difficult to treat.

Until recently, the cause of dystonia has been assumed to involve a dysfunction of the basal ganglia. However, it is now known that most patients with lesions of the basal ganglia show no evidence of dystonia while those patients with dystonia exhibit little biochemical or anatomical change in basal ganglia function. More recently, there is clinical evidence that dystonia is associated with lesions of the brain stem and the cerebellum. The cerebellum is closely linked to the red nucleus which contains a high density of sigma receptors but few dopamine, serotonin or glutamate receptors. The brain stem region is also implicated in the hereditary mutant mouse model of dystonia in which the symptoms are known to be associated with both brain stem and cerebellar lesions.

The presence of sigma receptors in anatomical structures that control movement and posture provides indirect evidence for the link between sigma receptors and dystonia. Further support for the involvement of these receptors is provided by the effects induced by the direct administration of sigma ligands into the red nucleus of rats; the degree of dystonia produced is directly proportional to the affinity of the drug for the sigma receptors. Additional experimental support for the involvement of sigma receptors in idiopathic dystonias comes from studies on a strain of rats which can develop a lethal dystonia but which are free of any identifiable anatomical lesions. It would appear that the density of sigma receptors is dramatically reduced compared to their non-affected litter-mates.

Regarding neuroleptic-induced dystonias, it is well known that typical neuroleptics cause catalepsy in rats and movement disorders in man. By contrast, the atypical neuroleptics clozapine and sulpiride have a low propensity to cause movement disorders in man even though they have established antipsychotic effects. These atypical neuroleptics, unlike many of the typical neuroleptics, have a low affinity for sigma receptors which lends support to the hypothesis that the dystonias produced by typical neuroleptics are related to their affinity for sigma receptors in the brain stem–cerebellar region.

Neurodegenerative disorders

So far all the evidence implicating the neuroprotective action of sigma ligands has been based on animal models of stroke or neurodegeneration. Several sigma ligands such as igmesine (JO 1784), NPC 26377, ifenprodil and eliprodil have been shown to protect gerbils against ischaemic insult resulting from the bilateral occlusion of the carotid arteries; this is a popular experimental model of stroke. Similarly, ifenprodil and eliprodil, which have high affinity for sigma receptors in rat brain, are effective in protecting the mouse against focal cerebral ischaemia when administered after the induction of ischaemia. It would appear that the neuroprotective action is due to modulation of the polyamine site on the NMDA-glutamate receptor. However, as sigma ligands such as DTG, 3-PPP and BM4 14802 (which lack affinity for the NMDA glutamate receptor), have no neuroprotective action in the mouse model of focal cerebral ischaemia, it is uncertain whether highly selective sigma ligands would be effective in focal ischaemia in man.

In other experimental studies, the potent sigma ligand igmesine has been shown to potentiate the potassium-evoked release or acetylcholine from rat hippocampal slices *in vitro*, an effect which is blocked by haloperidol. This suggests that igmesine may act as a sigma-1 agonist and may facilitate memory formation. Further evidence for this possibility is provided by the anti-amnestic action of igmesine in scopolamine-treated rats. These experimental studies suggest that sigma ligands, particularly sigma-1 agonists, may have therapeutic potential in the treatment of stroke and possibly in facilitating memory formation in the aged brain. Only double-blind clinical trials of drugs such as igmesine, which appear to be relatively devoid of peripheral organ toxicity, will determine whether the various animal models of memory deficit and neurodegeneration are really predictive of potential therapeutic activity.

Anxiety and depression

There is experimental evidence to show that representative drugs for most classes of antidepressants have a modest affinity for sigma-1 receptors *in vitro*. Some antidepressants, such as sertraline and the monoamine oxidase-A inhibitor clorgyline, are moderately potent ligands for their receptor site. However, more recent studies have indicated that the most important final common pathway for the action of antidepressants involves the modulation of the NMDA-glutamate receptor possibly via the sigma receptor. It therefore seems uncertain that potent and selective sigma ligands will form the basis of a new group of antidepressants. However, there is more convincing experimental evidence to suggest that sigma ligands could have anxiolytic or anti-stress activity. Thus igmesine and DTG have been shown to block environmentally induced stress or corticotropin-releasing factor induced colonic activity in the rat. Other experimental studies have shown that selective sigma ligands such as Lu 28-178 are potent anxiolytics in rodent models of anxiety.

The future of sigma receptor ligands

Besides the obvious need to develop highly potent and selective drugs for the sigma-1 and sigma-2 receptor sites, the precise structures of the sigma receptors is required in order to establish firmly their identity. The presence of sigma receptors in the brain, in the gastrointestinal tract and endocrine and immune systems suggests that there must be endogenous factors that act as agonists and antagonists for these receptors. To date the nature of these endogenous factors is unknown but there is experimental evidence to implicate some neuropeptides (such as neuropeptides-Y and PYY) and steroids such as progesterone and deoxycorticosterone as putative ligands.

In addition to the need for more detailed experimental studies to characterize the cellular mechanism of action of the different types of sigma receptors it is also essential to broaden the clinical profile of these drugs. So far, attention has been almost exclusively directed at the action of relatively non-selective sigma ligands in the treatment of psychotic disorders. The experimental findings that sigma compounds may have putative neuroprotective and anxiolytic/anti-stress effects will hopefully encourage the further development of the highly selective sigma compounds for their therapeutic application.

Appendix 1: Some Important Psychotropic Drug Interactions

Antidepressants and lithium			
	Interact with	Results of interaction	Possible mechanism
Tricyclic antidepressants	1. Directly acting sympathomimetics	Hypertension arrhythmias	Inhibition of neuronal uptake
	2. Guanethidine; clonidine	Decreased anti-hypertensive effect	Inhibition of neuronal uptake
Non-specific monoamine oxidase inhibitors	1. Tyramine-containing foods	Hypertensive crisis	Catecholamine release increased
	2. Sympathomimetic amines	Hypertensive crisis	Increased synthesis of noradrenaline and decreased metabolism
	3. Pethidine	Severe excitation, hypertension, coma, pyrexia, death	? 5-HT syndrome
Lithium	1. Tetracyclines	Lithium intoxication	Enhanced lithium absorption and impaired excretion?
	2. Succinylcholine (hexamethonium)	Prolonged muscle paralysis	Synergism at neuro-muscular junction
	3. Carbamazepine	Enhanced lithium effect	? Synergism
	4. Methyldopa, indomethacin	Enhanced lithium toxicity	Uncertain; may be due to increased tubular resorption of lithium

Sedative hypnotics and anxiolytics

	Interact with	Results of interaction	Possible mechanism
Alcohol and barbiturates	1. CNS depressants	CNS depression	Synergism
	2. Diphenylhydantoin (phenytoin)	(a) Decreased anticonvulsant effect	Liver enzyme induction
		(b) Enhanced diphenylhydantoin toxicity on stopping barbiturates	Return of liver enzyme oxidation to normal
	3. Oral anticoagulants	Decreased anticoagulant effect	Liver enzyme induction
Chloral hydrate	Oral anticoagulants	Enhanced anticoagulant effect	Metabolite of chloral hydrate displaces anti-coagulant from plasma proteins
Diphenylhydantoin (phenytoin)	Oral anticoagulants	(a) Enhanced diphenylhydantoin toxicity	Decreased diphenylhydantoin metabolism
		(b) Decreased anticoagulant effect	Diphenylhydantoin stimulates anti-coagulant metabolism
Benzodiazepines	Cimetidine	Enhanced benzodiazepine effect	Inhibition of benzodiazepine metabolism
Chlorazepate and prazepam	Antacids	Decreased benzodiazepine effect	Impaired absorption

Neuroleptics

	Interact with	Results of interaction	Possible mechanism
All neuroleptics	L-Dopa	Decreased L-dopa effect	Dopamine receptor blockade
Phenothiazines	1. Antacids	Decreased effects phenothiazines	Decreased absorption
	2. Vasodilators	Hypertension	Peripheral vasodilatation
	3. Antihypertensives	Hypertension	Peripheral vasodilatation
Chlorpromazine	Guanethidine; clonidine	Decreased antihypertensive effect	Chlorpromazine inhibits drug uptake into neurons
Haloperidol	Methyldopa	Dementia	Dopamine receptor blockade and decreased catecholamine synthesis

Appendix 2: Glossary of some Common Terms used in Psychopharmacology

This glossary should be used in conjunction with the Index.

Abuse liability　Capacity of a drug to produce physiological or psychological dependence and alter the behaviour in a manner detrimental to the individual.

Acetylator status　Refers to ability to acetylate organic compounds in the liver. A rapid acetylator refers to an individual whose N-acetyl transferase is hyperactive. Such individuals are more likely to require larger doses of drugs such as phenelzine. Conversely, slow acetylators have a genetically linked deficit in N-acetyl transferase and therefore require a lower dose of the drug.

Action potential　Wave of electrical impulses that travel down an axon to initiate the release of a neurotransmitter.

Addiction　State in which the individual is dependent on a drug of abuse. Term now replaced by *dependence*.

Adenylate cyclase　The intracellular enzyme associated with some types of receptor that on activation produces the secondary messenger cyclic adenosine monophosphate (cyclic AMP).

Affect　Mood or emotional state.

Affective disorder　Mental illness where the predominant abnormality is a disturbance of affect. Such disorders include depression and mania.

Affinity　The potency of a ligand to bind to a receptor or active site on an enzyme. This may be quantified by the affinity constant (K_m or B_{max}).

Age-associated memory　Disorder alleged to occur in those over 60 years of age in the absence of clinical evidence of dementia.

Agnosia　Loss of the ability to recognize sensory stimuli.

Agonist　A compound that acts on a receptor to produce similar effects to the natural ligand.

Agonist, partial　Drug that acts as an agonist at a low concentration but which, at higher concentrations, blocks the receptor thereby acting as an antagonist.

Agoraphobia　A phobia characterized by the need to avoid being trapped, usually in a public place.

353

Agranulocytosis   Usually an iatrogenic state in which the white blood cell count is less than 2000/cu.mm and the leucocyte count is less than 500/cu.mm.

Akathisia   Term used to describe a patient's restlessness and inability to sit still. Shortly after the introduction of neuroleptics, akathisia was recognized as one of the most common and distressing side effects. Propranolol is often useful in treating such symptoms.

Akinesia   Movement disorder characterized by reduction or loss of ability to initiate voluntary muscle movements. Often associated with side effects of neuroleptics: mask-like facial expression, absent arm swing, low voice.

Alcoholic dementia   An organic brain syndrome associated with prolonged, heavy ingestion of alcohol characterized by impairment of short- and long-term memory, abstract thinking and judgement.

Alkaloid   Complex nitrogen containing organic base of plant origin (e.g. morphine).

Alkyl group   A radical derived from an open chain hydrocarbon. Often referred to as an aliphatic group (e.g. a methyl or ethyl group).

Allele (allelomorph)   Alternative form of a gene found in the corresponding loci on homologous chromosomes, that determines alternative characteristics in inheritance.

Alpha electroencephalogram EEG that shows 8–13 Hz waves (alpha waves) in all recording leads from a resting subject with closed eyes.

Amnesia   Loss of memory, inability to recall past experience. *Anterograde* amnesia refers to an inability to recall events after a drug (e.g. a benzodiazepine or ECT). *Retrograde* amnesia refers to the loss of memory occurring prior to the incident that causes amnesia.

Anhedonia   Inability to derive pleasure from situations that usually induce pleasure. This is a characteristic feature of major depressive disorder.

Anorgasmia   Failure to achieve orgasm. Usually psychological or interpersonal but can be iatrogenic due to antidepressants (particularly selective serotonin reuptake inhibitors), neuroleptics or benzodiazepines.

Antagonist   A compound that blocks a receptor thereby preventing an agonist from eliciting a physiological response. An antagonist should have no biological activity of its own.

Antinociceptive   Having the action of reducing or abolishing a painful stimulus (e.g. an analgesic).

APUD cell   Amine precursor, uptake and decarboxylation cell from which the platelet is derived.

Arteriosclerosis   The thickening, hardening and loss of elasticity of arteries.

Aryl	Chemical group that is derived from, or related to, an aromatic hydrocarbon (e.g. a benzene-like molecule).
Ataxia	Loss of muscle co-ordination.
Autopsy	Post-mortem.
Autoreceptor	A receptor situated on the presynaptic nerve ending which responds to the transmitter released from the same nerve ending. Also termed a presynaptic receptor.
Autosome	Chromosome not determinant of sexual differentiation.
Aversive conditioning	Behavioural method whereby a sensory stimulus is paired with a painful, distasteful or unpleasant reinforcement. In behavioural therapy this method is used to produce an association between a negative experience and undesirable behaviour.
Axon	Part of the neuron consisting of a single fibre down which the action potential is transmitted to the nerve terminal.
Basal ganglia	A collection of nuclei in the brain concerned primarily with the initiation and control of movement consisting of the corpus striatum (globus pallidus and the putamen) and the substantia nigra.
Behavioural toxicity	Impairment of psychomotor and cognitive abilities by psychotropic drugs.
Binding site	Domain on receptor surface that has a characteristic arrangement of functional groups that recognize and bind specific ligands. Also sometimes called a recognition site.
Bipolar	Affective illness characterized by mood swings between mania and depression.
Blood dyscrasia	Abnormality ranging from a reduction in the white blood cells (leucopenia, agranulocytosis) to haemolytic anaemia.
Bradykinesia	Extrapyramidal disorder characterized by reduction in velocity of normal movements, paucity of movements and inability to initiate normal movements. Cardinal sign of Parkinson's disease.
Brain stimulation reward	Experimental procedure whereby an animal learns to receive brief, low intensity electrical stimuli to subcortical regions of the brain that elicit a reward.
Bulimia	Eating disorder that may be either a symptom or a syndrome. Manifested by insatiable hunger resulting in compulsive binge eating.
Carcinoid syndrome	Disease in which symptoms are due to a 5-hydroxytryptamine secreting tumour, usually located in the gastrointestinal tract.
Catalepsy	A state of rigidity with either resistance to alteration or ready adoption of a newly imposed posture.
Catatonia	A clinical symptom which is associated either with a marked reduction or increase in mobility or alternation between the two states. This term may also be used to describe automatism or stereotyped movements.

Catechol	A 1,2-dihydrobenzene structure, exemplified by the catecholamine transmitters noradrenaline and dopamine.
CD4 cell	T helper (Th) lymphocyte, a subset of lymphocytes identified by their differential function and specific cell surface markers.
cDNA library	Clones containing a single independent DNA molecule.
Cerebral insufficiency	State in the elderly characterized by difficulties in concentration and memory.
Cerebrospinal fluid (CSF)	Physiological fluid that bathes the brain and spinal cord and may be monitored by removing the fluid from the lumbar region of the spinal cord or occasionally from the lateral ventricles.
C-fos	Immediate early gene that serves as a transcription factor for the expression of other genes.
Chelating agent	Compound that sequesters a metallic ion, thereby inactivating it (e.g. EDTA).
Chorea	Repetitive involuntary jerky movements.
Chronic fatigue syndrome (CFS)	Symptom complex of extreme fatigue in combination with signs of an impaired immune and endocrine state. Frequently occurs after an acute, viral infection.
Circling	Behaviour initiated in animals by dopamine agonists following a unilateral lesion of the nigrostriatal pathway.
Classical benzodiazepines	1,4-Benzodiazepines that are structurally related to diazepam and that have qualitatively similar pharmacological profiles (e.g anxiolytic, anticonvulsant, muscle relaxant and sedative).
Clearance	The rate of elimination of a drug from the body.
Cofactor	A compound or ion that, while not being directly involved in a chemical reaction, facilitates an enzyme-catalysed reaction.
Comorbidity	Occurrence of more than one disease at the same time in the same patient (e.g. anxiety and depression).
Compartments	Areas of the body in which a drug or neurotransmitter have different kinetic characteristics.
Competitive inhibition	Inhibition of an enzyme or receptor that is dependent on the relative concentration of the inhibitor, substrate or agonist.
Corpus striatum	Part of the basal ganglia containing the caudate nucleus and the putamen.
Cytochromes	Part of the family of hepatic microsomal drug metabolizing enzymes. Two izozymes (P450 2D6 and 3A4) responsible for biotransformation of 90% of drugs used clinically.
Delirium	Transient organic mental syndrome characterized by global impairment of cognition, including memory and perception.
Delirium tremens (DTs)	Acute, sometimes lethal, brain disorder precipitated by total or partial withdrawal from excessive alcohol

	intake. Shown by confusion, disorientation, fluctuating or clouded consciousness, agitation and insomnia.
Delusion	A belief held without any supportive evidence.
Dementia	An acquired global impairment of intellect, memory and personality but without global impairment of consciousness.
Depersonalization	Subjective experience that the body is unreal.
Depolarization	The inside of a nerve cell becoming less negatively charged relative to the outside of the nerve membrane.
Desensitization	Reduction in the sensitivity of a receptor in response to excessive stimulation. Also termed *down regulation*. Such changes may be associated with a decrease in the number of receptors and/or their functional responsiveness. Desensitization is also a term used to describe the reduction in anxiety and panic states caused by controlled exposure to a specific anxiety-provoking stimulus.
Diencephalon	Anterior region of the brain that includes the thalamus, hypothalamus and pituitary gland.
Dissociation constant	Term used to describe quantitatively the separation of a ligand from a receptor. In ligand binding studies it may be expressed as the reciprocal of the affinity constant.
Dizygotic	In genetic studies this refers to twins who have developed from two ova and therefore have different genetic characteristics.
Down regulation	Reduction in response following the exposure of a receptor to a higher than normal concentration of an agonist.
Drug abuse	Use of any drug in a manner which is at variance with the approved use in that culture.
Drug dependence	Syndrome in which an individual continues to take a drug for its pleasurable effect despite the adverse medical and social consequences. The individual then continues to take the drug for his or her well-being.
Dyskinesia	Impairment of voluntary movements.
Dysphasia	Impairment of language.
Dysphoria	Acute, transient changes in mood (e.g. feelings of sadness, sorrow, anguish).
Dyspraxia	Impairment of ability to perform co-ordinated movement.
Dystonia	Neurological condition characterized by slow, tonic sustained muscle contractions often of the tongue, jaw, eyes, neck and occasionally the whole body.
Electrolytic lesion	Destruction of a specific nerve pathway by the passage of a current between electrodes inserted into the brain region which is innervated by the nerve pathway.
Enteroviruses	Small ribonucleic acid (RNA) containing viruses. For example, polio viruses, which destroy the anterior

horn cells leading to lower motor neuron paralysis, are of this type.

Enzyme induction Increase in enzyme activity in response to an increase in the amount of substrate available. For example, barbiturates increase the activity of the hepatic microsomal enzyme system following their repeated administration.

Eosinophilia myalgia syndrome (EMS) Toxic, potentially fatal disorder attributed to a contaminant of tryptophan.

Evoked potential (EP) Electrophysiological measurement in which a sensory (flight flash, tone) or cognitive signal stimulates a response that is detected from the scalp or cortex.

Exon Part of a gene that encodes information present in messenger RNA.

Extrapyramidal Motor control that does not involve the pyramidal tracts. It originates in the basal ganglia.

Extrapyramidal system Polysynaptic neuronal pathways involving the basal ganglia and related subcortical nuclei that influence motor behaviour.

Fatal toxicity index Number of deaths due to poisoning per million National Health Service prescriptions.

Fatigue The patient tires abnormally early during prolonged mental or physical activity or cannot sustain the same level of activity as normal.

Fetal alcohol syndrome Specific, recognizable pattern of malformation (brain, skull, heart) in offspring of alcoholic mothers.

Flashback Spontaneous occurrence of previously experienced drug effects (e.g. hallucinations, delusions, depersonalization) or distressing emotions originally associated with trauma. Generally associated with LSD-like drugs and occasionally cannabis.

Flight of ideas Rapid succession of thoughts without logical connections.

Gas chromatography Method whereby volatile compounds are separated by injecting them into a stream of inert gas which percolates over a solid or liquid stationary phase. The separated compounds are then detected and quantified by means of an electrochemical or fluorescent probe. GC-MS is a method whereby the gas chromatograph is linked to a mass spectrograph, thereby allowing very small quantities of the compound to be quantified.

Glia Supporting cells within the brain that act as a physical and metabolic buffer around nerve cells.

G proteins Family of proteins within neurons that link receptors to ion channels or secondary messengers.

Grand mal Major seizure disorder characterized by tonic and clonic muscular movements and loss of consciousness.

Guanylate cyclase The intracellular enzyme associated with some types of receptor that on activation produces the secondary

	messenger cyclic guanylate monophosphate (cyclic GMP).
Guillain–Barré syndrome	Acute idiopathic polyneuritis characterized by muscular weakness and paraesthesia.
Half-life	The time taken for the concentration of a compound in a tissue to decrease by 50%.
Hallucinations	Sensory perception that is not based on a real stimulus.
Hepatic encephalopathy	A progressive metabolic liver disorder that results in altered intellectual function and emotion.
5-HIAA	5-Hydroxyindoleacetic acid, the main metabolite of 5-hydroxytryptamine (serotonin) formed by monoamine oxidase.
High performance liquid chromatography (HPLC)	Form of chromatography in which mobile solvent passes through a column packed with a non-polar solid phase. The organic molecules are then detected fluorimetrically or electrochemically. Commonly used to determine trace concentrations of biogenic amines.
Hippocampus	Region of the temporal lobe that is thought to play a role in learning and memory.
HVA	Homovanillic acid, one of the main metabolites of dopamine formed by the actions of monoamine oxidase and catechol-O-methyltransferase.
Hyperbaric	Raised pressure.
Hyperkinetic	Increased movements or activity.
Hypertension	Raised blood pressure.
Hypnotic	Sleep inducing.
Hypochondriasis	Over-concern about health.
Hypofrontality	Hypofunction of prefrontal cortex as shown by positron emission tomography imaging or cerebral blood flow determinations. Hypofrontality occurs in both medicated and unmedicated schizophrenics.
Hypophysis	The pituitary gland. Hypophysectomy is removal of the pituitary gland.
Hypotension	Lowered blood pressure.
Hypothalamus	Region at the base of the brain concerned with the regulation of autonomic activity and some aspects of behaviour.
Hypothermia	Low body temperature.
Ideas of reference	Ideas that normal events have specific reference to the individual or are commenting on the individual.
Idiosynaptic drug reaction	Unpredictable side effects of a drug, including hypersensitivity reactions, that usually develop suddenly. Such reactions are often genetically determined and not related to the pharmacological properties of the drug.
Immunofluorescence	Fluorescence histochemistry using antibodies to identify the compounds under investigation.
Indoles	Compounds with a 2,3-benzpyrrole structure. The indoleamines, e.g. 5-hydroxytryptamine, are compounds containing the indole structure.

Infarct	An area of dead tissue caused by a reduced blood supply.
Intrinsic activity	The inherent ability of a ligand to elicit a biological response once it is bound to a receptor.
Inverse agonist	A substance that produces effects at a receptor that are the opposite to those produced by the usual agonist. Thus the inverse agonists at benzodiazepine receptors have anxiogenic, proconvulsant and promnestic properties.
Ion channel	Pore on the nerve membrane through which sodium potassium and other metal and non-metal ions (e.g. chloride) pass to produce changes in the electrical activity of the nerve membrane. These channels are controlled by receptors located in the nerve membrane.
Iontophoresis	Administration of compounds through micropipettes which are released by an electric current.
Isomerism	The existence of a molecule that possesses two or more structural forms. *Stereo-isomerism* refers to the existence of two or more compounds possessing the same molecular and structural formulae but having different spatial configurations.
Kindling	Consequences of repeated subthreshold electrical or chemical stimuli that progressively increase convulsive or behavioural responses, eventually resulting in a seizure. Subsequent application of a single subthreshold stimulus will also evoke a seizure.
Korsakoff's psychosis	An organic brain syndrome associated with prolonged, heavy ingestion of alcohol. It is characterized by amnesia for recent events and an inability to memorize new information.
Learned helplessness	Behavioural phenomenon consisting of passivity and withdrawal after exposure to an uncontrollable adverse event.
LD_{50}; ED_{50}	Dose of a compound which is lethal (LD_{50}) or effective (ED_{50}) in 50% of the test population.
Life events	Experiences which are part of normal life but which are stressful and thought to trigger a psychiatric disorder in a vulnerable individual.
Lifetime prevalence	Number of individuals who may have a disease any time during their lifetime.
Ligand	Compound which specifically binds to a receptor.
Ligase chain reaction (LCR)	Recently developed amplification method used to detect a gene mutation. The method uses the coupling of two adjacent synthetic oligonucleotides aligned on the template of the target deoxyribonucleic acid (DNA).
Limbic system	Area of the brain associated with small, involuntary functions, emotions and behaviour. Comprises the hypothalamus, parahippocampus, olfactory lobe, dentate gyrus, amygdala, anterior thalamus, fornix and stria terminalis.

Linkage analysis	Analysis of genetic markers linked to genes (e.g. genetic traits or phenotype markers such as enzyme deficiencies occurring in patients with mood disorders).
Liver enzyme induction	Increased liver enzyme activity due to chronic use of drugs such as barbiturates.
Lumbar puncture	The sampling of cerebrospinal fluid by insertion of a needle through the lumbar region of the spine into the space surrounding the spinal cord.
Malignant hyperthermia	Rare, familial hyperthermia (41 °C) associated with inhalation anaesthetics, muscle relaxants, tricyclic antidepressants, phenothiazine neuroleptics (particularly chlorpromazine) monoamine oxidase inhibitors and haloperidol.
Mass fragmentography	Quantitative analysis of compounds by measurement of specific fragments using mass spectrometry.
Mass spectrometry	Analysis of the chemical structure of a compound by measurement of the molecular weight of fragments formed by bombardment of the molecule by ions.
Medulla oblongata	Area of the brain lying below the pons.
Mesencephalon	Area of the brain also called the midbrain, which contains the tegmentum and the substantia nigra.
Mesocortical system	Part of the dopaminergic system with the cell bodies mainly in the ventral tegmental area which project to the prefrontal cortex, accumbens, septum and olfactory tubercles.
Mesolimbic system	Area of the brain containing the nucleus accumbens, olfactory tubercle and projections to the cortex.
MHPG	3-Methyoxy-4-hydroxyphenylglycol, the main brain metabolite or noradrenaline formed by the actions of monoamine oxidase and catechol-O-methyltransferase.
Microsomal ethanol oxidizing system	An enzyme complex in the liver that metabolizes alcohols and other compounds.
Microsomes	Subcellular particles occurring in most types of cell and involved in the metabolism of drugs as well as natural substances.
Migraine	A syndrome thought to involve 5-HT characterized by localized headache and often accompanied by nausea, vomiting and sensory disturbances.
Mitochondria	Rod-shaped subcellular particles involved in energy production (e.g. ATP) and metabolism.
Monoamine	General name for catecholamine and indoleamine neurotransmitters.
Monozygotic	In genetic studies this refers to twins who are derived from a single ovum and therefore have identical genetic characteristics.
Narcolepsy	Rare, disabling sleep disorder of unknown origin. Characterized by sudden attacks of flaccid paralysis

(cataplexy), extensive daytime sleepiness, sleep paralysis, hypnagogic hallucinations and rapid onset of rapid eye movement (REM) phase of sleep.

Natural killer cell (NKC) Any class of white blood cells that can spontaneously recognize and kill tumour or virus infected cells without previous exposure to an antigen. NKC cytotoxicity decreased in depression and in alcoholism.

Neuritic plaques Found in high density throughout the hippocampus and neocortex of patients with Alzheimer's disease. Density of plaques correlated with degree of cognitive impairment.

Neuroendocrine challenge test Any of a variety of tests used to examine the functional integrity of the monoamine pathways that control the secretion of pituitary hormones.

Neuromodulator A substance that modifies the function or effects of a neurotransmitter, e.g. peptides.

Neurons A nerve cell.

Neuroregulator A compound that has not been shown to fulfil the criteria of a neurotransmitter.

Neurosis Behaviour showing undue adherence to an unrealistic idea of things and showing an inability to take a rationally objective view of life.

Neurotransmitter A chemical messenger released by a neuron to excite or inhibit adjacent neurons.

Nigrostriatal pathway The neural projection from cell bodies in the substantia nigra to the striatum.

NMDA N-Methyl-D-aspartate, a synthetic amino acid that activates a subclass of excitatory amino acid (glutamate) receptors.

Novel anxiolytics Drugs chemically unrelated by diazepam that produce their anxiolytic effects by facilitating inhibitory transmission through mechanisms other than the GABA-benzodiazepine receptor complex (e.g. buspirone).

Nuclear schizophrenia The core symptoms of schizophrenia rather than the associated or social factors.

Obsessive–compulsive disorder (OCD) State characterized by recurrent, intrusive thoughts and compulsive stereotyped, repetitive behaviour or cognitions.

Oedema Swelling due to the presence of excess fluid in the intercellular spaces of the body.

Oligonucleotide Short (less than 30 nucleotides) piece of DNA.

Oncogene Gene involved in development and differentiation that causes cancer when mutated.

"On-off" phenomenon Occurs in patients with Parkinson's disease. The "on" phase (choreoathetotic dyskinesia) occurs at peak dose effect. In the "off" phase (akinesia), patients suddenly "freeze".

Palpitations	An unduly rapid heart beat which is noticed by the subject.
Panic attack	Sudden attack of fear or anxiety associated with one or more of 12 autonomic symptoms (e.g. shortness of breath, dizziness, palpitations, sweating).
Paper chromatography	Separation of a mixture of compounds on filter paper according to their relative solubility in organic solvents that diffuse through the paper by capillary action.
Paranoia	The occurrence of delusions that are frequently of a persecutory nature.
Particulate fraction	Usually applied to a fraction of a tissue homogenate which contains subcellular particles.
Passivity	A feeling of being under the control or will of an outside agency.
Penetrance	Genetic term referring to the degree to which an inherited characteristic is expressed.
Phobia	A persistent and unreasonable fear of some situation or object.
Phosphatidylinositol system (PI system)	G protein linked secondary messenger system which, by controlling the concentration of intracellular calcium, modulates the actions of some transmitters. The action of lithium may be mediated via the PI system.
Phospholipid	A phosphorus-containing lipid that comprises about 50% of the cell membrane.
Physical dependence	Phenomenon in which abnormal behavioural and autonomic symptoms occur following the abrupt withdrawal of a drug of dependence or when the effect of the drug is terminated by means of a specific antagonist.
Plasma	Blood from which the cells have been removed but without the blood being allowed to clot.
Platelet	Small blood constituents formed from APUD cells which are involved in blood clotting. Platelets are also called *thrombocytes*.
Polydipsia	Excessive drinking.
Polymerase chain reaction (PCR)	Technique using enzymes and specific primers to generate multiple copies of the original (usually viral) nucleic acid, thereby increasing its numbers so that it may more easily be detected.
Polymorphism	Occurrence of two or more gene structures in the same population.
Polypeptide	Protein-like molecule consisting of a chain of amino acids.
Polyuria	Voiding of excessive amounts of urine.
Pons	Area of the hindbrain under the cerebellum.
Postsynaptic	Part of the membrane lying adjacent to the nerve terminal that contains the postsynaptic receptors.
Post-traumatic stress	Anxiety disorder attributed to a severe, adverse life experience (e.g. threat to life) that is experienced again without the stimulus of the adverse experience.

Precursor	Usually used in reference to compounds which are metabolized in neurotransmitters (e.g. tryptophan is the precursor of 5-hydroxytryptamine).
Presynaptic	Events or structures occurring proximal to the synapse.
Protein kinases	A group of enzymes that transfer charged phosphate groups on proteins, thereby regulating intracellular processes in response to extracellular signals (see *PI system*).
Psychological dependence	Dysphoria and craving which arise following the abrupt withdrawal of a drug of abuse.
Psychosis	A psychiatric condition in which contact with reality and insight are lost.
Psychotropic drug	A drug acting on the brain to cause a change in mood or behaviour.
Purinergic	Neurons in the brain and heart that secrete purine neurotransmitters such as adenosine.
Putamen	Area of the brain within the corpus striatum.
Radioimmunoassay	Assay technique in which an antibody against a specific compound is used to measure the concentration of that compound.
Radiolabelled compound	Compound synthesized to contain one or more radioactive atoms (usually ^3H or ^{14}C).
Rapid eye movement (REM) sleep	Stage of sleep associated with high frequency, low voltage waves on the electroencephalogram. It is linked with dreaming, rapid movement of the eyes and pronounced changes in blood pressure and respiration.
Receptor	A protein-containing site in the neuronal cell wall to which a natural or synthetic ligand may bind to produce a physiological or pharmacological effect.
Reinforcement	The process by which a specific stimulus appears to increase the probability that a particular behaviour will occur.
Restriction enzyme	Enzyme that recognizes short stretches (4–8 base pairs) in a sequence-specific manner and cleaves the DNA at specific points.
Restriction fragment length polymorphism (RFLP)	Genetic tool from the direct analysis of the human genome to detect new genes that predispose to genetic disease.
Seasonal affective disorder (SAD)	Seasonal subtype of major depressive disorder characterized by an annual pattern of symptoms (e.g. depression occurring in the autumn or spring).
Secondary messenger	A molecule such as cyclic AMP, cyclic GMP or phosphatidylinositol that regulates intracellular processes in response to an extracellular signal.
Seizure	Uncontrolled or paroxysmal brain activity that is usually expressed through the motor system.
Selective 5-HT reuptake inhibitors	Antidepressants such as fluoxetine and fluvoxamine that show specificity in inhibiting the uptake of 5-hydroxytryptamine into platelets or brain tissue *in vitro* and *in vivo*.

Stereotaxic surgery	A method for accurately placing lesions in the brain by electrocoagulation, selective neurotoxins or radioactive pellets.
Stereotypy	The persistent repetition of body movements.
Subsensitivity	The decreased response of a receptor to a fixed concentration of an agonist, shown as a shift in the dose–response curve to the right. In behaviour, subsensitivity represents a decreased response to a fixed dose of a drug. *Supersensitivity* is the opposite of subsensitivity and the dose–response curve is shifted to the left.
Synapse	The gap separating adjacent neurons.
Synaptosomes	The pinched off and resealed nerve endings formed following the homogenization and high speed centrifugation of brain tissue in an isotonic medium.
Suprachiasmatic nucleus (SCN)	Collection of cells in the anterior hypothalamus acting as a biological clock or oscillator that maintains the circadian rhythm of the sleep–wake cycle.
Tachycardia	Rapid heart beat.
Tardive dyskinesia (TD)	Potentially irreversible, late onset, extra pyramidal hyperkinetic movement disorder often associated with the long-term administration of neuroleptics. Abnormal movements generally involve the mouth, lips and tongue.
Therapeutic index	The ratio between the dose of a drug needed to produce a therapeutic effect (assumed to be unity) and the toxic dose.
Tolerance	Reduced effect of an agonist or antagonist following its prolonged administration resulting from the increased metabolism (called *metabolic tolerance*) or decreased receptor sensitivity (termed *pharmaco-* or *tissue tolerance*).
Tuberoinfundibular system	The system connecting the hypothalamus with the pituitary gland.
Up-regulation	An increase in the number and/or sensitivity of receptors to compensate for the decreased effect of an agonist.
Vasoconstriction	Reduction in the diameter of blood vessels by contraction of the circular muscles in the vessel wall.
Ventral tegmental area (VTA)	Area of the midbrain dorsal to the substantia nigra.
Ventricles	Cavities within the brain containing the CSF.
Voltage-sensitive calcium channels	Ion channels for calcium uptake whose regulation is controlled by nerve impulses.
Volume of distribution	The apparent volume of the body in which a drug would be distributed if it was present throughout the body at the same concentration as that occurring in plasma.

Appendix 3: Generic and Proprietary Names of Some Common Psychotropic Drugs

This list of drugs is not intended to be entirely comprehensive and in most cases only the most frequently used proprietary names are given. For detailed coverage of the area the reader is referred to a local pharmacopoeia.

Approved name	European trade name	USA trade name
Acetazolamide	Diamox	Diamox
Alprazolam	Xanax	Xanax
Amantadine	Symmetrel	Symmetrel
Amitriptyline	Tryptizol; Lentizol	Elaril; Endep
Amoxapine	Asendin	Asendin
Amphetamine	Benzedrine	Benzedrine
Antipyrine (phenazone)	—	Auralgan
Baclofen	Lioresal	Lioresal
Benperidol	Anquil; Frenactil; Concilium	—
Benserazide	Madopar (with L-dopa)	Madopar (with L-dopa)
Benzhexol	Artane	Artane
Benztropine	Cogentin	Cogentin
Biperiden	Akineton	Akineton
Bromazepam	Lexotan	—
Bromocriptine	Parlodel	Parlodel
Brotizolam	Ladormin; Lendorm	—
Buprenorphine	Temgesic	—
Bupropion	Wellbutrin	Wellbutrin
Buspirone	Buspar	Buspar
Butorphanol	Torbutrol; Torate; Torbutesic	—
Captopril	Capoten; Capozide; Acepril	Capoten; Capozide
Carbamazepine	Tegretol	Tegretol
Carbidopa	Sinemet (with L-dopa)	Sinemet (with L-dopa)
Chlordiazepoxide	Librium	Librium; Limbitrol
Chlormethiazole	Heminevrin	—
Chlorpromazine	Largactil	Thorazine
Clobazam	Frisium	—
Clomipramine	Anafranil	—

Approved name	European trade name	USA trade name
Clonazepam	Rivotril	Klonopin
Clonidine	Catapres; Dixarit	Catapres; Dixarit
Clopenthixol	Clopixol	—
Clorazepate	Tranxene	Tranxene
Clozapine	Leponex; Lepotex; Clozaril	Leponex; Lepotex; Clozaril
Co-dergocrine	Hydergine	Hydergine
Debrisoquine	Declinax	—
Desipramine	Pertofran	Pertofran; Norpramin
Dexamphetamine	Dexedrine	Dexedrine; Desoxyn
Diazepam	Valium	Valium
Diethylpropion	Tenuate	Tenuate; Tepanil
Digoxin	Lanoxin	Lanoxin
Dihydrocodeine	DF 118; DHC Continus	—
Diphenylhydantoin – *see* Phenytoin		
Disulfiram	Antabuse	Antabuse
L-Dopa (levodopa)	Larodopa	Larodopa
Ethchlorvynol	Avinol; Serenesil; Normoson	Placidyl
Ethosuximide	Zarontin; Emeside	Zarontin
Ethytoin (ethotoin)	—	Peganone
Fenfluramine	Ponderax	Pondimin
Fentanyl	Thalamonal; Sublimaze	Innovar; Sublimaze
Flunitrazepam	Rohypnol	Rohypnol
Fluoxetine	Prozac	Prozac
Flupenthixol	Depixol; Fluanxol	—
Fluphenazine	Modecate	Prolixin; Permitil
Flurazepam	Dalmane	Dalmane
Fluvoxamine	Faverin	—
Haloperidol	Serenace; Haldol	Haldol
Heroin (diacetylmorphine)	Diamorphine	Diamorphine
Hydrocodone	—	Codinal; Codan
Imipramine	Tofranil	Tofranil
Iproniazid	Marsilid	Marsilid
Isocarboxazid	Marplan	Marplan
Ketamine	Ketalar	Ketalar
Ketanserin	Serefrex; Sufrexal	—
Levallorphan	Naloxiphan; Naloxifan	—
Levorphanol	Dromoran	Levo-Dromoran
Lithium	Priadel; Phasal; Camcolit	Lithonate; Lithane; Eskalith
Lofepramine	Gamanil	—
Loprazolam	Dormonoct	—
Lorazepam	Ativan	Ativan
Lormetazepam	Loramet	Noctamid
Loxapine	Cloxazepam; Oxilapine	Loxitane

Approved name	European trade name	USA trade name
Maprotiline	Ludiomil	—
Medazolam	Nobrium	—
Melperone	Buronil; Eunerpan	—
Meprobamate	Miltown; Equanil	Miltown; Equanil
Mesoridazine	Lidanar; Lidanil	Serentil
Methadone	Physeptone	Dolophrine
Methylphenidate	Ritalin	Ritalin
Mianserin	Tolvon; Bolvidon	—
Molindone	Lidone; Moban	—
Morphine	Duromorph; MST-Continus	Duromorph; Roxanol
Nabilone	Cesamet	Cesamet
Nalorphine	Allorphine; Anarcon	—
Naloxone	Narcan	Narcan
Nitrazepam	Mogadon	Mogadon
Nomifensine	Merital	Merital
Nortriptyline	Aventyl	Aventyl
Oxazepam	Serenid	Serax
Pargyline	Eutonyl	—
Paroxetine	Seroxat	—
Pemoline	Volital	Cylert
Penfluridol	Flupidol; Oraleptin	—
Pentazocine	Fortral; Fortagesic	Talwin; Talacem
Pentobarbitone	Nembutal	Nembutal
Pergolide	—	Permax
Perphenazine	Fentazin	—
Pethidine (meperidine in USA)	Pethilorfan (with levallorphan); Pamergan	Demerol
Phenazocine	Narphen	—
Phenelzine	Nardil	Nardil
Phenmetrazine	—	Adipost; Bontril
Phenobarbitone	Luminal	Luminal
Phentermine	Ionamine; Duromine	—
Phenytoin	Dilantin	Dilantin
Physostigmine	Eserine	Antilirium
Pimozide	Orap	Orap
Piribedil	Trivastal	—
Primidone	Mysoline	Mysoline
Prochlorperazine	Stemetil	Compazine
Promazine	Sparine	Sparine
Propranolol	Inderal	Inderal
Reserpine	Serpasil	Serpasil
Sertraline	Lustral	—
Sodium valproate (valproic acid)	Epilim	Depakene
Spiroperidol (spiperone)	Spiropitan	—

Approved name	European trade name	USA trade name
Sulpiride	Dogmatil; Sulpital	—
Sulthiame	Ospolat; Elisal; Trolone	—
Tacrine (THA)	Cognex	Cognex
Temazepam	Euhypnos; Normison	Levanxol; Cerepax
Thioridazine	Melleril	Melleril
Tranylcypromine	Parnate	Parnate
Trazodone	Molipaxin	Desyrel
Triazolam	Halcion	Halcion
Triclofos	Tricloryl	—
Trifluoperazine	Stelazine	Stelazine
Trimethadione (troxidone)	Tridione	Tridione
Trimipramine	Surmontil	—
Verapamil	Cordilox; Securon; Univer	Calan; Isoptin
Viloxazine	Vivalan	—
Yohimbine	Aphrodine; Corynine	Actibine; Aphrodyne
Zimelidine	Zelmid; Zelmidine	—
Zopiclone	Zimovane; Imovane	—

Appendix 4: Key References for Further Reading

No attempt will be made to give details of the experimental and clinical studies which have been surveyed in this text. I trust that the authors of these studies will forgive me for this deliberate omission, but my intention has been to create a readable text, not a detailed monograph, in which the flavour and excitement of the advances in psychopharmacology will encourage those interested to read further. With this in mind, a list of key monographs, review articles and textbooks is included merely as a guide for the reader. The choice of texts may seem idiosyncratic to some readers, but they include those which have appealed to the author because of their clarity, comprehensive nature or contribution to the advances in psychopharmacology.

General reading

Bloom, F. E. and Kupfer, D. J. (Eds) *Psychopharmacology: The Fourth Generation of Progress*. New York: Raven Press, 1995.

Cutler, N. R., Sramek, J. J. and Narang, P. K. *Pharmacodynamics and Drug Development*. Chichester: John Wiley & Sons, 1994.

Frazer, A., Molinoff, P. and Winokur, A. (Eds) *Biological Basis of Brain Function and Disease*. New York: Raven Press, 1994.

Nicholls, D. G. *Proteins, Transmitters and Synapses*. Oxford: Blackwell Scientific Publications, 1994.

Prien, R. F. and Robinson, D. S. *Clinical Evaluation of Psychotropic Drugs*. New York: Academic Press, 1994.

Revicki, D. A. and Murray, M. Assessing health-related quality of life outcomes of drug treatments from psychiatric disorders. *CNS Drugs* **1** (1994), 465 (review).

Riederer, P., Kopp, N. and Pearson, J. (Eds) *An Introduction to Neurotransmission in Health and Disease*. Oxford: Oxford University Press, 1990.

Spiegel, R. *Psychopharmacology: An Introduction* (Third Edition). Chichester: John Wiley & Sons, 1996.

Stahl, S. M. *Essential Psychopharmacology*. Cambridge: Cambridge University Press, 1996.

Stone, T. W. *Neuropharmacology*. Oxford: W. H. Freeman; Spektrum, 1995.

Strange, P. G. *Brain Biochemistry and Brain Disorder*. Oxford: Oxford University Press, 1992.

Trimble, M. R. *Biological Psychiatry* (Second Edition). Chichester: John Wiley & Sons, 1996.

Chapter 1—Functional Neuroanatomy of the Brain

Fitzgerald, M. J. T. *Neuroanatomy: Basic and Clinical* (Third Edition). London: W. B. Saunders, 1996.

Chapter 2—Basic Aspects of Neurotransmitter Function

Chuang, D. Neurotransmitter receptors and phosphoinositide turnover. *Annual Review of Pharmacology and Toxicology* 29 (1989): 71.

Collinridge, G. L. and Watkins, J. C. *The NMDA receptor* (Second Edition). Oxford: Oxford University Press, 1994.

Cooper, J. R., Bloom, F. E. and Roth, R. H. *The Biochemical Basis of Neuropharmacology* (Fifth Edition). Oxford: Oxford University Press, 1991.

Manning, D. R. G. Proteins: Linkage with amine receptors. *Neuropsychopharmacology* 3 (1990): 447.

McGeer, E. G. Neurotransmitters. *Current Opinion in Neurology and Neurosurgery* 2 (1989): 520.

Nicoll, R. A., Malenka, R. C. and Kauer, J. A. Functional comparison of neurotransmitter receptor subtypes in mammalian central nervous system. *Physiological Reviews* 70 (1990): 513.

Olney, J. W. Excitatory amino acids and neuropsychiatric disorders. *Biological Psychiatry* 26 (1989): 505.

Ring, H. A. The value of positron emission tomography in psychopharmacology (Review). *Human Psychopharmacology* 10 (1995): 79.

Vincent, S. (Ed) *Nitric Oxide in the Nervous System*. New York: Academic Press, 1995.

Webster, R. A. and Jordan, C. C. (Eds) *Neurotransmitters, Drugs and Diseases*. Oxford: Blackwell Scientific, 1989.

Chapter 3—Pharmacokinetic Aspects of Psychopharmacology

Bertilsson, L. and Dahl, M. L. Polymorphic drug oxidation: relevance to the treatment of psychiatric disorders. *CNS Drugs* 5 (1996): 200.

Catterson, M. O. and Preskorn, S. H. Pharmacokinetics of selective serotonin reuptake inhibitors: Clinical relevance. *Pharmacology and Toxicology* 78 (1996): 203.

Coutts, R. T. Polymorphism on the metabolism of drugs, including antidepressant drugs: Comments on phenotyping (Review). *Journal of Psychiatry and Neuroscience* 19 (1994): 30.

Javaid, J. I. Clinical pharmacokinetics of antipsychotics (Review). *Journal of Clinical Pharmacology* 34 (1994): 486.

Preskorn, S. H. Pharmacokinetics of psychotropic agents. *Journal of Clinical Psychiatry* 54 (Suppl) (1993): 141, 55.

Rowland, M. and Tozer, T. N. *Clinical Pharmacokinetics: Concepts and Applications.* (Second Edition) Philadelphia: Lea and Febiger, 1989.

Rudorfer, M. V. Pharmacokinetics of psychotropic drugs in special populations. *Journal of Clinical Psychiatry* 54 (Suppl) (1993): 50.

Spector, R. Therapeutic drug monitoring. *Clinical Pharmacology and Therapeutics* 43 (1988): 345.

Chapter 4—Molecular Genetics and Psychopharmacology

Barondes, S. H. *Molecules and Mental Illness*. New York: W. H. Freeman, 1993.
Heilig, M. Antisense technology: prospects for treatment in neuropsychiatric disorders. *CNS Drugs* 1 (1994): 405.
Mallet, J. Catecholamines: From gene regulation to neuropsychiatric disorders (Review). *Trends in Pharmacological Sciences* 17 (1996): 129.

Chapter 5—Psychotropic Drugs that Modify the Serotonergic System

Charney, D. S., Krystal, J. D., Delgado, P. L. and Henninger, G. R. Serotonin specific drugs for anxiety and depressive disorders. *Annual Reviews of Medicine* 41 (1990): 437.
Glennon, R. A. Serotonin receptors: Clinical implications. *Neuroscience and Biobehavioural Reviews* 14 (1990): 35.
Hoyer, D., Clarke, D. E., Fozard, J. R. *et al.* International Union of Pharmacology classification of receptors for 5-hydroxytryptamine (serotonin). *Pharmacological Reviews* 46 (1994): 157.
Le Marquand, D. Serotonin and alcohol intake, abuse and dependence—clinical evidence (Review). *Biological Psychiatry* 36 (1994): 326.
Leonard, B. E. Serotonin receptors and their function in sleep, anxiety disorders and depression. *Psychotherapy and Psychosomatics* 65 (1996): 66.
Pandey, S. C. Phosphoinositide system-linked serotonin receptor subtypes and their pharmacological properties and clinical correlates (Review). *Journal of Psychiatry and Neuroscience* 20 (1995): 215.
Pecknold, J. C. Serotonin 5-HTI$_A$ agonists—a comparative review. *CNS Drugs* 2 (1994): 234.

Chapter 6—Drug Treatment of Depression

Cassidy, S. L. and Henry, J. A. Fatal toxicity of antidepressant drugs in overdose. *British Medical Journal* 295 (1987): 1021.
Cortes, R., Soriano, E., Pazos, A., Probst, A. and Palacios, J. M. Autoradiography of antidepressant binding sites in the human brain: Localization using ^{3}H-imipramine and ^{3}H-paroxetine. *Neuroscience* 27 (1988): 473.
Den Boer, J. A. and Sitsen, J. M. A. *Handbook of Depression and Anxiety*. New York: Marcel Dekker, 1994.
Farmer, R. D. T. Suicide and poisons. *Human Psychopharmacology* 9 (Suppl 1) (1994): S11.
Feighner, J. P. and Boyer, W. F. (Eds) *Selective Serotonin Reuptake Inhibitors*. Chichester: John Wiley & Sons, 1995.
Healy, D. The circadian system and the therapeutics of the affective disorders. *Pharmacology and Therapeutics* 65 (1995): 241.
Holsboer, F. and Bardem, N. Antidepressants and hypothalamic pituitary-adrenocortical regulation. *Endocrine Reviews* 17 (1996): 187.
Jonsson, B. and Bebbington, P. E. What price depression? The cost of depression and the cost effectiveness of pharmacological treatments. *British Journal of Psychiatry* 164 (1994): 665.

Kane, J. M. Newer antidepressant drugs: A review of their pharmacology and therapeutic potential. *Drugs* 46 (1993): 585.

Kasper, S., Hoflich, G., Scholl, H. P. and Moller, H. J. Safety and antidepressant efficacy of selective serotonin reuptake inhibitors (Review). *Human Psychopharmacology* 9 (1994): 1.

Leonard, B. E. The comparative pharmacology of new antidepressants. *Journal of Clinical Psychiatry* 54 (1993): 3.

Leonard, B. E. Biochemical strategies for the development of antidepressants (Review). *CNS Drugs* 1 (1994): 285.

Leonard, B. E. Tricyclic antidepressants: Effective, cheap but are they safe? *Journal of Psychopharmacology* 10 (1996): 35.

Meyer, U. A. Antidepressants and drug-metabolizing enzymes. Expert group report (Review). *Acta Psychiatrica Scandinavica* 93 (1996): 71.

Norman, T. R. and Leonard, B. E. Fast acting antidepressants—can the need be met? (Review). *CNS Drugs* 2 (1994): 120

Spina, E. and Perucca, E. Newer and older antidepressants: A comparative review of drug interactions. *CNS Drugs* 2 (1994): 479.

Chapter 7—Drug Treatment of Mania

Belmaker, R. H. How does lithium work on manic depression? Clinical and psychological correlates of the inositol theory. *Annual Review of Medicine* 47 (1996): 47.

Finley, P. R. Clinical relevance of drug interactions with lithium (Review). *Clinical Pharmacokinetics* 29 (1995): 172.

Guscott, R. and Taylor, L. Lithium prophylaxis in recurrent affective illness. Efficacy, effectiveness and efficiency (Review). *British Journal of Psychiatry* 164 (1994): 741.

Harvey, N. S. and Merriman, S. Review for clinically important drug interactions with lithium. *Drug Safety* 10 (1994): 455.

Jefferson, J. W. and Greist, J. H. Lithium in psychiatry. *CNS Drugs* 1 (1994): 448.

Post, R. M. Time course of clinical effects of carbamazepine: Implication for mechanism of action. *Journal of Clinical Psychiatry* 49 (Suppl) (1988): 35.

Post, R. M., Uhde, T. W., Roy-Byrne, P. P. and Joffe, R. Correlates of anti-manic response to carbamazepine. *Psychiatry Research* 21 (1987): 71.

Chapter 8—Anxiolytics and the Treatment of Anxiety Disorders

Barbaccia, M. L., Berkovich, A., Guarneri, P. and Slobodyansky, E. Diazepam binding inhibitor: The precursor of a family of endogenous modulators of GABA-A receptor function. History, perspectives and clinical implications. *Neurochemical Research* 15 (1990): 161.

Burrows, G. D., Roth, M. and Noyes, R. (Eds) *Handbook of Anxiety, Volume 3: The Neurobiology of Anxiety.* Amsterdam: Elsevier, 1990.

Charney, D. S. Serotonin specific drugs for anxiety and depressive disorder. *Annual Reviews of Medicine* 41 (1990): 437.

Den Boer, J. A. and Westenberg, H. G. M. Serotonergic compounds in panic disorder, obsessive–compulsive disorder and anxious depression. A concise review. *Human Psychopharmacology* 10 (Suppl 3) (1995): S173.

Feighner, J. P. Serotonin 1A anxiolytics: An overview. *Psychopathology* 22 (Suppl 1) (1989): 37.
Haefely, W. The GABA–benzodiazepine interaction fifteen years later. *Neurochemical Research* 15 (1990): 169.
Hindmarch, I., Beaumont, G., Brandon, S. and Leonard, B. E. (Eds) *Benzodiazepines: Current Concepts*. Chichester: John Wiley & Sons, 1990.
Ko, S. M. Pharmacotherapy of obsessive–compulsive disorder (Review). *British Journal of Clinical Practice* 49 (1995): 36.
Malizia, A. L. and Nutt, D. J. Psychopharmacology of benzodiazepines: An update. *Human Psychopharmacology* 10 (Suppl. 1) (1995): S1.
Naranjo, C. A. Recent advances in geriatric psychopharmacology (Review). *CNS Drugs* 4 (1995): 207.
Piccinelli, M. Efficacy of drug treatment in obsessive–compulsive disorder: A meta-analytic review. *British Journal of Psychiatry* 166 (1995): 424.
Potokar, J. and Nutt, D. J. Anxiolytic potential of benzodiazepine receptor partial agonists (Review). *CNS Drugs* 1 (1994): 305.
Sieghart, W. Pharmacology of benzodiazepine receptors: An update (Review). *Journal of Psychiatry and Neuroscience* 19 (1994): 24.
Woods, J. H. Current benzodiazepine issues (Review). *Psychopharmacology* 118 (1995): 107.

Chapter 9—Drug Treatment of Insomnia

Balter, M. B. New epidemiologic findings about insomnia and its treatment. *Journal of Clinical Psychiatry* 53 (Suppl) (1992): 34.
Hartmann, P. M. Drug treatment of insomnia: Indications and newer agents. *American Family Physician* 51 (1995): 191.
Mendelson, W. B. Insomnia and related sleep disorders. *Psychiatric Clinics of North America* 16 (1993): 841.
Roth, T. Zolpidem in the treatment of transient insomnia. *Sleep* 18 (1995): 240.

Chapter 10—Drug Treatment of Schizophrenia and the Psychoses

Andersen, P. H., Gringrich, J. A., Bates, M. D., Dearry, A., *et al.* Dopamine receptor sub-types: beyond the D_1/D_2 classification. *Trends in Pharmacological Sciences* 11 (1990): 231.
Barnes, T. R. The present status of tardive dyskinesia and akathisia in the treatment of schizophrenia. *Psychiatric Developments* 5 (1987) 301.
Brunello, N. New insights into the biology of schizophrenia through the mechanism of action of clozapine (Review). *Neuropsychopharmacology* 13 (1995): 177.
Carlsson, A. The current status of the dopamine hypothesis of schizophrenia. *Neuropsychopharmacology* 1 (1988): 179.
Coyle, J. T. The glutamatergic dysfunction hypothesis for schizophrenia (Review). *Harvard Reviews of Psychiatry* 3 (1996): 241.
Den Boer, J. A., Westenberg, H. G. M. and van Praag, H. M. (Eds) *Advances in the Neurobiology of Schizophrenia*. Chichester: John Wiley & Sons, 1995.
Johnson, D. A. Pharmacological treatment of patients with schizophrenia: past and present problems and potential future therapy. *Drugs* 39 (1990): 481.

Kapur, S., 5-HT$_2$ antagonism and EPS benefits: Is there a causal connection? *Psychopharmacology* 124 (1996): 35.

Kinan, B. J. and Lieberman, J. A. Mechanism of action of atypical antipsychotic drugs—A critical analysis. *Psychopharmacology* 124 (1996): 2.

Tamminga, C. A. and Schulz, S. C. (Eds) *Schizophrenia Research: Advances in Neuropharmacology and Psychopharmacology. Volume 1.* New York: Raven Press, 1991.

Weller, M. (Ed) *International Perspectives in Schizophrenia.* London: John Libby, 1990.

Chapter 11—Drug Treatment of the Epilepsies

Albini, F. Carbamazepine: Clinical pharmacology—A review. *Pharmacopsychiatry* 28 (1995): 235.

Bleck, T. P. Convulsive disorders: Mechanisms of epilepsy and anticonvulsant drugs. *Clinical Neuropharmacology* 13 (1990): 122.

Chadwick, D. The modern treatment of epilepsy. *British Journal of Hospital Medicine* 39 (1988): 104.

Joffe, R. T. and Calabrese, J. R. *Anticonvulsants in Mood Disorders.* New York: Marcel Dekker Inc, 1994.

Meldrum, B. S. GABAergic mechanisms in the pathogenesis and treatment of epilepsy. *British Journal of Clinical Pharmacology* 27 (1989): 3S.

Mikati, M. A. Comparative efficacy of antiepileptic drugs. *Clinical Neuropharmacology* 11 (1988): 130.

Vermeulen, J. and Aldenkamp, A. P. Cognitive side effects of chronic antiepileptic drug treatment: A review of 25 years' research. *Epilepsy Research* 22 (1995): 65.

Chapter 12—Drug Treatment of Parkinson's Disease

Carlsson, M. and Carlsson, A. Interactions between glutaminergic and monoaminergic systems within the basal ganglia—implications for schizophrenia and Parkinson's disease. *Trends in Neuroscience* 13 (1990): 272.

Freed, W. J., Poltorak, M. and Becker, J. B. Intracerebral adrenal medulla grafts: A review. *Experimental Neurology* 110 (1990): 139.

Jellinger, K. Overview of morphological changes in Parkinson's disease. *Advances in Neurology* 40 (1987): 1.

Kopin, I. J. MPTP toxicity: Implications for research in Parkinson's disease. *Annual Review of Neuroscience* 11 (1988): 81.

Marsden, C. D. and Fahn, S. (Eds) *Movement Disorders.* Butterworth, 1987.

Robertson, D. R. Drug therapy for Parkinson's disease in the elderly. *British Medical Bulletin* 46 (1990): 124.

Chapter 13—Alzheimer's Disease and Stroke

Allen, N. H. P. The treatment of Alzheimer's disease (Review). *Journal of Psychopharmacology* 9 (1995): 43.

Benesova, O. Neuropathology of senile dementia and mechanism of action of nootropic drugs (Review). *Drug Aging* 4 (1994): 285.

Byrne, T. Tetrahydroaminoacridine in Alzheimer's disease. *British Medical Journal* 298 (1989): 845.

Crook, T. Pharmacotherapy of cognitive defects in Alzheimer's disease and age associated memory impairment. *Psychopharmacology Bulletin* 24 (1988): 31.

Eagger, S. A. Tacrine and older anticholinesterase drugs in dementia. *Current Opinion in Psychiatry* 8 (1995): 264.

Gottfries, C. G. Neurochemical aspects of dementia disorders. *Dementia* 1 (1990): 56.

Johnson, J., Sims, R. and Gottlieb, G. Differential diagnosis of dementia, delirium and depression: Implications for drug therapy (Review). *Drug Aging*, 5 (1994): 431.

Kumar, V. Advances in pharmacotherapy for decline of memory and cognition in patients with Alzheimer's disease. *Psychiatry Services* 47 (1996): 249.

Mohr, E., Mendis, T. R., Rusk, I. N. and Grimes, J. D. Neurotransmitter replacement therapy in Alzheimer's disease (Review). *Journal of Psychiatry and Neuroscience* 19 (1994): 17.

Mondadori, C. The pharmacology of the nootropics: New insights and new questions (Review). *Brain Behavior Research* 59 (1993): 1.

Soares, J. C. and Geshon, S. Advances in the pharmacotherapy of Alzheimer's disease. *European Archives of Psychiatry and Clinical Neuroscience* 244 (1994): 261.

Terry, R. D., Katzman, R. and Bick, K. L. (Eds) *Alzheimer's Disease*. New York: Raven Press, 1994.

Wagstaff, A. J. and McTavish, D. Tacrine: A review of its pharmacodynamic and pharmacokinetic properties and therapeutic efficacy in Alzheimer's disease. *Drug Aging* 4 (1994): 510.

Chapter 14—Psychopharmacology of Drugs of Abuse

Green, A. R. Review of the pharmacology and clinical pharmacology of 3, 4, -methylene dioxmethamphetamine (MDMA "Ecstasy"). *Psychopharmacology* 119 (1995): 247.

Koob, G. F. and Bloom, F. E. Cellular and molecular mechanisms of drug dependence. *Science* 242 (1998): 715.

Kuriyama, K. Alteration in the function of central neurotransmitter receptors during the establishment of alcohol dependence. *Alcohol and Alcoholism* 25 (1990): 239.

Lader, M. H. Anxiolytic drugs. Dependence, addiction and abuse (Review). *European Neuropsychopharmacology* 4 (1994): 85.

Littleton, J. Alcohol intoxication and physical dependence: A molecular mystery tour. *British Journal of Addiction* 84 (1989): 267.

Meyer, R. E. Prospects for a rational treatment of alcoholism. *Alcohol and Alcoholism* 25 (1989): 239.

Rush, C. R., Higgins, S. T., Bickel, W. K. and Hughes, J. R. Abuse liability of alprazolam relative to other commonly used benzodiazepines—a review. *Neuroscience and Biobehavioral Reviews* 17 (1993): 277.

Simonds, W. F. The molecular basis of opioid receptor function. *Endocrinology Review* 9 (1988): 200.

Vogtsberger, K. N. Designer drugs. *Texas Medicine* 85 (1989): 30.

Chapter 15—Paediatric Psychopharmacology

Berlin, C. M. Advances in pediatric pharmacology and toxicology. *Advances in Pediatrics* 36 (1989): 431.

Brown, C. S. and Cooke, S. C. Attention deficit hyperactivity disorder—clinical features and treatment options. *CNS Drugs* 1 (1994): 95.

Campbell, M. and Cueva, J. E. Psychopharmacology in child and adolescent psychiatry: A review of the past seven years. *Journal of the American Academy of Child and Adolescent Psychiatry* 34 (1995): 1124.

Devane, C. I. and Sallee, F. R. SSRIs in child and adolescent psychopharmacology. *Journal of Clinical Psychiatry* 57 (1996): 55.

Dodson, W. E. Medical treatment and pharmacology of antiepileptic drugs. *Pediatric Clinics of North America* 36 (1989): 421.

Chapter 16—Geriatric Psychopharmacology

Chiu, E. and Ames, D. (Eds) *Functional Psychiatric Disorders of the Elderly*. Cambridge: Cambridge University Press, 1994.

Knegtering, H. Effects of antidepressants on cognitive functioning of elderly patients. *Drug Aging* 5 (1994): 192.

Shorr, R. I. and Robin, D. W. Rational use of benzodiazepines in the elderly (Review). *Drugs Aging* 4 (1994): 9.

Tsujimoto, G. Pharmacokinetic and pharmacodynamic principles of drug therapy in old age. *International Journal of Clinical Pharmacology, Therapeutics and Toxicology* 27 (1989): 102.

Volz, H. P. and Moller, H. J. Antidepressant drug therapy in the elderly: A critical review of the controlled clinical trials conducted since 1980. *Pharmacopsychiatry* 27 (1994): 93.

Zaleon, C. R. and Guthrie, S. K. Antipsychotic drug use in older adults (Review). *American Journal of Hospital Pharmacy* 51 (1994): 2917.

Chapter 17—The Inter-relationship Between Psychopharmacology and Psychoneuroimmunology

Ader, R., Cohen, N. and Felten, D. Psychoneuroimmunology: Interactions between the nervous system and the immune system. *Lancet* 345 (1995): 99.

Bell, D. S. and Concemi, P. T. Chronic fatigue syndrome: Psychotropic or immunological therapy (Review). *CNS Drugs* 1 (1994): 348.

Friedman, M. J., Charney, D. S. and Deutch, A. Y. *Neurobiological and Clinical Consequences of Stress*. Philadelphia: Lippincott-Raven, 1995.

Hanish, U-K. and Quirion, R. Interleukin-2 as a neuroregulatory cytokine. *Brain Research Reviews* 21 (1996): 246.

Kreutzberg, G. W. Microglia: A sensor for pathological events in the CNS. *Trends in Neurosciences* 19 (1996): 312.

Leonard, B. E. and Miller, K. (Eds) *Stress, the Immune System and Psychiatry*. Chichester: John Wiley & Sons, 1995.

Maes, M. Evidence for an immune response in major depression. A review and hypothesis. *Progress in Neuro-Psychopharmacology and Biological Psychiatry* 19 (1995) 11.

McCubbin, J. A., Kaufmann, P. G. and Nemeroff, C. B. (Eds) *Stress, Neuropeptides and Systemic Disease*. New York: Academic Press, 1991.

Merrill, J. E. and Benveniste, E. N. Cytokines in inflammatory brain lesions: Helpful and harmful. *Trends in Neurosciences* 19 (1996): 331.

Chapter 18—Possible Function and Therapeutic Role of Sigma Receptors

Itzhak, Y. (Ed) *Sigma Receptors*. San Diego: Academic Press, 1994.
Junien, J.-L. and Leonard, B. E. Drugs acting on sigma and phencyclidine receptors: A review of their nature, function and possible therapeutic importance. *Clinical Neuropharmacology* 12 (1989): 353.

Index

Index compiled by C. Purton